000174

WHEEL KICK

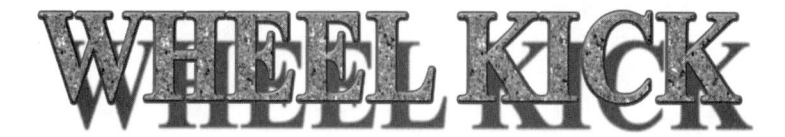

Achieving Kicking Excellence™

Shawn Kovacich

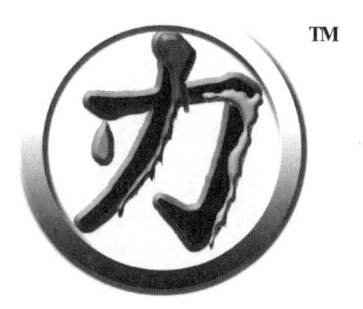

AUTHOR APPROVED FIRST EDITION

All Rights Reserved © 2005 CHIKARA KAN—SHAWN KOVACICH

No part of this book may be reproduced or transmitted in any form or by any means, graphic, electronic, or mechanical, including photocopying, recording, taping, or by any information storage retrieval system, without the express written consent of the author.

Printed in the United States of America

Library of Congress Card Number: 2004090159

ISBN #0-9707496-1-9

Table of Contents

Introduction
    Disclaimer 3
    Acknowledgments 4
    About the Author 5
    Preface 6
    What is a Wheel Kick? 7
    How to Use This Book 8
Chapter One: Basic Anatomy of the Wheel Kick
    Bones and their function relating to the Wheel Kick 11
    Muscles and their function relating to the Wheel Kick 14
Chapter Two: Warm Up and Stretching
    The Do's and Don'ts of Stretching 23
Chapter Three: Basic Principles of Kicking Movement
    Striking Surface 25
    Target Areas 26
    Stability 28
    Balance 30
    Alignment 30
    Sequence of Movement 31
    Accuracy 31
    Strength 32
    Speed 32
    Distance and Timing 33
    Impact 33
    Follow Through 33
    Visualization 34
Chapter Four: Primary Kick
    Turning Wheel Kick 35
Chapter Five: Variations of the Turning Wheel Kick
    Step-Back Wheel Kick 63
    Spinning Wheel Kick 73
    Hop/Slide Forward Wheel Kick 82
    Hop/Slide Backward Wheel Kick 91
    Front Leg Wheel Kick 100

  Back Leg Wheel Kick 108
  Switch Wheel Kick 116
  Off-Setting Wheel Kick 125
  Jump Turning Wheel Kick 136
  540 Degree Jump Turning Wheel Kick 144
  Spinning Wheel Kick (with the left leg) 153
Chapter Six: Training and Practice Methods
  Skill Training
    Training Partner 162
    Three Dimes 162
    Wall Practice 163
    Chair Practice 164
  Strength Training
    Hack Squat Machine 166
    Seated Calf Machine 168
    Side-to-Side Squats with weights 169
    Cable Machine Leg Raises to the Side 170
    Seated Leg Curls 171
    Side-to-Side Squats 172
    Plyometric Ski Jumps 174
  Speed Training
    Ankle Weights 176
    Quick Draw 176
    Water Training 177
  Power Training
    Force Bag 178
    Kicking Paddles 178
    Running 179
Chapter Seven: Trouble Shooting Guide 180
Chapter Eight: Kicking Applications 183
Chapter Nine: Awards & Accomplishments
  World Record Certificates 200-201
Chapter Ten: Preview Volume 3
  Axe Kick 202
Recommended Reading 205
Index 207

Disclaimer

Please note that the author and/or publisher of this instructional book are **Not Responsible** in any manner whatsoever, for any injury, which may occur by reading and/or following the instructions located within this book. The techniques described within this book are sophisticated in nature and have the potential to cause serious damage to the reader or readers, if performed incorrectly. Therefore, it is essential that the reader or readers of this book consult a qualified and competent physician before following any of the activities, physical or otherwise, which are described within this book. This book is intended to be used as a supplemental training aid, and should be used as such, under the guidance of a qualified and competent martial arts instructor.

Copyrights & Trademarks

Please note that no part of this book including text, photographs, and illustrations may be reproduced or transmitted in any form or by any means, graphic, electronic, or mechanical, including photocopying, recording, taping, or by any information storage retrieval system, without the express written consent of the author.

Chikara Kan, the **Chikara Kan "symbol"** (which is shown on the title page and the back cover), and **Achieving Kicking Excellence** are all trademarks of Chikara Kan, Inc.

Acknowledgments

I would like to take this opportunity to thank the following individuals, whose participation in helping me to achieve one of my life long goals on April 16th, 1999 will never be forgotten, nor held in anything less than the highest regards.

Shihan Dennis Dallas

Steve Humphries

Chris Eamon

Shem Wold

Conrad Donovan

This book would never have been published without the assistance of the following people who have contributed their time, energy and skill in the creation of this book.

Doug and Cassie Bender for the use of their facility used in principle photography.

The staff and owners of Sports West Gym for the use of their facility and equipment used in principle photography.

Jessica Bronder for her photographic and editing skills, and Ron Dunlap for his participation in this book.

"Before I studied the art, a punch to me was just a punch, a kick was just a kick. After I studied the art, a punch was no longer a punch, a kick was no longer a kick. Now that I understand the art, a punch is just a punch, a kick is just a kick." —Bruce Lee

About the Author

Watching Shawn Kovacich teach is like watching a college professor explaining quantum physics in such a way, that it is as easily understandable as a current episode of Sesame Street. With his unique ability to analyze and break down any kick to its most basic level, he then explains in exacting detail, the important aspects of each and every component in the kick. This gives the student a complete and detailed analysis of every movement in the kick from beginning to end.

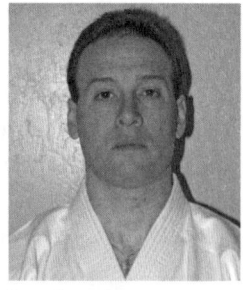

Mr. Kovacich started his martial arts training at the age of seventeen, and took to it like the proverbial duck to water, earning his first-degree black belt after two years and nine months of training. His teaching ability became evident early on in his training and he often assisted his instructors with newer students.

The most influential moment of Mr. Kovacich's early martial arts training came when he was privileged to not only witness, but also to participate in two of his instructors, Shihan Brian Knechtges and Sensei Ben Hunn's, third degree black belt test, in which Shihan Knechtges and Sensei Hunn had to fight continuously for 100 minutes each against a fresh opponent every minute. Punches and kicks were not pulled and the two men were pushed beyond all normal standards of human endurance. Both men not only prevailed and were awarded their third degree black belts, but they also became a source of inspiration for Mr. Kovacich. Years later, he would take this test not once, but twice, emerging triumphant both times.

Shortly after testing for and receiving his first-degree black belt, Mr. Kovacich accomplished another prestigious goal while participating in a charity fund-raiser. That goal, which he easily reached, was the first of what was to become two world records for endurance high kicking certified by The Guinness Book of World Records.

Mr. Kovacich has been an active instructor, teaching in as many as three schools at a time since 1985. He has taught students of all ages from six to sixty-eight, and from all walks of life, including law enforcement personnel, military personnel, correctional officers, mental health professionals, etc. Since the early 90's, he has also been an active competitor in bare knuckle full-contact karate. Competing in such prestigious tournaments throughout the United States such as the Sabaki Challenge, the Great Northwest Sabaki Satellite, the U.S. Shidokan Open, and the Shidokan Team USA. Mr. Kovacich still actively competes in these tournaments as well as being one of the top Instructor/Coaches for USTU (United States Tae Kwon Do Union) national and international tae kwon do competition.

Mr. Kovacich is currently a fourth-degree black belt in both karate and tae kwon do. Powerful and intelligent, he is constantly analyzing every movement in a kick in order to get the most speed and power available. He is one of only a handful of instructors who can improve anyone's kicking ability regardless of their physical ability or non-ability, or their martial arts style. Unyielding power is what makes Shawn Kovacich a world-class fighter, but what makes him truly unique is his analytical and innovative teaching ability.

Preface

In an unarmed self-defense encounter, your kicking skills or lack thereof, can be the deciding factor between victory and defeat. I can still remember back in my high school days when kicking was considered dirty fighting, and seldom if ever used. Things certainly have changed since the late 70's and early 80's. Today kicking is not only used more frequently, but it also ranks as perhaps the most versatile and underrated weapon that you have in your personal arsenal. With the noted exception of your head, and I don't mean as a physical weapon, but in your ability to intelligently avoid the threat, and if you are unable to avoid it, to overcome it as quickly and efficiently as possible.

Presented here are several different reasons why you should learn and practice the kicking skills presented not only in this book, but also from a certified and competent martial arts instructor.

1. The majority of people do not know how to kick, and therefore tend to rely mainly on their hands, giving them only two weapons. By learning how to kick, you have doubled your available weapons from two (your hands) to four (your hands and feet).
2. Your legs are the most powerful physical weapons that you have in your arsenal. They are several times stronger than your arms and have a greater reach.
3. Kicking can be your "Ace in the Hole" when fighting. Used properly, your opponent will not expect it and will never know what hit him.
4. Kicking adds another dimension to your fighting abilities by allowing you to kick at the same time your hands are defending, attacking or grabbing your opponent.
5. If you wind up on the ground, kicking can give you that extra split second in order to keep your opponent at bay while you regain your standing position.
6. Kicking helps keep you in shape by constantly strengthening and stretching the legs and lower torso. It is all too easy to forget that your legs are carrying you around everyday. Without them where would you be?

The exact reason why you have decided to begin utilizing the kicking skills taught in this book depends upon your own personal needs and interests. You may enjoy it because of the stress reduction and physical fitness benefits, or simply because you enjoy the physical challenge that kicking correctly presents. While others enjoy the sporting, or competition aspects of the tournament arena. However for most people, their primary reason for practicing these kicking skills is for self-defense.

Irregardless of the reason, the materials presented in this book are beneficial to anyone who wants to improve their kicking ability, whether it is the martial artist, tournament competitor, aerobic kick-boxing enthusiast, or the self-defense advocate.

While this book and the material presented within it are invaluable to the individual who does not have the opportunity to learn in a formal setting, it is also a tremendous benefit to those who are fortunate enough to have access to a qualified and competent instructor. A privilege and an honor one should never take for granted.

It is my hope that every person who picks up this book and studies it, walks away with an in-depth understanding of how to correctly perform all of the intricate aspects of the Turning Wheel Kick and its 10 most common variations. As the individual becomes increasingly proficient at performing their kicking and fighting skills, their need to exercise self-discipline, self-control, and responsibility increases dramatically.

What exactly is a Wheel Kick?

I am often asked this question and the best response that I have come up with is simply this, "A properly executed Wheel Kick performed by a man (or woman), is likened to the swing of a professional golfers golf club as he hits a golfball off a tee."

Note:

All of the kicks shown in this book were executed with the right leg. Therefore, in order to execute these kicks with the left leg, simply switch each kicks description from left to right and vice versa where appropriate. I have included a complete description of Spinning Wheel Kick utilizing the left leg at the end of the Turning Wheel Kick Variations chapter. Use this as a guideline for switching the description of the other kicks for use with the left leg.

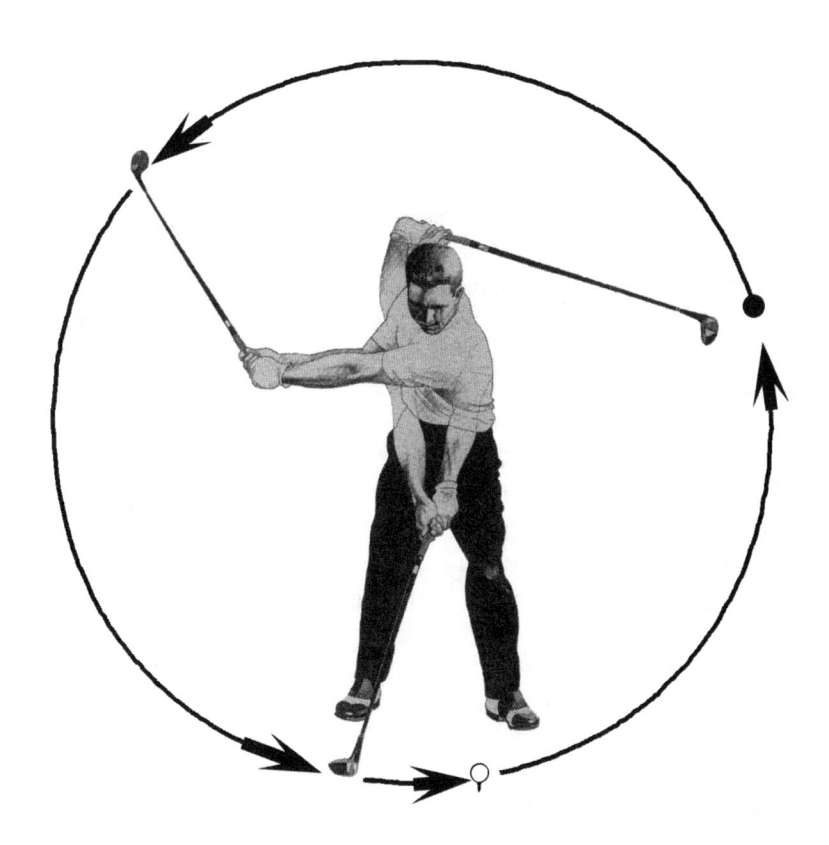

How To Use This Book

Although you can learn all of the techniques shown in this book on your own, there are many different subtleties and variables present within each of the kicks shown that true mastery of any of these kicks can only be gained under the knowledgeable eye of a qualified and competent instructor. This book is designed to be a reference manual for the instructor, and a textbook for the student. In order to learn from this book, you must first grasp a basic understanding on how to learn. In explaining this, I like to use the story of learning how to walk.

Every one of us, you included, came into this world as a baby. Did you run marathons as a baby? Of course not. You weren't even able to do anything for yourself, except for maybe making messes. And everybody has been through that, no matter whom or what they are, we all started out as babies. Now how does a baby first get around? Does he walk or run? No of course not, a baby first gets around by being carried. Then as the baby's muscles get stronger and he gets a little older he starts to crawl. And in no time at all, he gets pretty good at it and watch out, he is all over the place and seemingly faster than greased lightning. After awhile crawling gets kind of old and he begins to start learning how to walk. Mom and Dad are their holding his hand as he staggers across the room like a drunken sailor on a Saturday night.

Of course there are the falls and spills that happen as he tries walking on his own, but such is the process of learning. After a while he starts walking on his own and then comes the baby run, which if you are a parent or have ever baby sat a small child you know exactly what I am talking about. It begins with you looking away for just a second and then bang, he's off like a thoroughbred at the Kentucky Derby going for the Triple Crown, and almost as fast. Eventually the baby grows into a child and learns how to run and jump and do all kinds of things.

Of course none of these would have been possible if he hadn't first been carried, then taught to crawl, and had his hand held as he learned to walk, and perhaps just as important, received all those bumps and bruises from falling down and getting back up and trying it again.

The key to learning from this book is to be patient, start slow and take it in steps. Don't skip steps or rush the learning process. Years went into the making of this book in order to give you the best possible source of information on how to correctly execute the kicks presented within.

Go to the Doctor:

You should always consult with a qualified and competent physician before trying any of the techniques described in this book.

Read:

Take this book and read it cover to cover several times, before attempting to execute any of the techniques presented in this book.

Study and Learn:

Learn the who, what, where, when, why and how's of the anatomy and principles behind the kicks presented in this book. Remember that ignorance may be bliss, but knowledge truly is power.

Warm-up and Stretching:

Always warm-up and stretch thoroughly and properly before participating in any physical activity. An ounce of prevention is worth a pound of cure.

Take One Step at a Time:

When writing this book, I designed it so that each kick was broken down into several different sections with several technical points in each section. All of this was done so that you could full understand how to correctly execute each of the 11 kicks presented. With the understanding that once you had learned all of the technical points in each section, that you would then put them all together until you were able to perform each movement in every section of the kick as one continuous movement.

Let's use the primary kick Turning Wheel Kick as an example, now the best way to understand this is to look at it on a mathematical level. By this I mean that you are going to learn this kick on a 1 + 1 = 2 level. Each number one is representative of a technical point that is included in each section. For example Fighting Position has seven technical points. Here is what I mean.

1. Position of your feet = 1
2. Position of your knees = 1
3. Position of your upper body = 1
4. Position of your hand and elbows = 1
5. Position of your back = 1
6. Position of your head = 1
7. Position of your eyes = 1

For a total of 7 technical points.

Now when you look at all of the technical points in each section of a Turning Wheel Kick, it would look like this.

Fighting Position = 1 + 1 + 1 + 1 + 1 + 1 + 1 = 7
Turn Back = 1 + 1 + 1 + 1 + 1 + 1 = 6
Begin Trajectory = 1 + 1 + 1 + 1 + 1 + 1 + 1 + 1 = 8
Peak of Trajectory = 1 + 1 + 1 + 1 + 1 + 1 + 1 + 1 = 8
Impact = 1 + 1 + 1 + 1 + 1 + 1 + 1 + 1 = 8
Follow Through = 1 + 1 + 1 + 1 + 1 + 1 + 1 + 1 = 8
End of Trajectory = 1 + 1 + 1 + 1 + 1 + 1 + 1 + 1 = 8
Return to Fighting Position = 1 + 1 + 1 + 1 + 1 + 1 + 1 = 7

For a total of 60 technical points.

What this book was designed to do was to have you fully practice each section until each of the technical points in each section becomes second nature to you. Then you will go onto the next section and do the same thing until you have learned each of the technical points in each section. After that has been accomplished, you will then put each of the sections together one at a time until you are able to perform the entire sequence of movements correctly. For example:

1. Fighting Position
2. Fighting Position + Turn Back

3. Fighting Position + Turn Back + Begin Trajectory
4. Fighting Position + Turn Back + Begin Trajectory + Peak of Trajectory
5. Fighting Position + Turn Back + Begin Trajectory + Peak of Trajectory + Impact
6. Fighting Position + Turn Back + Begin Trajectory + Peak of Trajectory + Impact + Follow Through
7. Fighting Position + Turn Back + Begin Trajectory + Peak of Trajectory + Impact + Follow Through + End of Trajectory
8. Fighting Position + Turn Back + Begin Trajectory + Peak of Trajectory + Impact + Follow Through + End of Trajectory + Return to Fighting Position

Ideally you should execute any kick without conscious thought and in one single fluid motion. The execution of the kick should be instinctive in nature rather than an action or reaction, which in both cases are infinitely slower than acting instinctively. However just like a baby, you must first go through the entire learning process until executing the kick becomes as natural and without thought as breathing.

Learn the Primary Kick First:

This is pretty much self-explanatory, since everything else is based on the Turning Wheel Kick. Once you learn this primary kick, all of the other variations will be much easier to learn and execute.

Practice, Practice, Practice:

I have heard it said that one must practice any given technique 1,000 times before they know it. I totally and completely disagree. You should correctly practice any technique 3,000 to 5,000 times to learn it, 10,000 times correctly to know it, and a lifetime of practice to master it.

Read this book regularly:

Use this book as a reference guide on a regular basis. As a rule of thumb, every time you practice a Wheel Kick 1,000 times you should have read this book at least once.

Quality Supervision:

Whenever possible, you should always practice under the watchful eye of a qualified and competent martial arts instructor.

Basic Anatomy of the Wheel Kick

In this chapter I will attempt to give you a basic understanding of the primary muscular groups and bones in the skeletal system that form the anatomical basis of a Wheel Kick. I will do this by listing each of the muscle and bones separately and then at the end of each description, I will provide an explanation as to their role in the correct execution of a Turning Wheel Kick. Although the entire body is utilized in the correct execution of a Wheel Kick, I will only be concentrating on the muscle and skeletal structure of the lower back, hips, legs and feet.

BONES:

The skeleton of the leg is composed of the femur (thigh bone), tibia and fibula (calf bones), and the patella (kneecap). These bones have three primary sites of articulation; the hip joint, formed by the head of the femur and the acetabulum of the pelvis, the knee joint, formed by the joining of the lower end of the femur, the patella, and the superior end of the tibia and fibula, and the ankle, formed by the articulation between the tibia and the tarsus. The legs are responsible for bearing a great deal of weight and are subjected to intense vertical and lateral stresses, especially at the knee joint. Consequently, the bones of the leg are often cracked or broken, and the knee, hip and ankle joint are particularly susceptible to fracture, strain, sprain, and dislocation.

Each foot is made up of twenty-six bones, which form the ankle, top and bottom of the foot, and toes. These bones are articularly specialized, allowing a wide range of flexibility, while being able to withstand the incredible amounts of stress placed upon them. It is estimated that each stride of an adult places 900 pounds of pressure per square inch on the bottom of the foot. Seven of these bones form the compact arrangement of the ankle, or tarsus, and the heel.

Calcaneus:

The calcaneus bone forms the lower, outer part of the ankle and extends downward to form the heel. It is responsible for bearing much of the immediate stress placed upon the foot during walking and running. **The back of the calcaneus or heel, is the striking surface used when executing a Wheel Kick.**

Femur:

The femur is the longest bone in the body, and composes the upper leg, or thigh. The upper portion of the femur articulates with the acetabulum, the large circular cavity on each side of the pelvis, to form the ball and socket joint at the hip. The bottom portion of the femur articulates with the tibia and fibula, and the patella (knee cap) to form the knee joint. Each femur directly bears the weight of the entire upper body. **The femur provides support to the lower leg bones (tibia and fibula), at the junction of the knee joint, which lend direct support to the calcaneus bone. The head of the femur also connects to the pelvis.**

Fibula:

The fibula is the smaller of the two bones of the lower leg. It articulates at each end with the parallel tibia, at its upper portion with the femur to form the knee joint, and at its lower portion with the bones of the ankle, or tarsus. The fibula is so named

Bones of the Feet and Ankle

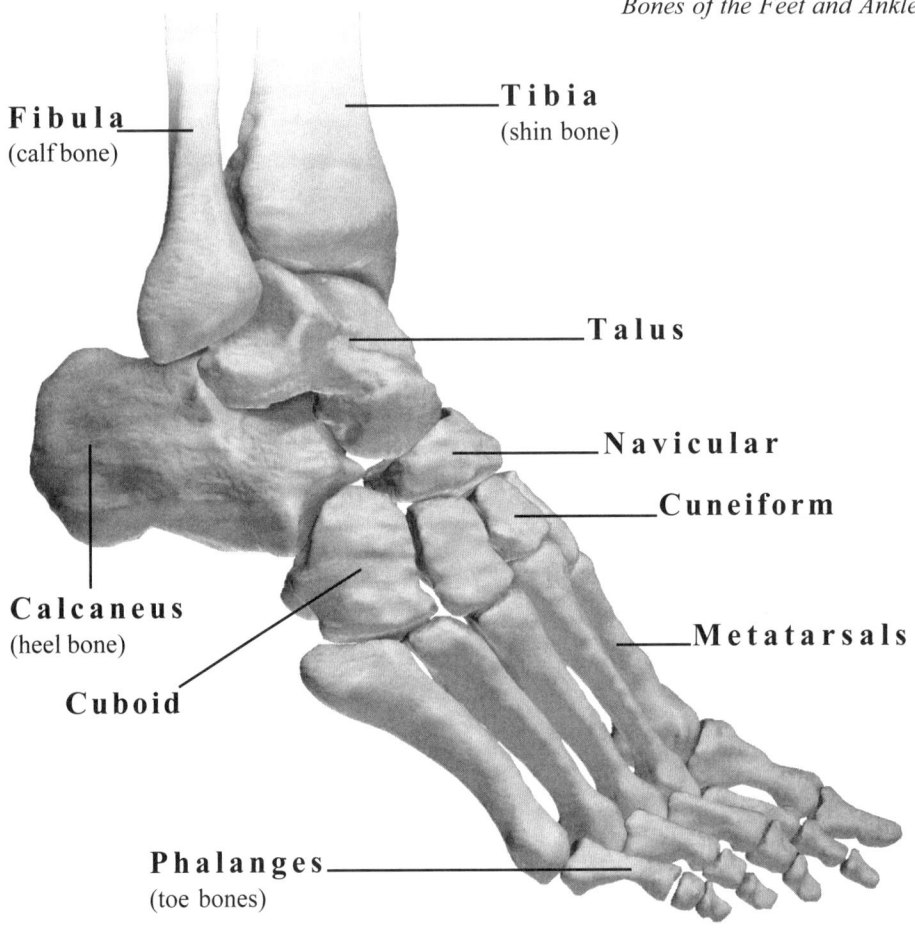

Fibula (calf bone)
Tibia (shin bone)
Talus
Navicular
Cuneiform
Calcaneus (heel bone)
Metatarsals
Cuboid
Phalanges (toe bones)

because it serves as a brace for the lower leg. **The fibula along with the tibia, lend direct support to the calcaneus bone, which is the striking implement used in a Wheel Kick.**

Knee:

The knee is the hinge like joint formed by the lower end of the femur, the upper ends of the tibia and fibula, and the patella (kneecap). The knee is a joint, which is subjected to tremendous lateral stress during normal activity and is guarded by a number of ligaments to help lend it support. Even so, however, the increased stresses placed upon this joint during extreme athletic activity, which require the individual to alter directions rapidly, the knee often bears the brunt of intolerable shearing forces. Such incidences often result in torn ligaments within the knee, which require corrective surgery. Proper technique and attention to detail must be utilized at all times in order to avoid injuring yourself during the execution of any technique. **Both the base leg knee and the kicking leg knee, can be easily damaged if proper technique is not used throughout the entire execution of a Wheel Kick.**

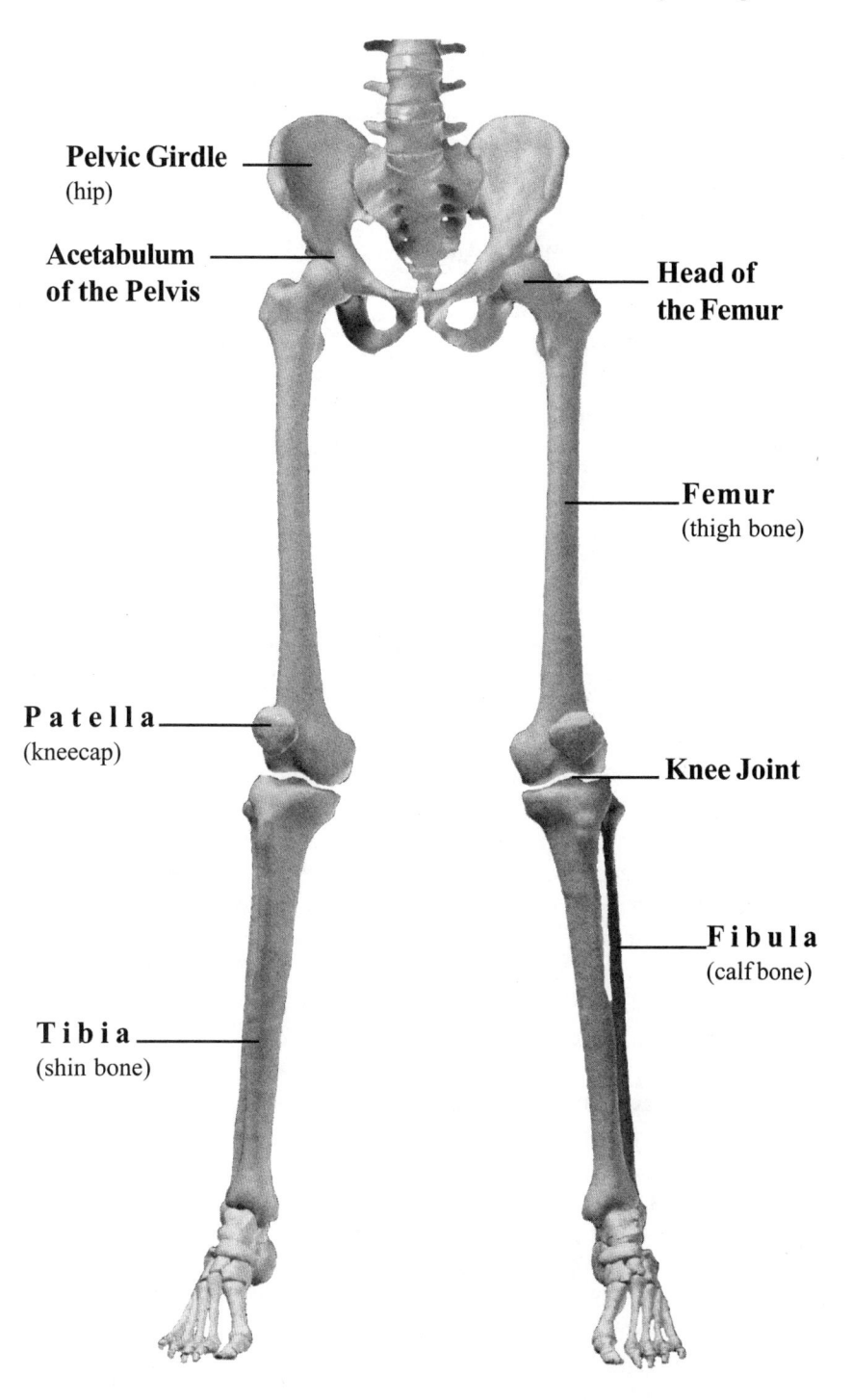

Bones of the Leg and Pelvis

- **Pelvic Girdle** (hip)
- **Acetabulum of the Pelvis**
- **Head of the Femur**
- **Femur** (thigh bone)
- **Patella** (kneecap)
- **Knee Joint**
- **Fibula** (calf bone)
- **Tibia** (shin bone)

Patella:
The patella or kneecap is a small bone of the knee joint, which resembles an inverted teardrop. The patella is connected to the joint by a series of ligaments.

Pelvis:
The pelvis creates the basin of the lower abdominal cavity. It articulates with the sacrum in the back, and thereby connects to the rest of the vertebral column, and also to the legs through the ball and socket joint formed by the two acetabula of the pelvis and the head of each femur. **The pelvis is the connecting link between the actions of the upper and lower body.**

Phalanges:
The bones of the toes are known as phalanges. Each toe has three phalanges, with the exception of the large toe, which has only two. Toes and ankles are the most common self-inflicted injuries when kicking. Keeping your toes back, and out of the way, and your foot tight upon impact will greatly reduce the risk of injury. **The toes provide balance and stability in all activities that involve moving on your feet.**

Tibia:
The tibia is the primary bone of the two in the lower leg. Also called the shinbone, the tibia bears most of the weight. Its upper portion articulates with the parallel fibula, patella and the femur at the knee joint. Its lower portion articulates with the fibula and the talus of the ankle. **The tibia along with the fibula lend direct support to the calcaneus bone, which is the striking implement used in a Wheel Kick.**

MUSCLES:
The muscles and joints of the legs provide strength and stability for the body. These muscles serve to transmit the weight of the body and provide power for such common activities as walking, running and jumping. They also absorb the cumulative impact of those activities. The leg bones are girded on all sides by sets of powerful muscles that allow the legs to bend (flexion) and straighten (extension) as well as move outward from the body (abduction) and inward (adduction). Some of these muscles are relatively long and participate in more than one type of movement. The thigh consists of the body's largest bone, the femur, which is bound on all sides by sets of powerful muscles.

The calf, ankle and foot are controlled largely by a series of muscles and tendons that function as a single biomechanical unit. These muscles work together to lift or lower the heel for virtually any activity that involves locomotion. All of the parts of the lower leg are interconnected. For example, when you stand on your toes, you can feel the muscles in the back of your calf doing most of the work. Because of its structure, and because it absorbs the impact from activities like running and jumping, the lower leg is subject to more exercise related injuries than any other area of the body. These problems range from bunions and blisters to stress fractures and ankle sprains, the most common sports injury of all.

The feet and toes are essential elements in body movement. They bear and propel the weight of the body during walking and running, and help to maintain balance during changes of body position. The foot can adapt itself to different surfaces and

Muscles of the Lower Abdomen and Pelvis

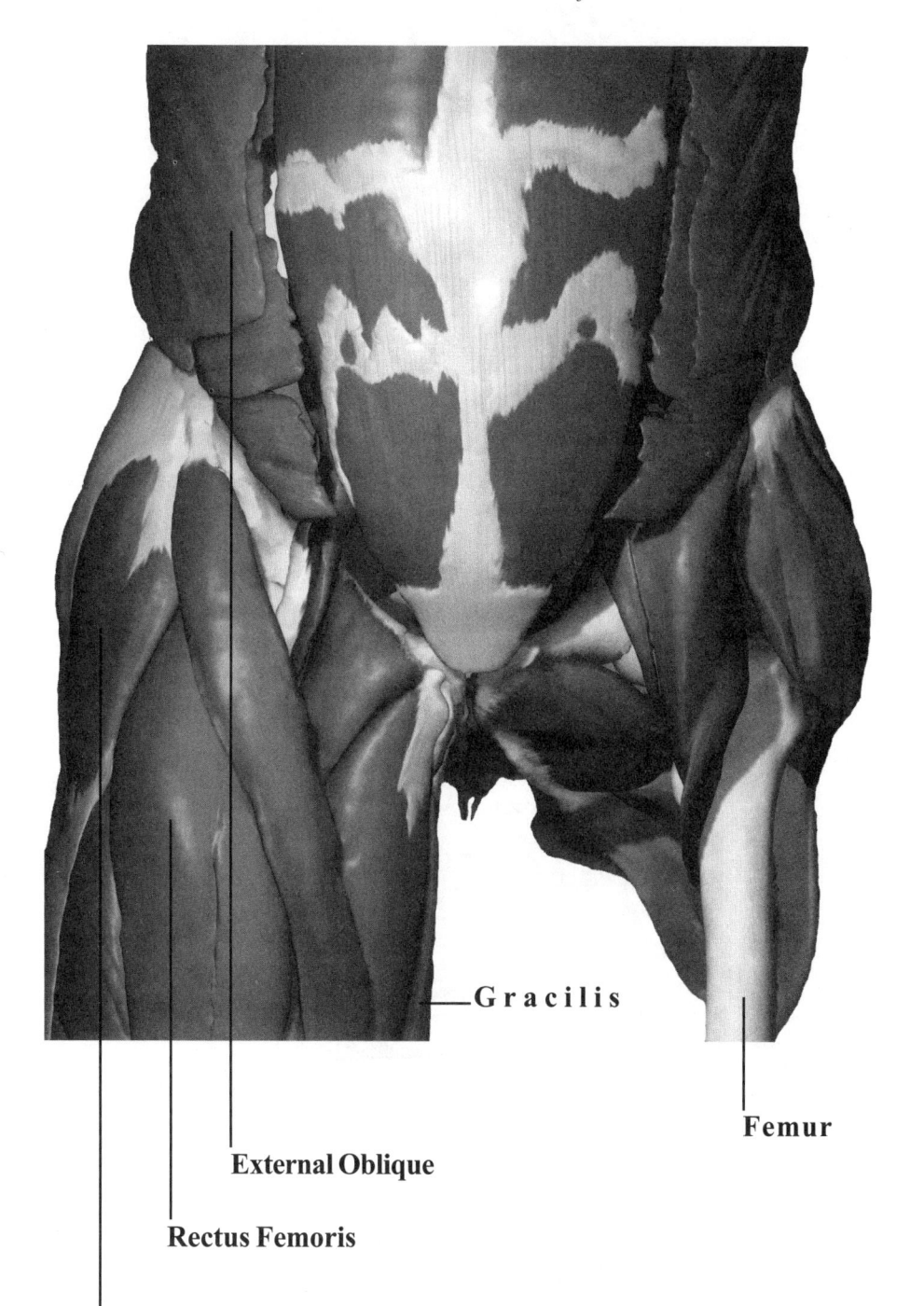

- Gracilis
- Femur
- External Oblique
- Rectus Femoris
- Tensor Fascia Latae

Muscles of the Leg (Front View)

- Pectineus
- Illiotibial Tract
- Gracilis
- **Rectus Femoris** (quadriceps)
- **Vastus Medialis** (quadriceps)
- **Vastus lateralis** (quadriceps)

16

Muscles of the Leg (Back View)

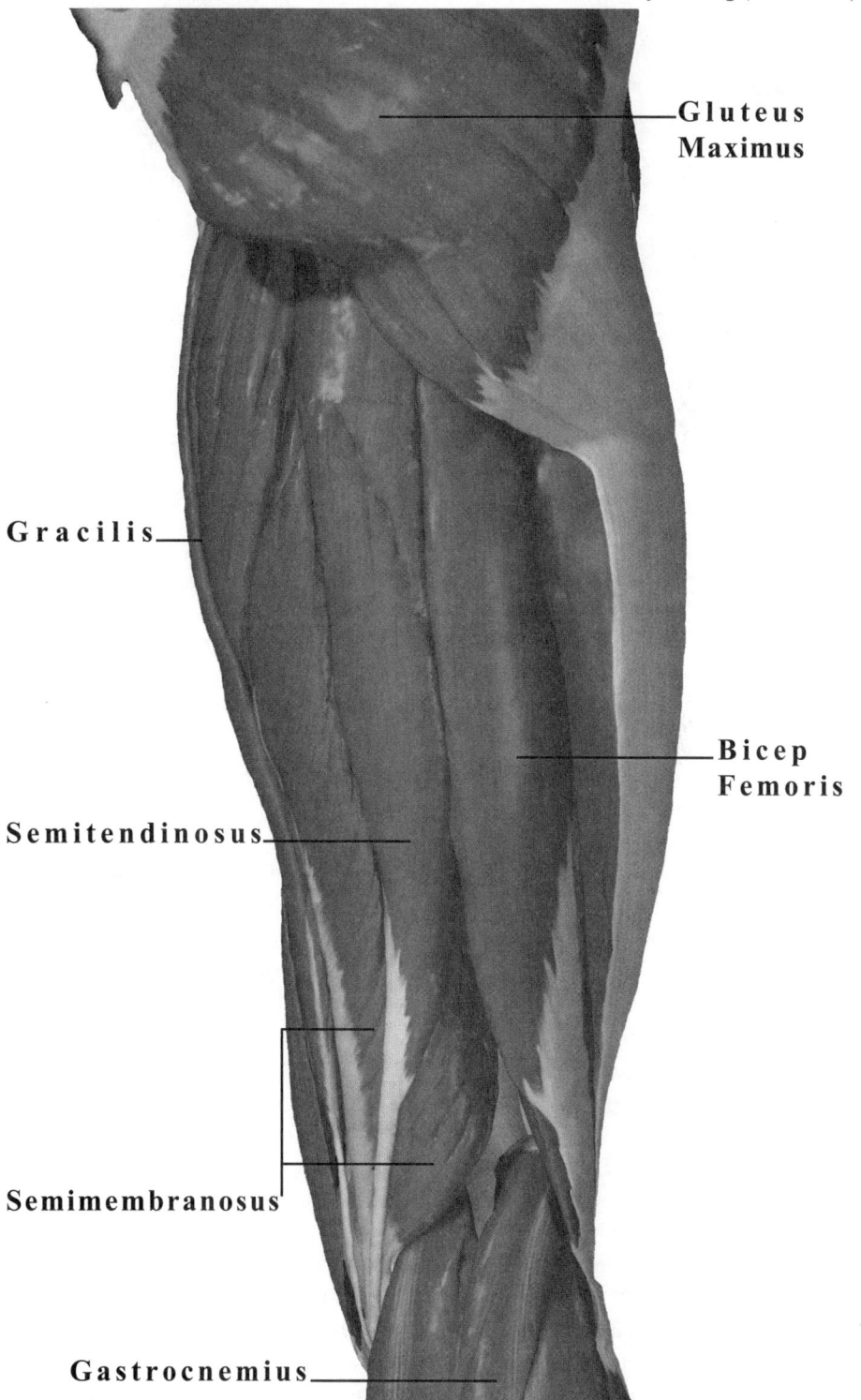

- Gluteus Maximus
- Gracilis
- Bicep Femoris
- Semitendinosus
- Semimembranosus
- Gastrocnemius

Muscles of the Lower Leg and Feet

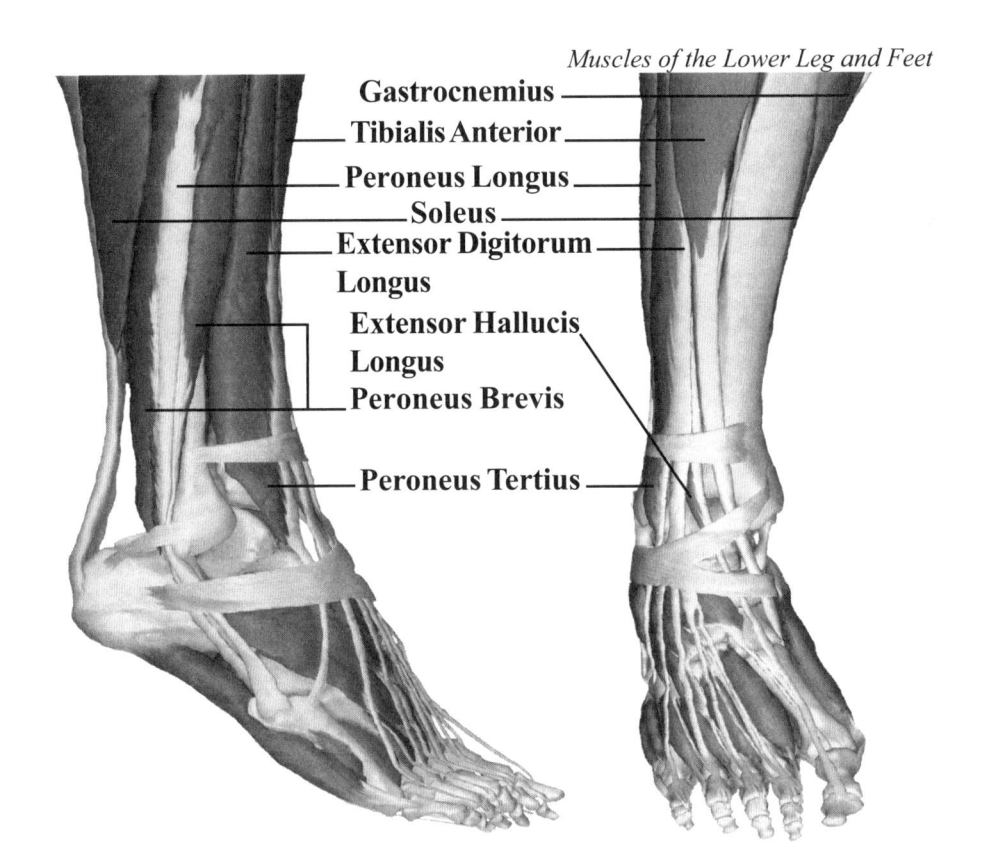

Gastrocnemius
Tibialis Anterior
Peroneus Longus
Soleus
Extensor Digitorum Longus
Extensor Hallucis Longus
Peroneus Brevis
Peroneus Tertius

absorb mechanical shocks as well. Each foot has about thirty-three muscles, some of which are attached to the lower leg.

Bicep Femoris:
The bicep femoris muscle runs from the tuberosity of the ischium down to the back of the head of the fibula. This muscle flexes the lower leg at the knee joint and also abducts or rotates the tibia outward. **This muscle helps extend the leg from the "Peak of Trajectory" position to "Impact" and continuing through to the "Follow Through" position.**

Extensor Digitorum Longus:
The extensor digitorum longus muscle arises from the tibia and the front of the fibula, and runs down into the foot and the toes. This muscle extends the toes and flexes the foot toward the leg. **This muscle assists in pushing off the floor with your toes during the "Begin Trajectory" phase of executing a Wheel Kick. It also flexes the foot toward your knee in order to obtain the proper foot position for the Wheel Kick.**

Extensor Hallucis Longus:
The extensor hallucis longus muscle lies deep in the lower leg and extends down to the big toe. This muscle extends the big toe and assists in flexing the foot. **As with the extensor digitorum longus, this muscle assists in pushing off the floor with your big toe during the "Begin Trajectory" phase of executing a Wheel**

Kick. It also flexes the foot toward your knee in order to obtain the proper foot position for the Wheel Kick.

External Oblique:

The external oblique muscle runs along the side of the torso and partially on the front from the lower ribs to the rectus, the pubis bone, and iliac crest of the hip. This muscle assists the rectus abdominus muscle in flexing the spine when the trunk twists or turns. **This muscle assists with the flexing of the spine and twisting of the upper body when turning to execute the Wheel Kick.**

Flexor Digitorum Longus:

The flexor digitorum longus muscle runs deep in the lower leg from the middle of the tibia to underneath the foot to the toes. This muscle assists to flex the toes during the final push off in walking or running. **As with the extensor digitorum longus and the extensor hallucis longus, this muscle assists in pushing off the floor with your toes during the "Begin Trajectory" phase of executing a Wheel Kick.**

Gastrocnemius:

The gastrocnemius muscle runs from the back of the knee to the ankle to form the calf muscle. This muscle propels the body when walking, running or jumping. It raises the heel, which lifts the body. It also assists, though minimally, in flexing the knee joint. **This muscle assists the bicep femoris in raising the heel of your foot off the ground when you begin to initiate a Wheel Kick.**

Gemelli:

The gemelli are two small muscles of the hip. The muscles arise from the spine and insert into the upper edge of the thighbone. These muscles help rotate the thigh. **This muscle helps rotate the thigh when turning to initiate a Wheel Kick.**

Gluteus Maximus:

We sit on the largest and most powerful muscle in our body, the gluteus maximus. This muscle powerfully extends the thigh at the hip joint and moves it away from the body, as when walking or running. **This muscle helps raise the leg up to the "Peak of Trajectory" position, as well as extending the leg from there to "Impact" and continuing through to the "Follow Through" position. Proper utilization of this muscle will greatly increase the power in your Wheel Kick.**

Gluteus Medius:

The gluteus medius runs from the outer portion of the pelvis, up to the crest of the pelvis. The gluteus medius is partially covered by the gluteus maximus. It moves the thigh outward and rotates it, as when walking or running. It keeps the torso upright during walking when one foot is touching the ground and the other is not. **This muscle assists in raising the leg up to the "Peak of Trajectory" position.**

Gracilis:

The gracilis muscle lies on the inside of the femur and begins at the pubic arch and runs down towards the inside of the tibia or shinbone. This muscle brings the knee up and pulls it across the front, toward the middle of the body. It also assists in rotation of the leg. **This is the primary muscle utilized when bringing the kicking leg back down to its original position after executing the Wheel Kick.**

Iliopsoas:
The iliopsoas runs from deep in the back of the abdomen towards its insertion on the back of the femur. This muscle flexes the hip and assists in abduction and outward rotation of the hip. **This muscle assists in flexing the thigh towards the abdomen and assists in raising the leg up to the "Peak of Trajectory" position.**

Iliotibial Tract:
The iliotibial tract begins at the upper edge of the femur and ends where it inserts into the condyle of the tibia. It acts almost like a ligament, by helping mainly to stabilize the knee joint, but also acts in flexing (bending) and extending (straightening) the knee. **This muscle assists in straightening and stabilizing the knee during the execution of the Wheel Kick.**

Pectineus:
The pectineus muscle lies on the front of the upper and middle part of the thigh. This muscle flexes and moves the thigh towards the body and rotates it towards the center. **This muscle helps flex the hip creating added force (not speed) to the Wheel Kick. It also assists with bringing the kicking leg back down to its original position after executing the Wheel Kick.**

Peroneus Brevis:
The peroneus brevis muscle runs along the outside of the lower half of the fibula or lower leg. This muscle works with the peroneus longus to extend the foot. **This muscle helps extend the foot as when pushing off the floor to move into the "Begin Trajectory" position.**

Peroneus Longus:
The peroneus longus muscle runs along the upper part of the outside of the fibula or lower leg. This muscle works with the peroneus brevis to extend the foot. **This muscle, along with the peroneus brevis, helps extend the foot as when pushing off the floor to move into the "Begin Trajectory" position.**

Peroneus Tertius:
The peroneus tertius runs from the lower third of the fibula downward and slightly forward, across the ankle and inserts into the little toe. This muscle provides dorsiflexion and eversion of the foot. **This muscle helps the foot maintain its proper position in order to execute the Wheel Kick.**

Plantaris:
The plantaris muscle runs from the lower end of the femur down to a small area on the bottom of the calcaneus or heel bone. This muscle works with the gastrocnemius to extend the ankle if the foot is free, and bend the knee if the foot is fixed, as when walking. **This muscle helps extend the foot as when pushing off the floor to move into the "Begin Trajectory" position.**

Popliteal Region:
The popliteal muscle starts from the femur and the ligament behind the knee joint and extends down to the shaft of the tibia or shinbone. This muscle assists in rotating the tibia and is used when bending the knee. **This muscle is used to slightly bend the knee on the kicking leg prior to impact.**

Quadriceps:

The quadriceps consists of four separate muscles. The rectus femoris, which runs from the ilium or hipbone down to the knee. This muscle flexes the hip joint and helps with hip joint abduction. The vastus lateralis is located halfway down the outside of the thigh, this muscle extends the knee, but it needs the vastus medialis in order to give a straight pull to the knee. The vastus intermedius lies between the vastus medialis and the vastus lateralis, and beneath the rectus femoris. This muscle extends the knee with its pull directly upward on the patella. And finally the vastus medialis, which is located above the knee, on the top of the thigh. This muscle extends the knee with the assistance of the vastus lateralis. These muscles cover the front and sides of the femur or thigh, and work together as a primary extensor of the knee. The rectus femoris muscle extends the leg at the knee joint and flexes the thigh at the hip joint. **The rectus femoris primarily flexes the thigh towards the abdomen and assists in raising the leg up to the "Peak of Trajectory" position. All four-quadriceps muscles work together to straighten the knee when executing the Wheel Kick.**

Semimembranosus:

The semimembranosus muscle begins in the tuberosity of the ischium or underneath and back of the pelvis, and runs two-thirds of the way down the back of the thigh to the outer condyle of the femur or upper leg, just above the knee. This muscle extends the thigh and assists with the inward rotation of the hip joint. It also provides flexion and inward rotation for the knee. **This muscle along with the semitendinosus assists in extending the thigh from the "Peak of Trajectory" position to "Impact" and continuing through to the "Follow Through" position.**

Semitendinosus:

The semitendinosus muscle begins in the ischium or bottom and back of the pelvis, and runs two-thirds of the way down the middle of the back of the thigh. It is considered one of the hamstring muscles. This muscle flexes the lower leg and extends the thigh at the hip joint. It also provides flexion and inward rotation for the knee. **This muscle along with the semimembranosus assists in extending the thigh from the "Peak of Trajectory" position to "Impact" and continuing through to the "Follow Through" position.**

Soleus:

The soleus muscle is located on the back of the lower leg and runs from the upper part of the fibula down to the middle portion of the calcaneus or heel bone. This muscle is used to point the foot or raise the heel, which lifts the body. **This muscle raises the heel off the floor when you begin to initiate a Wheel Kick.**

Tensor Fascia Latae:

The tensor fascia latae muscle is located on the outer front corner of the ilium or hipbone. It connects the ilium to the tissues of the outer thigh. This muscle flexes, abducts, and medially rotates the thigh. **This muscle assists in the raising of the leg up to the "Peak of Trajectory" position.**

Tibialis Anterior:
The tibialis anterior muscle sits on the front of the tibia, and originates from the outside of the tibia below the knee and runs down into the foot. This muscle controls the descent of the foot during walking after the heel strikes the ground. **This muscle assists in keeping your foot in the proper position in order to execute the Wheel Kick.**

Tibialis Posterior:
The tibialis posterior muscle originates from the back of the tibia, behind the knee, and runs down into the foot. This muscle flexes the foot and, working with the tibialis anterior, turns the sole of the foot inward. It is the strongest support for the arch of the foot. **This muscle is responsible for adding "spring" to your foot when stepping or running.**

Warm Up and Stretching

Although stretching is perhaps the single greatest activity that you can perform to improve your kicking (other than utilizing proper technique), I am not going to go into great detail on the types of stretches to perform. Instead I will try and give you a firm understanding on the do's and don'ts of proper stretching. So without further delay, let's get started.

It is a well-known fact that active people tend to lead fuller more productive lives due to better health. Their endurance and stamina are greater not only during exercise, but also during normal everyday activities; such as climbing stairs, walking, doing normal household chores, etc. Medical research has shown us over the years that poor health is directly related to our increasingly sedentary life-style.

Research has also shown us that exercise, done at any age, retards the aging factor and allows our bodies to become healthier and more resistant to disease. It is obvious that as we become less active, we begin to lose not only our physical strength, but our mental strength as well. Therefore, our ability to utilize our bodies potential is greatly diminished. However, we can regain that potential and more through a correct and consistent stretching and training program.

Without a daily regiment of stretching and physical conditioning, our bodies become atrophied and weak with stored up tension, both physical and mental. Let's face it, regardless of how out of shape you are from lack of physical activity and poor eating habits, your body's potential to recover from this mistreatment and in fact flourish to new levels of health and increased physical abilities, is nothing short of phenomenal.

What does stretching do for your body? Well primarily it keeps your muscles and connective tissue flexible and more resilient to injury. It also prepares your body for more vigorous activity. Similar to starting your automobiles engine in cold weather and allowing it to idle for several minutes before driving. This idling period allows the engine of your car to warm up before the more strenuous demands of driving are placed upon it. Stretching is the idling period for your body. Stretching is essential to any martial art or combat sport, if you wish to perform at your optimum level, whether that is in the dojo, on the street, or in competition. Stretching in and of itself is easy to do, when performed correctly and consistently, and should take you between 25 to 35 minutes depending upon your level of fitness.

However, when performed incorrectly, it can actually cause injuries and impede your progress. It is for this reason that I recommend that you utilize your head when stretching and take your time. Perform the stretches correctly and slowly for the best results. Stretch at your own pace, not someone else's.

A regular program of correct stretching, will help you avoid injuries and will allow you to perform to the best of your abilities. Stretching, when performed correctly should not be painful. You should be able to feel the stretch, as it is performed in a slow, relaxing manner. Your body should not be tense nor should you force your body when stretching. Stretching should be a relaxing and warming up process, which takes place before performing a strenuous exercise.

Do Not make stretching a strenuous exercise. Your goal to achieve when stretching should be to reduce tension in the muscles, which will allow you to stretch further. Which in turn improves your level of flexibility. For the best results, stretch before and after participating in any strenuous activity, in addition to a daily stretching routine. A good stretching program can be adjusted to suit the needs of the individual. Certain characteristics to keep in mind when developing a stretching program are; type of activity involved in, personal goals, body type, current level of flexibility, and most important, your current physical condition.

Anyone who actively participates in a correct stretching program on a regular basis can become more flexible and improve their overall physical conditioning. You don't have to be able to perform the splits or be the reincarnation of Bruce Lee in order to gain flexibility, but you do have to have the desire and the willingness to train on a daily basis, and perhaps more importantly, you must learn to be patient with yourself.

Do's and Don'ts of Stretching:

Do's:
1. Wear loose fitting, yet comfortable clothing that will not impede movement and will keep your body warm in cold or inclement weather.
2. Perform a light exercise to get your body warmed up such as jumping rope, running in place, etc.
3. Hold each stretch for 10 to 30 seconds. Relax. Then go a little farther into your stretch and hold for another 10 to 30 seconds.
4. Keep your breathing slow and under control.
5. Keep track of the time during each stretch by slowly counting to yourself.
6. When your are performing the stretch correctly, you should feel a mild tension in the muscles. It should not be painful.
7. Take your time when stretching.
8. Stretch every day for 25 to 35 minutes.
9. Pay attention to your body and what it tells you.

Don'ts:
1. Bounce up and down while stretching.
2. Over stretch to where it becomes painful.
3. Hold your breath while stretching.

Perhaps the greatest example of what a daily program of stretching can do for you is brought to us from the animal kingdom. The most dangerous and skillful hunters are without a doubt the cats. From the regal "king of the beasts" on the plains of Africa, to our own domestic house cats. No other animal displays such a tremendous combination of flexibility, agility and strength as the cat. Watch them and learn. Remember that Rome wasn't built in a day, and neither shall you.

Basic Principles of Movement for the Turning Wheel Kick

In this chapter I will give you a basic understanding of the kicking principles involved in the correct execution of a Wheel Kick. Although a lot of these principles are the same for the other primary kicks and their variations, there are others that are exclusive only to the Wheel Kick and its variations. Study each one of these in detail until you know them inside and out. The more you know about a kick, the better you will be able to execute it.

Striking Surface:

The striking surface utilized in executing any Wheel Kick, is the back center of the heel or calcaneus bone. This bone extends down from the ankle to form the heel.

When a Wheel Kick is properly executed, with the back of the heel as the striking surface, the bones and muscles of the ankle, lower leg, upper leg and hip provide additional support upon impact with the target. As you can see, in the photographs on the right, hitting with the sole of the foot or your Achille's Tendon, would result in little more than a push or hard slap, when executing a Wheel Kick.

Remember, the idea is not to inflict damage upon yourself, but rather to your intended target when executing a Wheel Kick. Therefore, you must constantly be aware of your foot position and proper striking surface every time you kick, even if you are only kicking air.

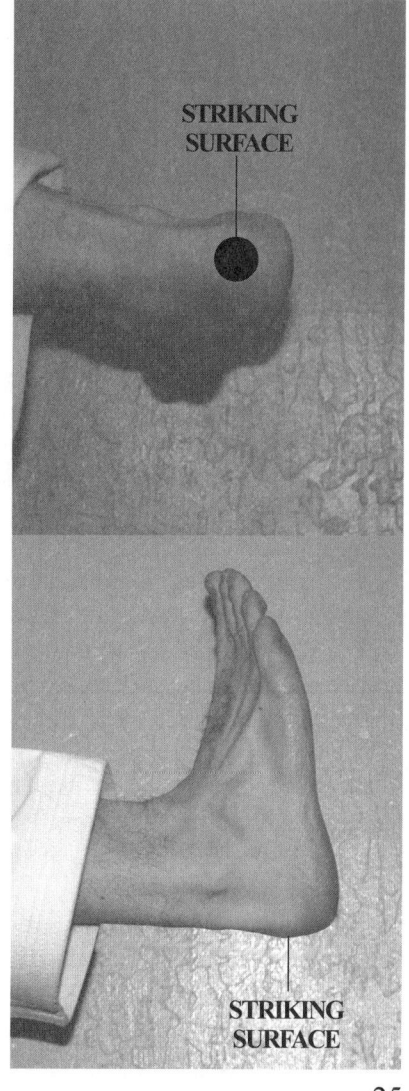

One way to produce a greater amount of force is to utilize a smaller surface area when striking your intended target. Let's say for the sake of argument that you can deliver a total of 100 lbs. of force to your target, and that the surface area of your heel is equal to 2 square inches. If you strike the target correctly with your heel, you will be able to deliver 50 lbs. of pressure per square inch. If however you strike the target incorrectly with your entire foot or leg, which has a surface area of say 20 square inches, then you would be striking your target with 5 lbs. of pressure per square inch. Do you see what the difference is between striking with the correct surface area of the foot and the incorrect surface area? Not quite sure, let me put it to you this way. Try hammering a nail into a piece of wood using the pointed end of the nail to make contact with the board first, and then hammering on the head of the nail. Then take another nail and lay it on its side and try hammering it into the wood?

Now do you see the relevancy of striking with the correct surface area? Although the amount of force exerted against your opponent in both cases are equal, the pressure exerted upon the target struck correctly with the heel is five times greater than if you used the entire surface area of your foot. When you strike the intended target with to large a surface area, you are dissipating the force over a wider surface area resulting in a push or surface strike rather than a penetrating impact. This greatly reduces the effectiveness of your kick.

Target Areas:

I define the target area as, the general location of a vital or vulnerable point on the human body. For the greatest effectiveness with the Wheel Kick in combat, you want to strike a particular vital or vulnerable point every time you strike your opponent. This will most likely deter any continued attack from your opponent by causing pain and/or injury. However this is not always possible as very few individuals are going to stand there and let you take shots at them. They are going to be moving, blocking, dodging and perhaps more importantly trying to hit you back. Therefore, you want to be able to strike your opponent the most effective and efficient way that you can.

One component of that is a thorough knowledge of the vital or vulnerable points of the human body. Not only is this knowledge important to inflict damage upon your opponent (only when absolutely necessary), but also to enable you to avoid such damage being inflicted upon yourself. I am not going to discuss in detail the vital or vulnerable points in this book. However, I am going to list the general target areas and the vital or vulnerable points that lie within those areas that you will want to strike with the Wheel Kick.

For more detailed information on vital or vulnerable points, please refer to the recommended reading section at the back of this book.

The effects of striking each vital or vulnerable point vary drastically depending on the accuracy, direction, speed and power utilized when striking them. Another factor that has to be taken into consideration is the human factor. Each individual is vastly different from the next and each person is going to react differently when struck. Some people may go down from the lightest of blows, while still others will merely shake off your strongest blows and keep coming at you. Which is a very good reason why you should have a thorough understanding of vital or vulnerable areas.

Be prepared for any and all eventualities. Because serious injury or even death may result from forceful blows to these target areas, you must exercise extreme caution when practicing with a partner, and you should never actually strike any of these areas with even the lightest blows in practice. If you are called upon to strike these areas in self-defense, you should only use full force to save one's life. Along with this knowledge comes great responsibility, not only to one's self, but also to

Facial Area (1)

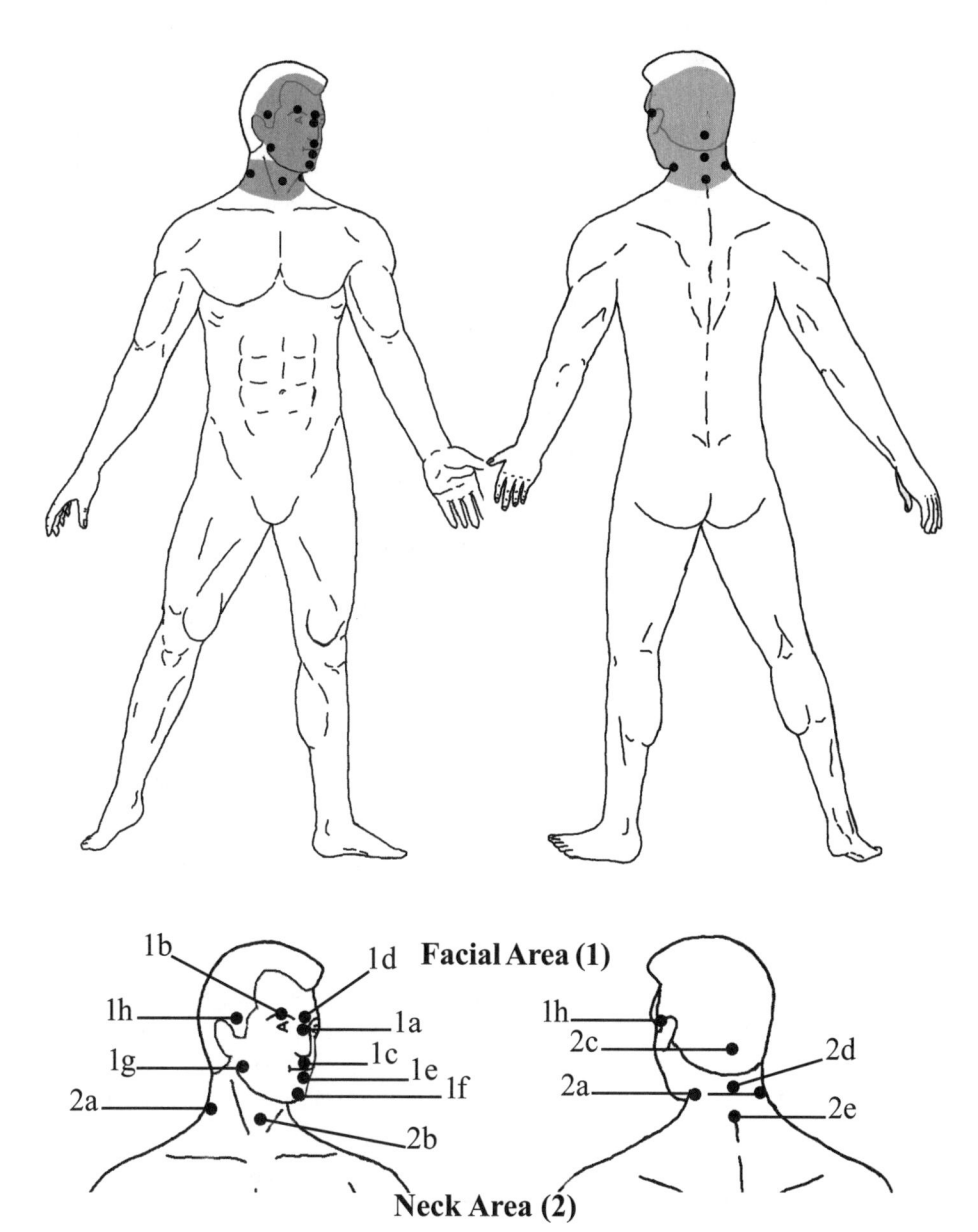

Neck Area (2)

those around you. **Never Use Excessive Force!**

1. **Facial Area:** This target area encompasses the nose (1a), orbital bones (1b), the philtrum (1c), glabella (1d), mouth (1e), point of chin (1f), the jaw (1g), and the temple (1h).
2. **Neck Area:** This target area encompasses the sides of the neck (2a), throat (2b), occipital bone (2c), 3rd intervertebral space (2d), and the spine (2e).

Each one of these vital or vulnerable areas can be struck separately utilizing the Wheel Kick.

Stability:
For the purpose of the material presented in this book, stability is defined as, "A person's ability to stand upon any given surface in a controlled and capable manner." For example you would have an easier time executing a kick on a hard flat surface such as cement or pavement, than you would if you were standing on gravel or ice. Sometimes it is necessary to create a very stable position or stance, such as when delivering a powerful kick.

Other times it is important to be in an unstable position, such as moving quickly in order to avoid being hit. Therefore a thorough understanding of the following principles will give you the ability to apply them on a daily basis, whether it be in practice, self-defense, or in competition. Several different factors contribute to one's stability such as your weight, height, center of gravity, equilibrium or balance, and your base of support. Let's take a look at each one of these factors.

Weight:
With all other factors being equal, a heavier person is generally speaking more stable than a lighter person. Consequently, a heavier person such as World Heavyweight Boxing Champion George Foreman would be harder to push off balance than a lighter person such as World Boxing Champion Oscar De LaHoya. It also stands to reason that Foreman is able to punch harder from his heavier and more solid position than De LaHoya is from his lighter and less solid position.

However, no one would argue the fact that De LaHoya, being a lighter weight fighter, has the advantage of being able to move and change direction quicker than the heavier Foreman. This is of course taking into consideration that all other factors involved are equal. I have seen some very big men that could move a lot faster and a lot smoother than their smaller counterparts.

Height and Center of Gravity:
Your center of gravity is defined as being located approximately 2 to 3 inches below your belly button and in the center of your body when standing perfectly straight with correct posture, and your feet flat on the floor. This of course varies from person to person and also upon their general body type. Women tend to have a lower center of gravity than men, and individuals with heavier legs have a lower center of gravity than someone with lighter legs. The closer one's center of gravity is to the ground or base of support, the greater their increase in stability.

You can easily change your center of gravity by bending your knees and squatting down to lower it, or by standing on your toes to raise it. You can even move your center of gravity outside your body by bending over at the waist and touching your toes. Generally speaking, the taller you are the less stability you have, while the shorter you are the more stability you have. Ask yourself this question, which has more stability the giraffe or the hippopotamus?

Equilibrium:
Equilibrium is defined as a state of balance between opposing forces. A prime example of equilibrium is a figure skaters ability to stand upon the toes of their skates while spinning their entire body into a tightly controlled blur of motion and then stopping without any outwards signs of loss of balance or equilibrium. For equilib-

rium to exist, your center of gravity must be centered over your base of support throughout the entire sequence of events involved when executing the Wheel Kick, or any other athletic endeavor. Failure to maintain equilibrium will result in a loss of balance, and can result in a slight case of disorientation. Either of which could prove disastrous in a self-defense or tournament situation.

Base of Support:

Your base of support is described as the area of the feet upon which the weight of your body is supported, along with the space between your feet. For example,

(A) if you were standing flat footed with both feet on the ground and directly beneath your shoulders, your base of support would not only include both feet, but also the space between them.

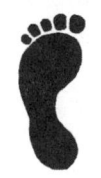

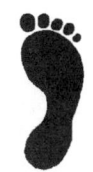

(B) If you were standing on the toes of both feet, your base of support would include the surface area of your feet that are in direct contact with the ground and the space between them.

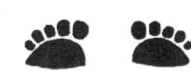

And

(C) if you were balancing on the ball of one foot, your base of support would be the surface area covered by the ball of your base foot.

Generally speaking, the greater the surface area of your feet that is in direct contact with the ground, and the wider the stance, the greater your base of support.

Therefore, after taking all of these factors into consideration, it stands to reason that the heavier, shorter individual is more stable during the execution of a punch when both feet are on the ground, than the lighter taller individual is when executing a kick and balancing on one leg. Does this mean that you are better off punching than kicking? Of course not, it simply means that the skills needed to kick effectively take a lot more time, effort, and attention to detail than those skills needed to punch effectively.

This is one of the reasons why so many people tend to neglect their kicking skills in favor of the easier learned punching and grappling skills. Your stance when fighting should be unstable in that you should not be set in one position, you should be constantly moving in order to avoid an attack while positioning yourself to effectively attack your opponent.

If your stance is too wide, you will sacrifice mobility as well as telegraphing any kick that you may attempt. This in effect makes you a sitting duck. If your stance is too short, you will have lost balance and stability. The ideal stance is to keep your feet shoulder width apart in length and about 4 to 8 inches apart in width.

Balance:

Although the previous section on stability also included information on equilibrium or balance, this section is devoted to balance as it applies to the execution of a kick. If you do not have good balance when kicking, not only is your kick going to be ineffective, but you may have put yourself in a dangerous situation by overextending your kicking leg, losing your balance all together, and possibly even falling to the ground. In order to prevent this, you must follow these few simple points when executing your kick.

1. Your center of gravity must be centrally located over your base foot throughout the entire kicking sequence from start to finish.
2. In order to execute your kick, you are going to pivot on the ball of your base foot. However, the entire base foot must be in direct contact with the ground at the moment of impact, with your center of gravity in the middle of the foot, not over the ball, heel, inner or outer edge of the foot. After the initial contact is made, you will continue with the "Follow Through" and then return the kicking foot to the starting position by once again pivoting on the ball of the base foot. You should never make contact with your target while balancing on the ball of your base foot. This incorrect technique is not only unstable, but it also causes a dramatic decrease in the effectiveness of the kick.
3. The position of your base foot is directly related to the effectiveness of maintaining your balance when kicking. For example the inside edge of your base foot is facing directly toward your opponent during the Impact Phase of a Wheel Kick. Try performing the Wheel Kick with the toes of your base foot pointed at your opponent; now try it with the heel pointed at your opponent. Did they work? How does your knee and hips feel?
4. And finally, don't forget the importance of that area of the body above your waist. I always find it amazing how many people forget about how important proper upper body position is to achieving and maintaining balance when kicking. Keep your head up and looking at your opponent, keep your back straight, and stop moving your arms around like a bird flapping its wings.

You'll be surprised at how much your kicks have improved by simply paying attention to these few things.

Alignment:

Your entire body should be aligned properly at the moment of impact in order to generate the maximum amount of power into the delivery of your kick upon its target. The proper body alignment at the moment of impact for the Wheel Kick is as follows. The kicking foot is parallel with the ground, and the back of the heel should be the only part of the foot in contact with the target. The toes should be in a vertical position, and pulled back toward the kicking leg knee, which not only exposes the heel for better contact, but also tightens the ankle.

The lower leg, knee and upper leg should all be in a straight line and supporting one another in order to increase the overall effectiveness of the kick. The kicking leg hip, shoulder, back, and the head should all be in a straight line with the heel. The inside edge of the base leg foot is facing toward your opponent and the supporting base leg is straight. This will have the effect of putting your entire body behind the kick, where the culmination of muscular speed, strength and proper technique combine to deliver the generated force into your target along a straight line of trajectory.

Sequence of Movement:

What this means is that the correct sequence of movements from the beginning stages of the kick, to impact and subsequent follow through, should be followed in one smooth continuous motion in order to achieve the maximum effectiveness in your kick. In order to do this however, you must first work upon each individual section of the kick until you can effectively flow from one section of the kick to the other, without any noticeable pauses or breaks between them. Even though the Wheel Kick should be performed in one fluid motion, there are three distinct and separate sections to this kick. The first is the delivery of the kick to the "Peak of Trajectory," the second is the straight "Path of Trajectory," which begins with the "Peak of Trajectory" through "Impact" and continues to "Follow Through." The third is the recovery after delivering the kick. Combine the three, but keep them separate.

Accuracy:

No matter how perfectly you execute your Wheel Kick, it isn't going to do you one ounce of good unless you can hit your intended target. Imagine going out to war and being equipped with the biggest most powerful rifle you can get, and then not being able to hit your target. Now combine that with the fact that the guy you are fighting against is equipped with a .22 caliber rifle and the ability to hit a dime at 100 yards. Who do you think is going to survive that encounter? There are several factors involved in obtaining accurate kicks such as eye contact, proper technique, muscular control or coordination, breath control, conditioning, and most importantly, proper practice.

Eye Contact:

Your eyes should remain in constant contact with your opponent at all times. The focus of your attention should be like a flashlight on your opponent's chest, while your peripheral vision encompasses everything else from his head to his hands and down to his feet. Be careful not to focus your eyes like a laser beam on one single point, this can cause a delayed reaction time to incoming attacks and can also telegraph your intentions to your opponent.

Practice Proper Technique:

The ability to kick proficiently is not instinctive, it is a learned activity that takes years of study and constant practice to perfect. I cannot stress this simple fact enough, "Pay Attention To Detail and Practice!" The kicks presented in this book have been explained in precise detail so that you can learn the proper technique for executing them as efficiently and as accurately as possible. Practice and study the material in this book until it becomes second nature.

Muscular Control or Coordination:

This is the ability to control ones own body during physical activities such as kicking. This is not an easy skill to learn, and it takes a considerable amount of practice in order to utilize it effectively. The best method that I know of to improve your muscular control for kicking, is to perform the entire kicking sequence in slow motion until the point of impact, at which point you hold that position for approximately five seconds tensing your entire body during that time. After the five seconds are over, relax the entire body and slowly continue with the "Follow Through" returning to your original starting position. This should be performed at least 10 times prior to and at the end of every kicking session. Another variation of this technique is to tense all of your muscles during the entire time you are performing this exercise. This is called Dynamic Tension training and is very effective.

Breathing:

You should never hold your breath when fighting. Breathing should be done normally by inhaling through your nose and exhaling through your mouth. Remember to keep your mouth closed when fighting. Don't open it or you may get a broken jaw for your trouble. At the exact moment that you make impact with your target, you will exhale sharply, and tighten your entire body, this will add power to your kick.

Conditioning:

Physical conditioning is an absolute must if you want to perform these kicks to the best of your abilities. The better condition that you are in, the more that you will be able to do for a longer period of time before becoming fatigued. The harder you train, the easier it will become.

Strength:

Strength is the amount of muscular force that you can apply at any given time to a particular target. Don't confuse strength with power. Speed and strength are two sides of the same coin which when combined together create power. Pivoting of the hips and the turning of the body are two methods of applying strength to a kick with minimal muscular effort. I am sure you have heard of a boxer who uses only his arms when he punches rather than utilizing his entire body. The same is also true of kicking, in that the majority of individuals kick only with their legs, rather than with their entire body.

Leg strength alone does not give any real strength to the kick. Granted there is some strength present, however it is minimal compared to the strength that can be delivered if the entire body is utilized in the execution of the kick. The positioning of your head, arms, hands, and upper body are also instrumental in increasing the strength of your kick.

Speed:

The only drawbacks to kicking are that although the leg is longer than the arm, it is relatively slower, and if you don't practice your kicking skills regularly they tend to deteriorate and lose their speed. Speed and strength are two side of the same coin, which when combined together creates power. To best explain this principle I like to use the analogy of a Lamborghini and a bulldozer.

Which one of the two is faster yet not very forceful? Which one is more forceful yet slower? Obviously the Lamborghini is faster and the bulldozer is more forceful. Yet if both of these vehicles started at the same time from one mile away and they both drove as fast as they could until they hit a brick wall at the end of that mile, which one would hit first, and second? And what would happen to them? Obviously the Lamborghini traveling in excess of 200 plus miles per hour would strike the wall long before the much slower bulldozer. However, when it hit the wall it would totally destroy the car and I am sure would cause some minor damage to the wall.

The bulldozer on the other hand, would take a considerably longer amount of time to cover that distance in order to reach the wall. However, once it reached the wall, its greater strength would easily, but slowly go through it. My whole point being that your body should be like the blinding speed of the Lamborghini as your foot travels to reach its target. However, at the moment of impact, your foot and entire body should transform itself instantaneously from the blinding speed of the Lamborghini into the wall-crushing strength of the bulldozer.

Immediately after impact, your entire body should return to the blinding speed of the Lamborghini in order to facilitate a faster "Follow Through" and completion of the 360-degree circular motion, which would result in you returning to your original starting position. A relaxed muscle is faster, while a tense or contracted muscle is slower yet stronger. Utilize this to your best advantage when executing these kicks.

Distance and Timing:

If the opponent is too far away, how are you going to hit him? If you execute a kick too slow or too fast, and your opponent moves, how are you going to hit him? If you attempt to execute a kick and your opponent is too close to you and jams the kick, how are your going to hit him? These are just a few of the problems that can be solved by creating the proper distance between you and your opponent and the utilization of proper timing. You cannot leave it up to chance or fate to create the perfect kicking distance between you and your opponent; you have to control the distance, and therefore the fight. Don't allow your opponent that opportunity.

Impact:

Impact is the culmination of all of the other principles and techniques performed correctly, in order to generate the maximum amount of force, and to transfer that power into your opponent at the precise moment of impact. If any one technique or principle is neglected, or applied improperly, then you will not be able to produce the maximum amount of force upon impact that you are capable of.

Follow Through:

Proper "Follow Through" of the foot and leg after kicking is perhaps one of the most important movements you can make during the kicking sequence. To begin with, the faster your follow through is after striking your target, the more effective your kick is going to be. This is primarily due to the transfer of energy that is being delivered from your entire body through your leg and foot into the intended target at the moment of impact. The longer your striking implement is in contact with its target, the more energy that is reflected back into you rather than being transferred into the target.

Secondly, the longer you have your foot in the air, the longer it is going to take you to follow up with another technique. It also allows your opponent the opportunity to grab your foot or leg and put you in a world of hurt. Unlike the movies where an actor can kick ten opponents all at once and never put his foot back on the ground, you should never attempt such a foolish stunt. Multiple kicks with one leg in the air can be effective, but only after years and years of devoted practice, and a cooperative opponent. As a general rule of thumb, as fast as your kick leaves the ground, it should be just as fast if not faster getting back down on the ground.

Visualization:

"**Any sport is 95 percent mental, and anyone who tells you differently, doesn't know what he's talking about,**" Joe Fields, center for the New York Jets.

"**Mind is everything, muscles are pieces of rubber,**" Paavo Nurmi, Olympic Gold Medallist.

Like I stated before, your mind controls your body. Therefore you have to believe in yourself and your abilities, if you ever want to become more proficient than what you currently are. There are three separate and unique times that one should utilize visualization as an effective training tool. They are; before, during and after every practice.

Before:

When you use visualization before practice you want to envision yourself performing the fastest, most powerful, most technically perfect kick you have ever done. Do not envision anything other than perfection. If you see yourself making mistakes or performing a kick poorly, then you will. If you see yourself doing your best then you will do your best. This is also referred to as positive thinking. It works, so use it. This should take anywhere from 5 to 15 minutes.

During:

As you are performing the kick, envision an imaginary opponent in front of you that you want to kick. Aim your kick to hit a certain target. Be aware of your body movement and position throughout the entire kicking sequence. Imagine your opponent being totally devastated by your kick. Concentrate.

After:

Use this time to reflect upon your workout and how well you did. Envision yourself doing even better the next time you practice. Answer this question, "If you don't believe in you, who will?"

Turning Wheel Kick

The Turning Wheel Kick is one of the ten primary kicks associated with Karate and/or Tae Kwon Do. Although it goes by many different names, the Wheel Kick, is perhaps the most misunderstood and least used kick in the martial artist's arsenal. This section will go into minute detail over all areas and phases of executing the Turning Wheel Kick. Once this primary kick is mastered, all of the other variations of this primary kick will fall into place. Without any further ado, let's get started.

Fighting Stance:

Your fighting stance should be approximately shoulder width apart (1a) with the toes of your front or lead foot pointed directly at your opponent. The heel of your lead foot should be in a direct line (1b) with the heel of your rear foot. This allows for you to facilitate a faster turn when executing this kick. Remember that the foot positions in this stance will actually change after you become comfortable executing this kick. At that time your feet will still be approximately shoulder width apart in length, however the heels will be about 4 to 8 inches apart, rather than in a straight line with one another.

The toes of your back or rear foot (1b) should be pointed away from your body at a 45-degree angle. For example, if your right foot were in the rear position, then the toes of that foot would be pointed to the right at a 45-degree angle. If the left foot were in the rear position, then the toes of your left foot would be pointed to the left at a 45-degree angle.

Your weight should be distributed over the balls of both feet and not over the entire surface area of the feet. This way your mobility is increased and you will be able to facilitate a faster turn when executing the kick. The weight distribution over your feet should be approximately 55% over the lead leg and 45% over the rear leg. This also allows for faster movement when kicking or when evading your opponent's attack.

Your knees (2) should be slightly but not noticeably bent. The lead leg knee should be slightly bent over the lead leg foot in the direction of the toes. The same also holds true for the rear knee in the fact that it too should be slightly bent over the rear foot in the direction of the rear toes. The bending of the knees contributes to faster movement with the legs as they are not locked straight or rigid and have better mobility when slightly bent rather than straight.

Your body (3) is facing at a 45-degree angle to your opponent. This presents a smaller target area facing toward your opponent. It also allows you better mobility moving forward toward your opponent, or backward away from your opponent. Additionally it allows you quicker access to offset your opponent by moving in the direction your body is facing.

Your hands (4a) and elbows (4b), should be held up like a boxer's, that is with the lead hand held up at head level and away from your face about 8 to 12 inches (toward your opponent). Your lead elbow should be tucked in along your side in order to protect your ribs and stomach area. Your rear hand is held up alongside your cheek or neck, with the palm of that hand facing toward your cheek. Your rear elbow is also tucked in along your side in order to protect your ribs and stomach area.

Your back (5) should be straight but not rigid and your lead shoulder should be raised up slightly in order to protect your chin.

Your head (6) is facing toward your opponent with the chin tucked down behind your upraised lead shoulder.

Your eyes (7) should focus like a flashlight on your opponent's chest to center your vision. At the same time, allow your peripheral vision to scan the rest of your opponent's body and therefore any movements he will make. A word of caution, **do not** become fixated on a particular spot or point of focus on your opponent. This becomes more of a hindrance than an asset when fighting.

Additionally, you should **never** take your eyes off your opponent for any reason. This mistake is quite common when turning in order to perform this kick. Always turn your head first in order to maintain eye contact with your opponent. Remember the old saying, "Look before you leap"?

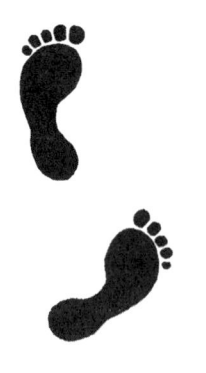

Fighting Position Foot Position (Beginning)

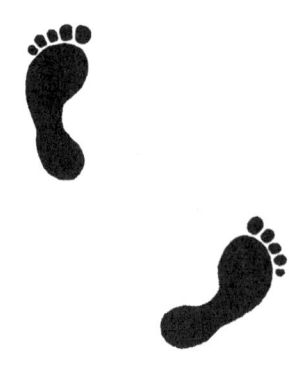

Fighting Position Foot Position (Advanced)

Note: To better understand the visual aspects of a Turning Wheel Kick, imagine that you have an overhead view of yourself standing on the clock image which is shown on the right. Your base leg foot is represented by the pivot point in the center of the clock, while the minute hand represents your kicking leg. In the advanced fighting position, the toes of your base leg foot are pointing at the 12 o'clock position while your kicking foot is at the 5 o'clock position (6 o'clock in the beginning fighting position).

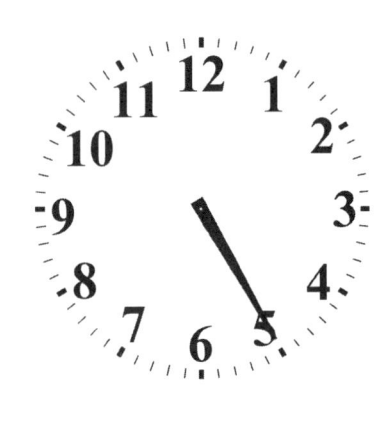

Overhead View

36

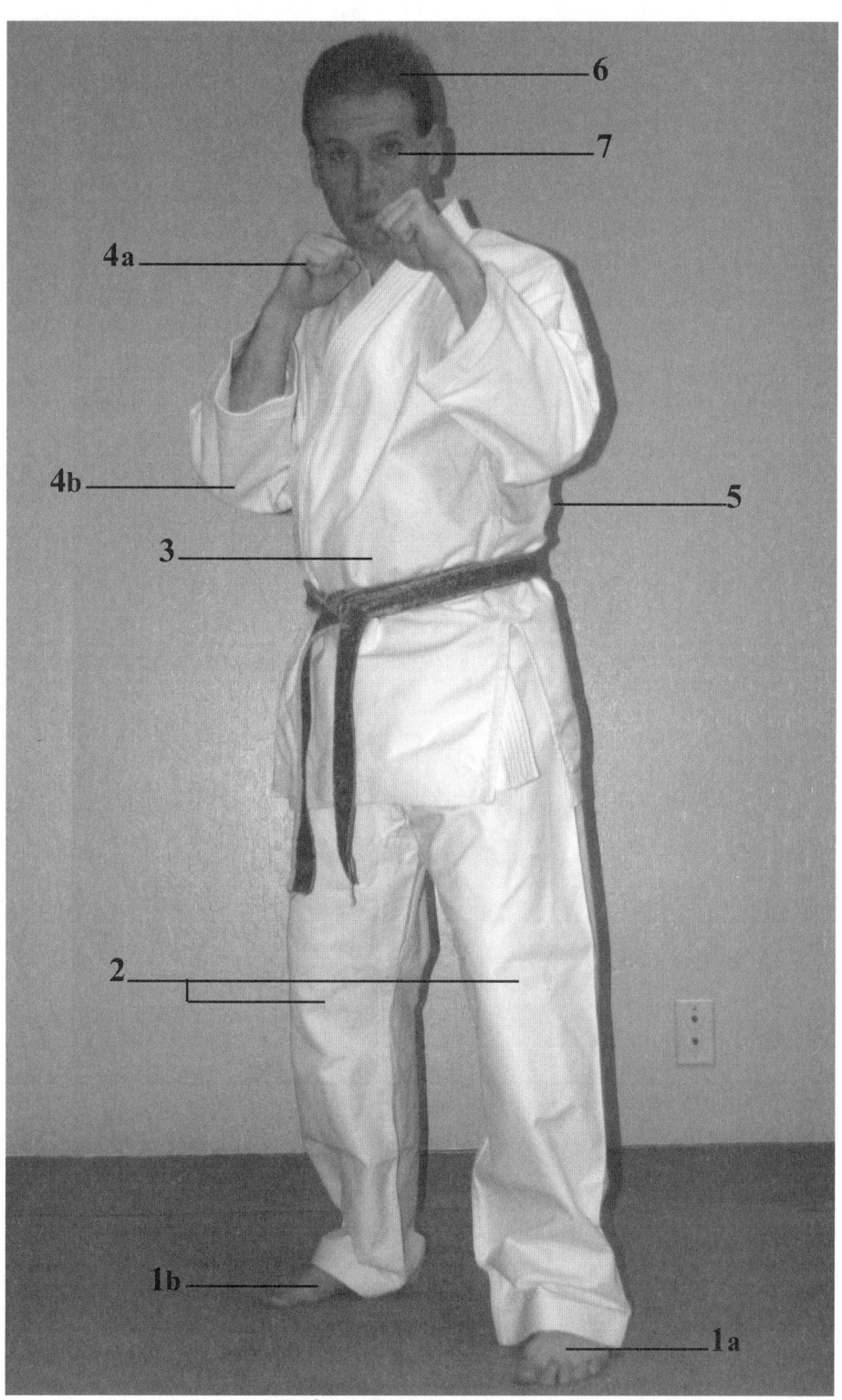

Fighting Position Front View

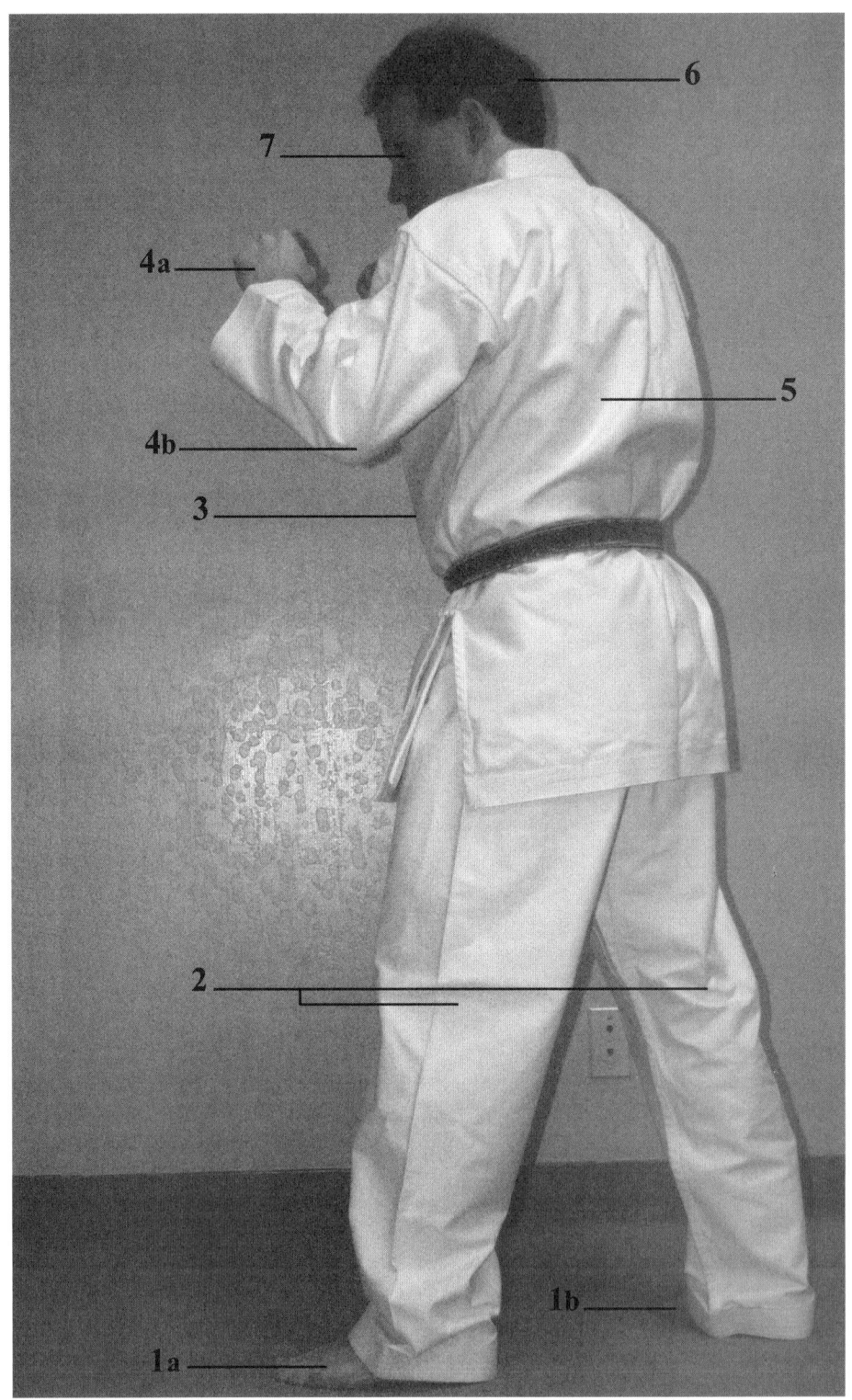

Fighting Position Side View

Turning:

The turn itself is easy to perform if all of the components of the turn are performed correctly. Your lead foot (8a) is going to pivot 180-degrees clockwise on the ball of the foot so that your lead foot heel is now pointed directly at your opponent. While you are doing this your rear foot (8b) is going to slide over approximately 8 inches while also turning 135-degrees clockwise so that the rear or kicking leg heel is also pointed directly at your opponent. Both heels are now pointed directly at your opponent, while the toes of both feet are facing directly away from your opponent.

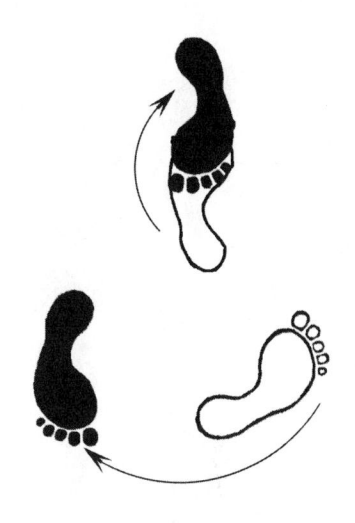

Turning Back Foot Position

Both knees (9) are slightly, but not noticeably bent. The knees are bent in the direction of the toes of each respective foot. Your back (10a) and (10b) should be straight and facing directly toward your opponent (at the 12 o'clock position), with the shoulder of your kicking leg slightly forward and toward your opponent. Your hands (11a) and elbows (11b) should still be in relatively the same position as they were in fighting position.

Your head (12) is turned so that you are looking over your kicking leg shoulder. Your chin is tucked down behind your kicking leg shoulder, and your eyes (13) should still be centered on your opponent's chest.

Note: When you execute the turn, you will pivot on the ball of your base foot in a clockwise motion resulting in your base foot heel now pointing at the 12 o'clock position, while your kicking foot moves from the 5 o'clock position (1) to the 7 o'clock position (2). Your kicking leg will momentarily remain in relatively the same position as you initiate the "Begin Trajectory," phase of the Turning Wheel Kick. Although, it will no longer be in contact with the ground.

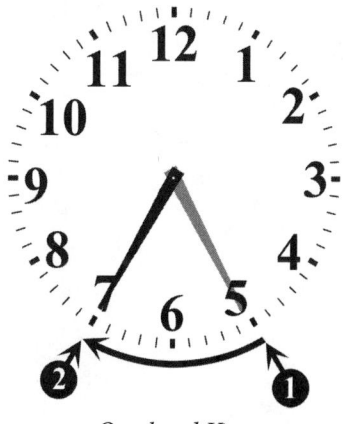

Overhead View

39

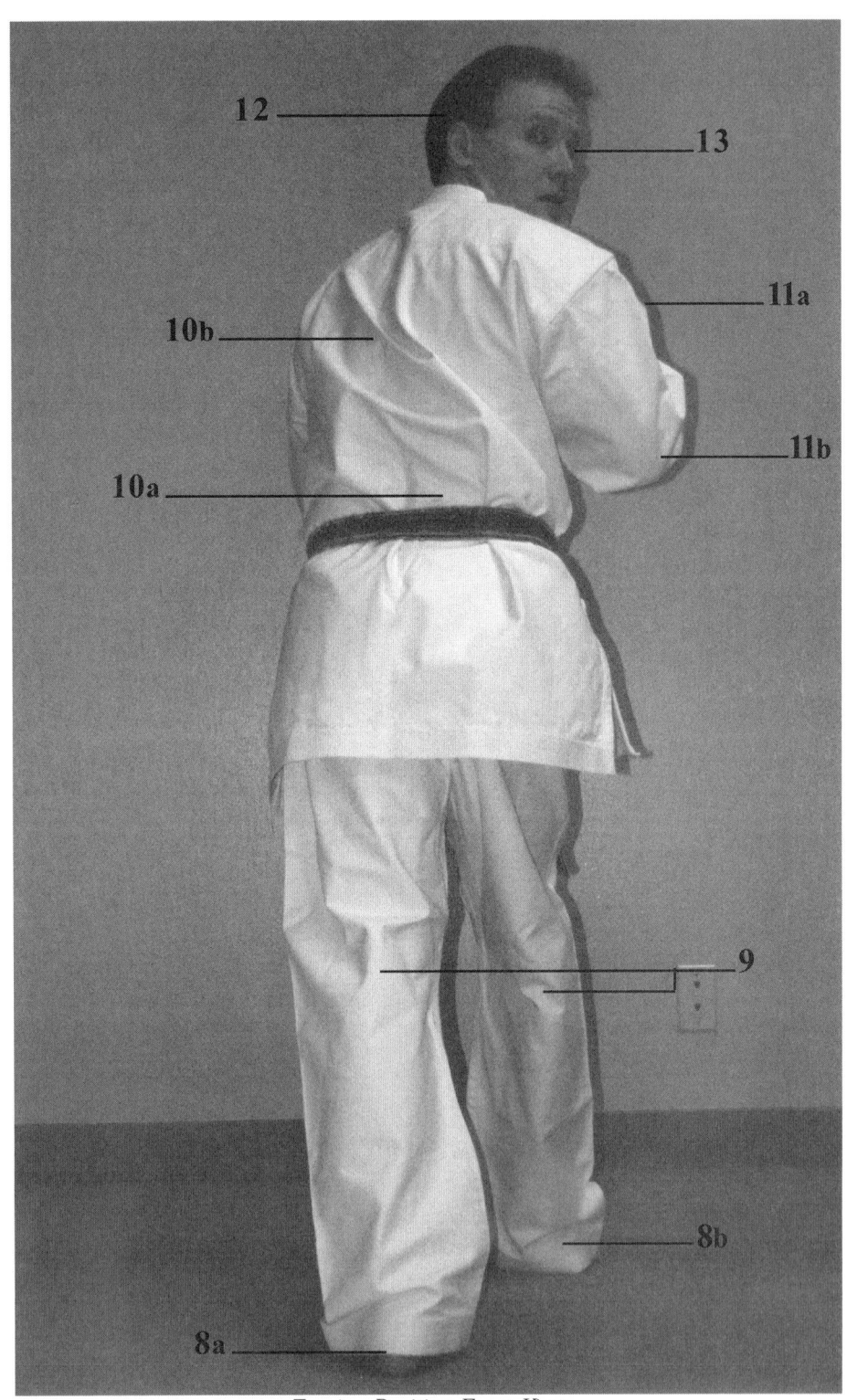

Turning Position Front View

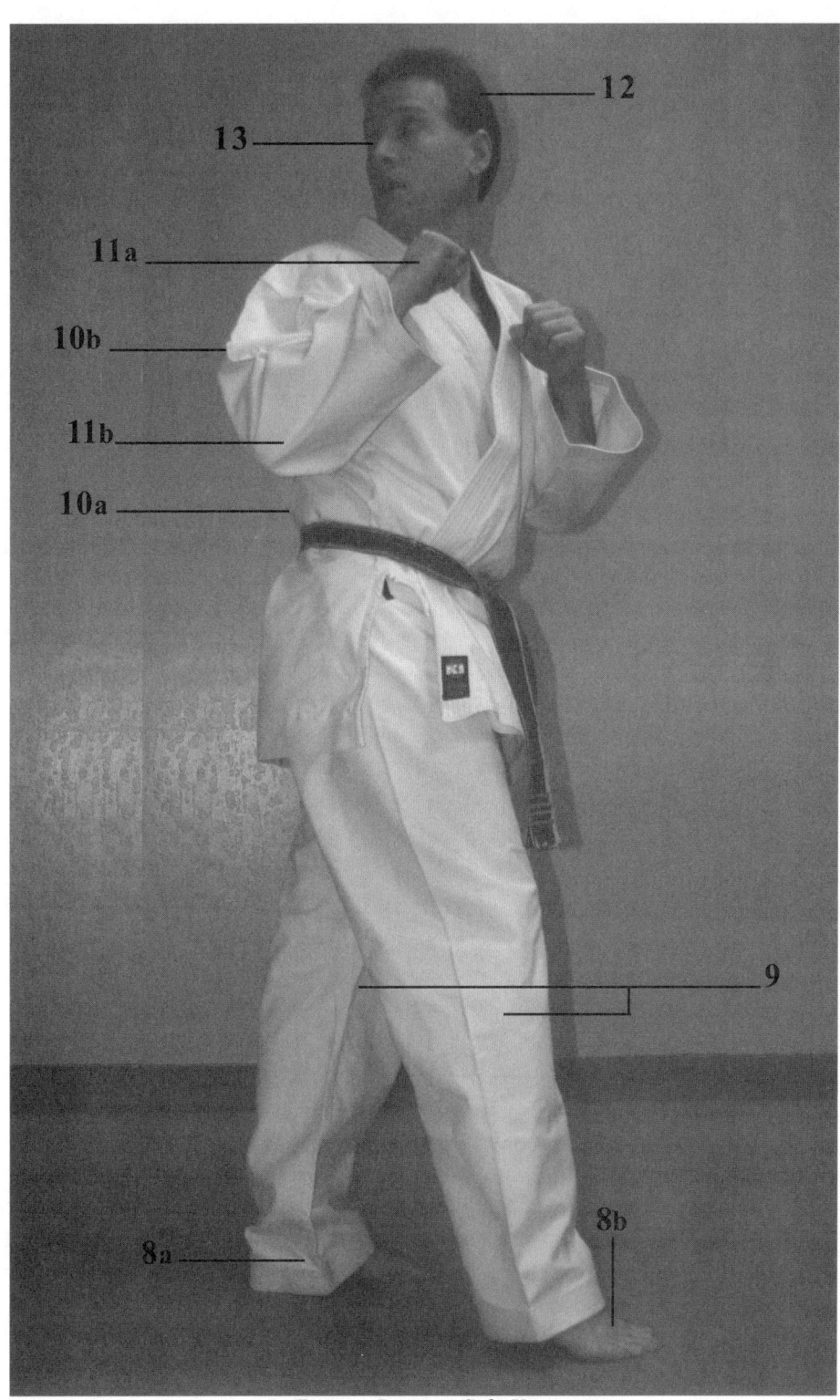

Turning Position Side View

Begin Trajectory:

Your base leg foot (14) is still in the same position as (8a), although it will now bear 100% of the weight as you shift all of your weight onto it, while raising your kicking leg up in order to execute the Turning Wheel Kick.

The base leg knee (15) remains slightly bent in the direction of the toes on your base leg foot. Using your kicking leg foot (17), push off the ground bringing your kicking leg up at approximately a 45-degree angle (midway between the 7 and 8 o'clock positions). This is done by first raising the heel of your kicking foot (17) as you quickly push off the ground using the toes of your kicking foot. After your kicking foot has left the ground, the muscles on the top of your kicking leg thigh contract to bring your leg up into this position. Your kicking leg should be straight, with a slight bend in the kicking leg knee (16).

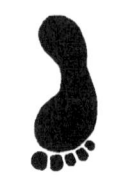

Begin Trajectory Foot Position

Your kicking foot (17) should be at approximately the same height as your base leg knee and parallel with the ground. Your kicking foot and toes, are flexed back towards your kicking leg knee, exposing the back of your heel as the striking surface, rather than your toes or the sole of your foot. The thigh muscles on the top of your kicking leg should be flexed like a piece of spring steel, so that your kicking leg is brought towards your abdomen. While simultaneously, the muscles in the back of your kicking leg thigh are stretched like a giant rubber band. This results in the creation of more tension and subsequently more potential power available to you, during the execution of this kick.

Too many martial artists are sacrificing proper technique in order to get the kick to the target faster. Although it is true to a certain extent that a kick will get to the target faster without utilizing proper technique, it is incorrect and can prove potentially harmful to the individual kicker. Proper technique should never be sacrificed for the sake of speed.

Your back (18a) and (18b), should already have begun turning clockwise from the 12 o'clock position, to the 1 o'clock position with your kicking leg shoulder and hip being the closest to your opponent at the 12 o'clock position. Your back should be straight but not rigid, and does not bend over at the waist at this time. Your hands (19a) and elbows (19b), are also in relatively the same position as in (11a) and (11b).

Your head (20) remains in the same position as in (13). Your eyes (21) are still focused on your opponent's chest like a flashlight, not a laser beam.

Note: The primary key to the successful execution of not only a Turning Wheel Kick, but any kick especially a 360-degree circular kick, is the proper pivoting on the ball of the base leg foot throughout the entire execution of the kick.

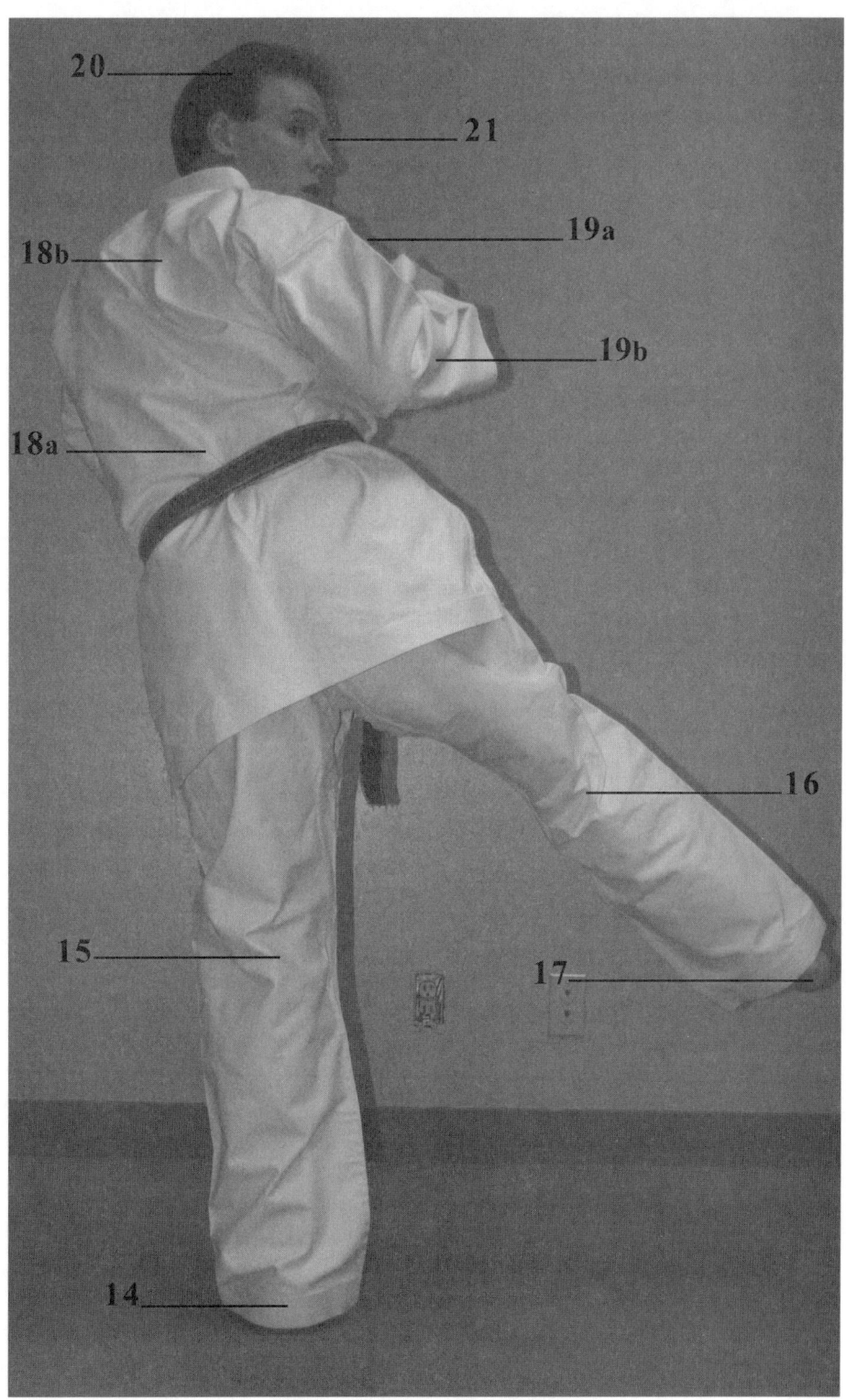

Begin Trajectory Front View

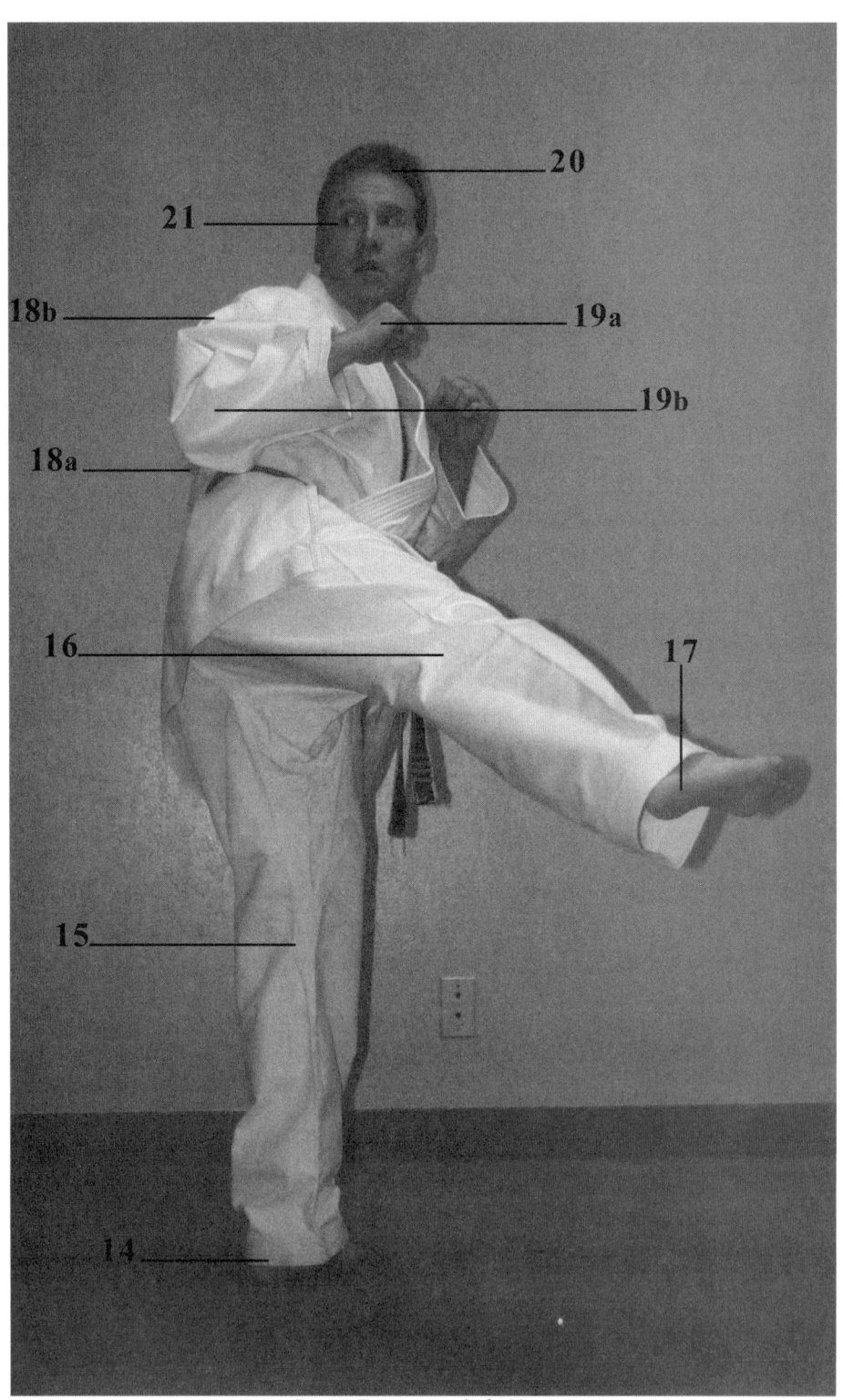

Begin Trajectory Side View

Peak of Trajectory:

Begin by pivoting clockwise on the ball of your base leg foot (22) approximately 45-degrees from the 12 o'clock position to midway between the 1 and 2 o'clock positions. Your base leg knee (23) is still slightly bent as you begin to raise your kicking leg foot up to the correct target height. This is determined by the height of the target you choose, and the height of your opponent. The toes of your kicking foot (24) continue to be flexed back toward your kicking knee in order to fully expose the back of the heel as the striking surface. Although your toes and foot are flexed towards the kicking leg knee, do not flex them to the point of having your foot and ankle too tight. It should be a relaxed tension or flexion.

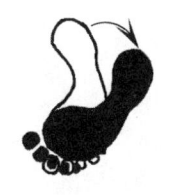

Peak of Trajectory Foot Position

Your kicking leg and kicking foot (24), continue to travel in a circular (clockwise) motion, while simultaneously increasing in height, to the correct target height of your choosing from the previous "Begin Trajectory" position, to this current position, at approximately a 45-degree angle to the left of your opponent. Your kicking leg knee (25) should remain slightly bent throughout the entire execution of this kick. It should not be locked straight as this can prove to be potentially harmful to the individual kicker.

Your back (26a) and (26b), which has continued to move in a clockwise direction, is now facing at the 2 o'clock position, it remains straight but not rigid, and is now bent over at the waist at approximately a 75-degree angle, which allows for an increased range of motion in order to properly execute the kick.

Your hands (27a), and elbows (27b), are still in relatively the same position as they were in the "Begin Trajectory" position. That is with your hands up high around your chest and chin, and your elbows along side your ribcage.

Your head (28) continues to turn toward your opponent with your chin tucked in behind the kicking leg shoulder. Your eyes (29) should be looking over your kicking leg shoulder and focused on your opponent's chest like a flashlight, not a laser beam.

Note: As you continue to pivot on the ball of your base leg foot in a clockwise motion, the heel of your base leg foot is now pointing midway between the 1 and 2 o'clock positions. While your kicking leg (2) continues its circular motion as it increases in elevation to the correct target height. This is called the "Peak of Trajectory" (3) and is located midway between the 10 and 11 o'clock positions.

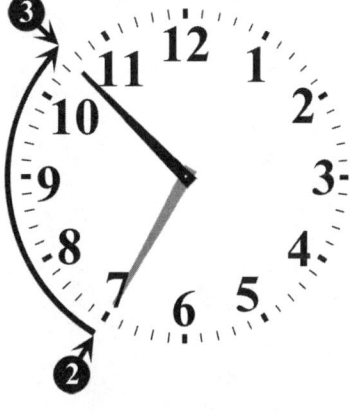

Overhead View

45

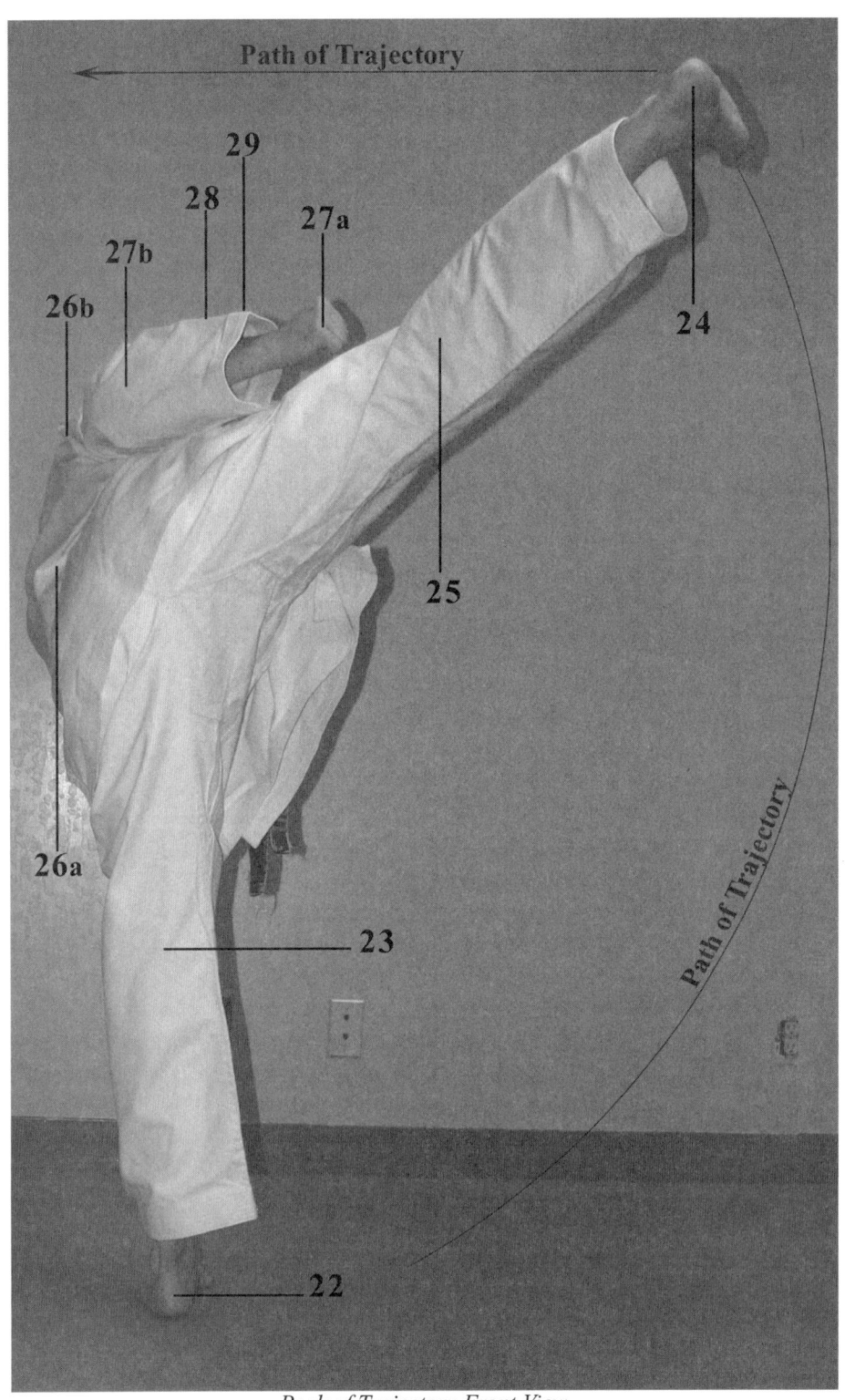

Peak of Trajectory Front View

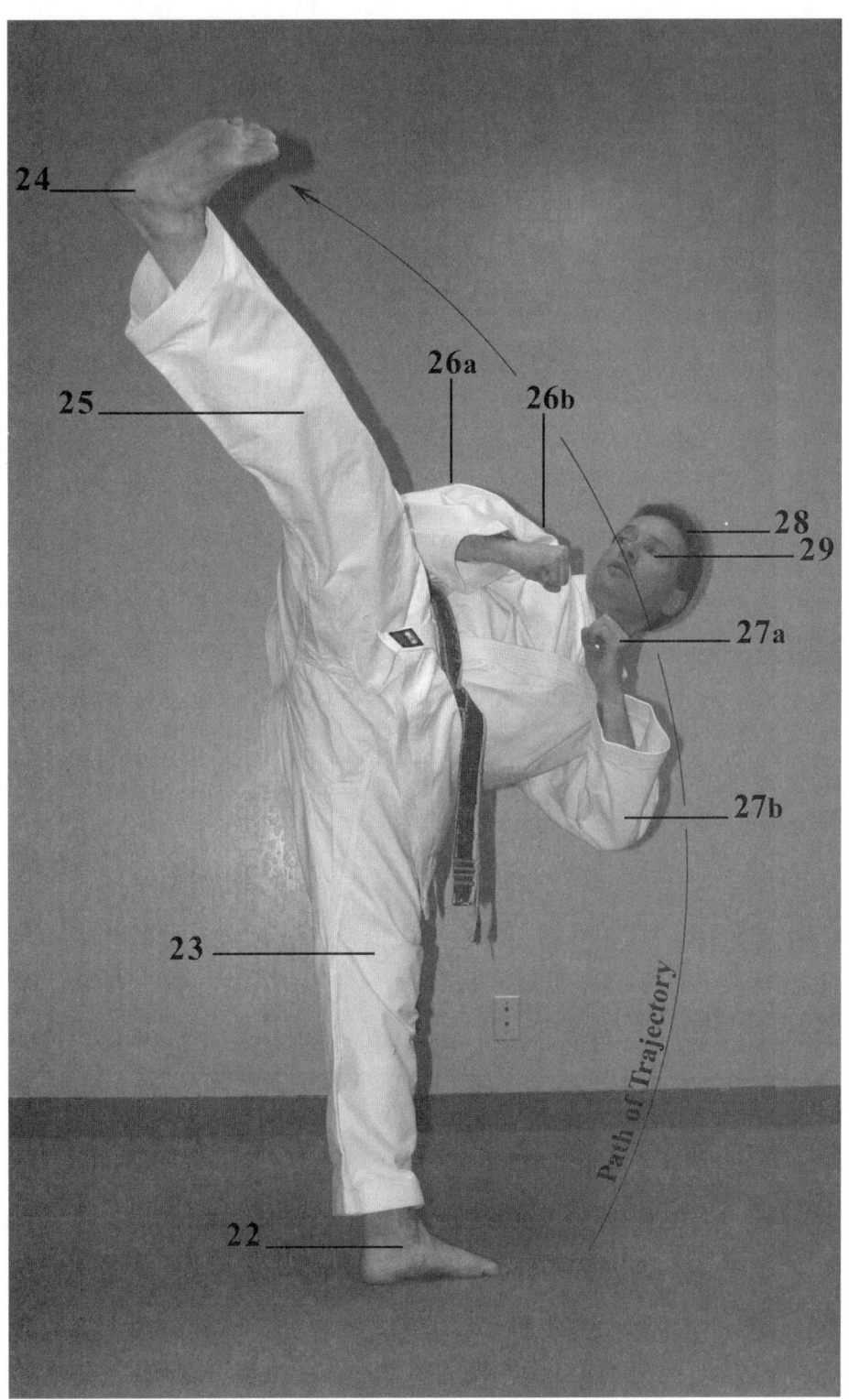

Peak of Trajectory Side View

Impact:

Continue pivoting clockwise on the ball of your base leg foot (30) approximately 45-degrees from the previous position to the 3 o'clock position. After your foot has reached this position, it should now be pushing against the floor, while simultaneously gripping the floor with the entire foot. In other words, your entire foot should be in solid contact with the ground while the heel remains pointed at the 3 o'clock position. Your base leg knee (31) is now straightened at the moment of impact to add power to the kick.

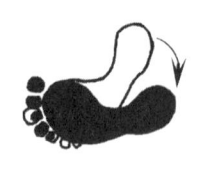

Impact Foot Position

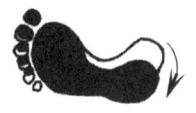

The heel of your kicking foot (32) should now be making contact with the appropriate, vital or vulnerable point, in one of the selected target areas on your opponent. Remember that the contact time between your striking surface and the opponent's target area is minimal. Do not hit the target area and bounce off, or slow down. Strike through the target in an explosive, penetrating manner. Like a bullet!

Impact (ADVANCED) Foot Position

At the moment of impact, your kicking leg knee (33) should be slightly bent in order to absorb the initial shock of impact. The entire kicking leg as well as; your shoulders, back, hips, base leg and head, should all be in a straight line. Upon initial impact, your entire body will tighten up to add power to the kick, and then immediately relax again, in order to facilitate a faster more explosive follow through. Your kicking foot (32) and kicking knee (33), remain parallel to the ground, and continue to travel along the straight even line of trajectory from the "Peak of Trajectory" to "Impact" and continuing through to the "Follow Through" position.

Your back (34a) and (34b), which has continued to move in a clockwise direction, is now facing at the 3 o'clock position, it remains straight but not rigid, and continues to remain bent over at the waist at approximately a 75-degree angle. Your shoulders are basically at the same angle as your back, with the kicking leg shoulder up higher and more toward your opponent.

Your hands (35a) and elbows (35b), should still be up in relatively the same position as before in (27a) and (27b). Do not let them fly all over like a bird flapping its wings. Keep the elbows in to protect the ribcage and your hands up to protect your head. Your head (36) is still up with the chin tucked in behind the kicking leg shoulder. Your eyes (37) should still be looking over your kicking leg shoulder and focused on your opponent's chest.

Overhead View   *Overhead View*

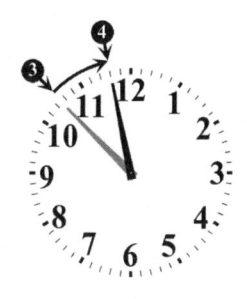

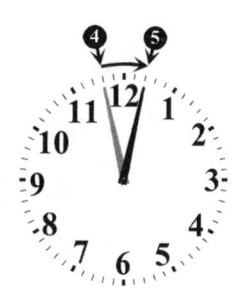

Note: As you continue to pivot on the ball of your base leg foot in a clockwise motion, the heel of your base leg foot is now pointing at the 3 o'clock position, while the toes of your base leg foot are pointing at the 9 o'clock position. From the "Peak of Trajectory" (3), your kicking leg and foot, travels on a straight and level path to the initial "Impact" (4) and subsequent "Strike Through" (5) of your target. The impact side of your target is represented by the outside edge of the number 1 (at the 12 o'clock position), while the strike through side of your target is represented by the outside edge of the number 2 (at the 12 o'clock position).

Note: Look closely at the front and side view photographs from the Peak of Trajectory to the End of Trajectory, do you see anything out-of-place or incorrect? Look again! Notice how my base leg foot seems to lag behind the rest of my body as I execute the kick. This is perhaps the most common error committed by a person when executing a kick, and especially a 360-degree circular kick. If you pivot incorrectly when kicking, you are not only going to have an improper kick, but more importantly you are risking serious injury to yourself and your base leg knee in particular. I have purposely demonstrated this throughout this entire book to point out this most common error, and to emphasize the importance of <u>pivoting correctly on the ball of your base leg foot throughout the entire kicking process.</u>

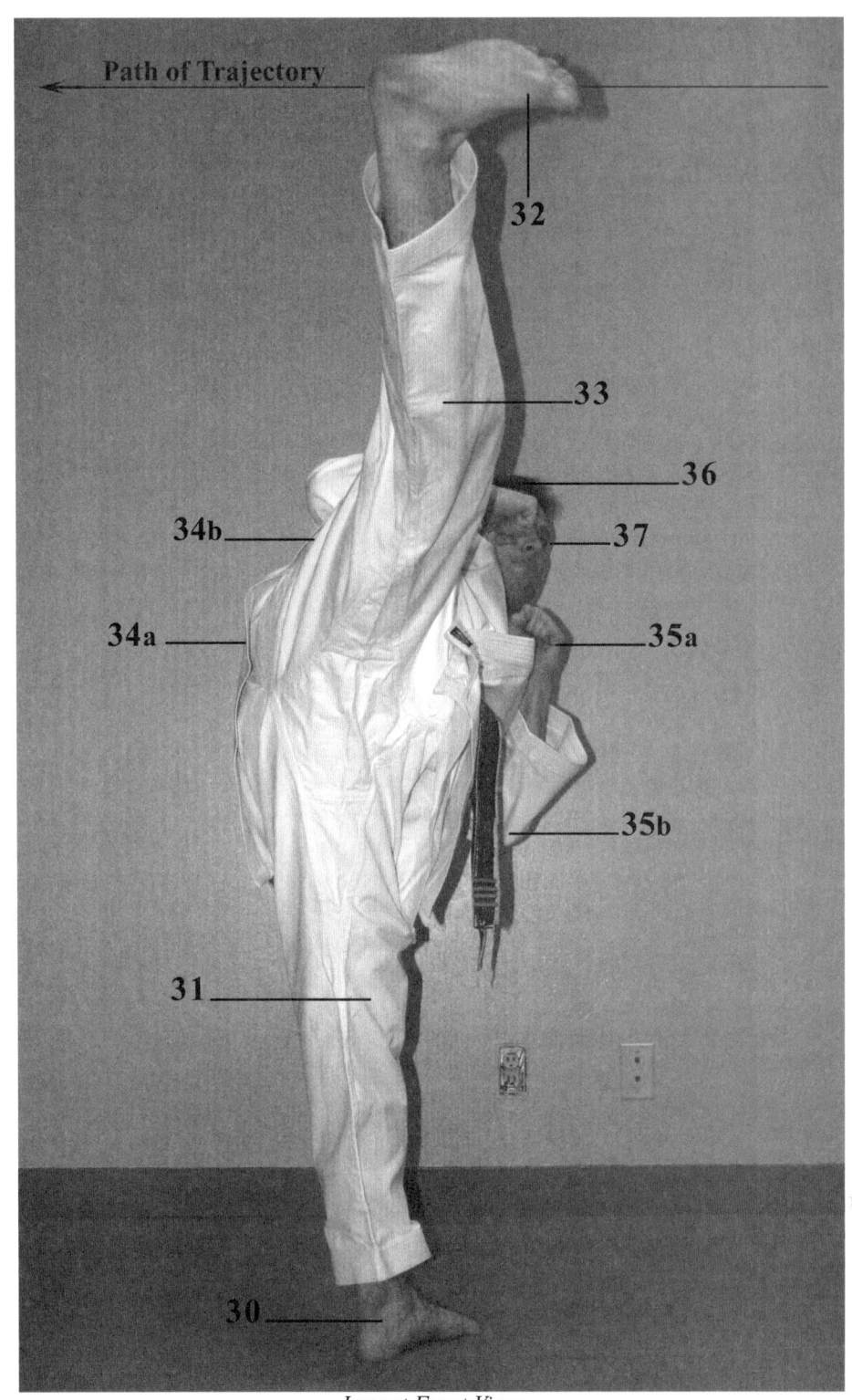

Impact Front View

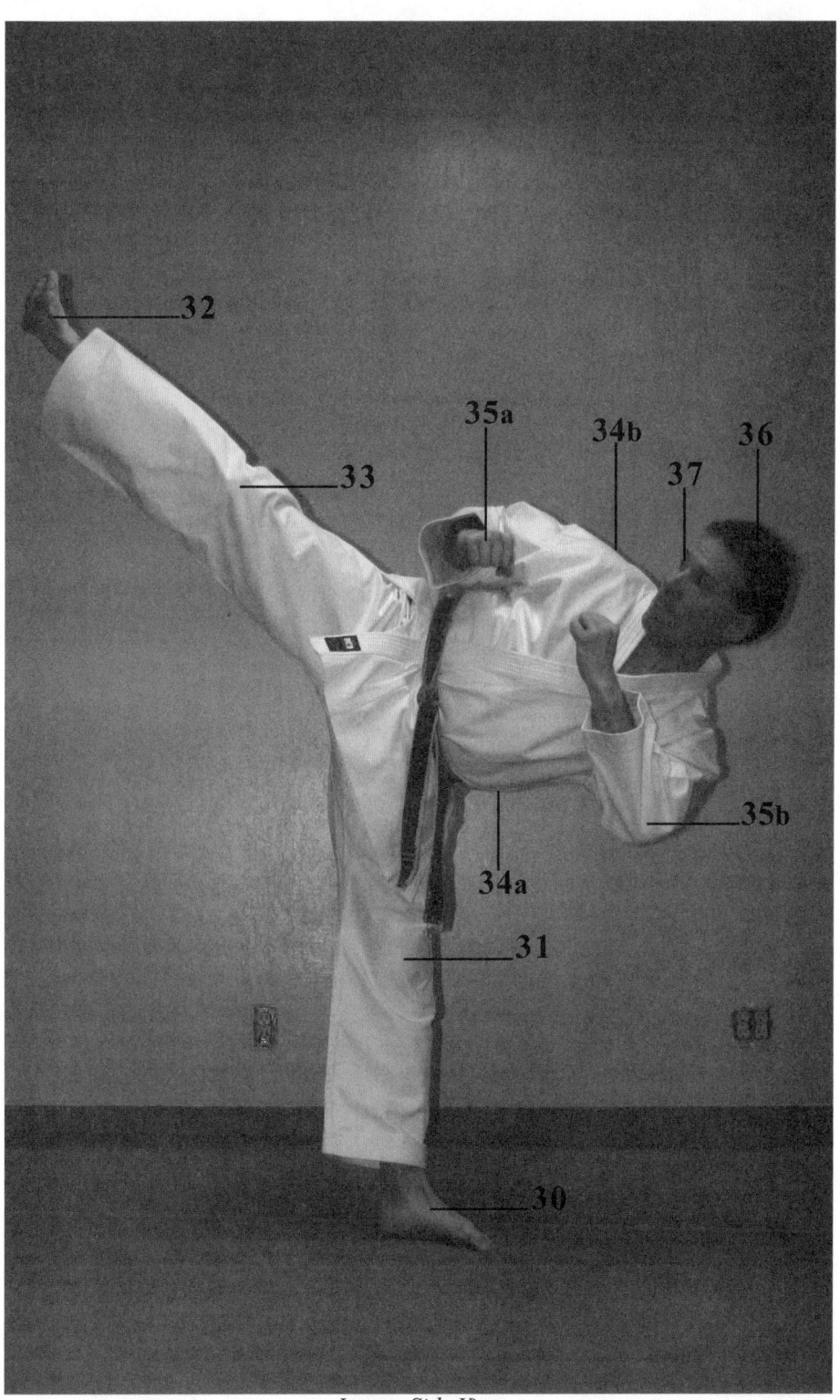

Impact Side View

Follow Through:

Continue pivoting clockwise on the ball of your base leg foot (38) approximately 45-degrees from the previous position to midway between the 4 and 5 o'clock positions. The base leg knee (39) returns to the slightly bent position, with it bending once again in the direction of the toes of the base foot. The kicking leg knee (40) remains slightly bent, and as with your kicking leg foot (41), should be approximately 45-degrees past your opponent, as well as remaining parallel with the ground as it finishes traveling along the straight even line of trajectory. The toes on your kicking foot (41) should still be flexed towards your kicking leg knee, and perpendicular to the ground. This can clearly be seen in both the front and side view photographs of the Follow Through Position.

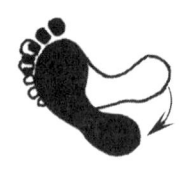

Follow Through Foot Position

Too many martial artists are sacrificing a proper follow through in order to get the kick back on the ground faster. Although it is true to a certain extent that a kick will get to the ground faster without a proper follow through after impact, it can lead to potential problems. **Proper technique should never be sacrificed for the sake of speed. Remember the fable about the tortoise and the hare!**

Your back (42a) and (42b), which has continued to move in a clockwise direction, is now facing at the 4 o'clock position, it remains straight but not rigid, and continues to remain bent over at the waist at approximately a 75-degree angle. Your shoulders remain at basically the same angle as your back, with the kicking leg shoulder up higher and closer to your opponent.

Your hands (43a) and elbows (43b), are also in relatively the same position as they were in (35a) and (35b).

Your head (44) remains in the same position as in (36), however you will no longer be looking over your kicking leg shoulder. Your eyes (45) should be still be on your opponent, although they may not be focused on your opponent's chest if you have knocked him backward or down. However, if you look closely at the front view photograph, you will see that I am looking at my kicking foot instead of my opponent, this is incorrect and a very bad mistake to make. **Never take your eyes off of your opponent!**

Note: As you continue to pivot on the ball of your base leg foot in a clockwise motion, the heel of your base leg foot is now pointing at the 5 o'clock position. After the initial "Impact" and "Strike Through" (5) of your target, your kicking leg and foot should continue traveling along a straight and level path to the "Follow Through" position (6), which is located midway between the 1 and 2 o'clock positions.

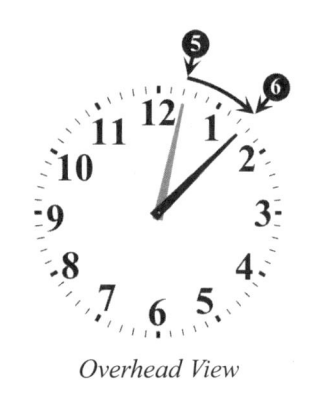

Overhead View

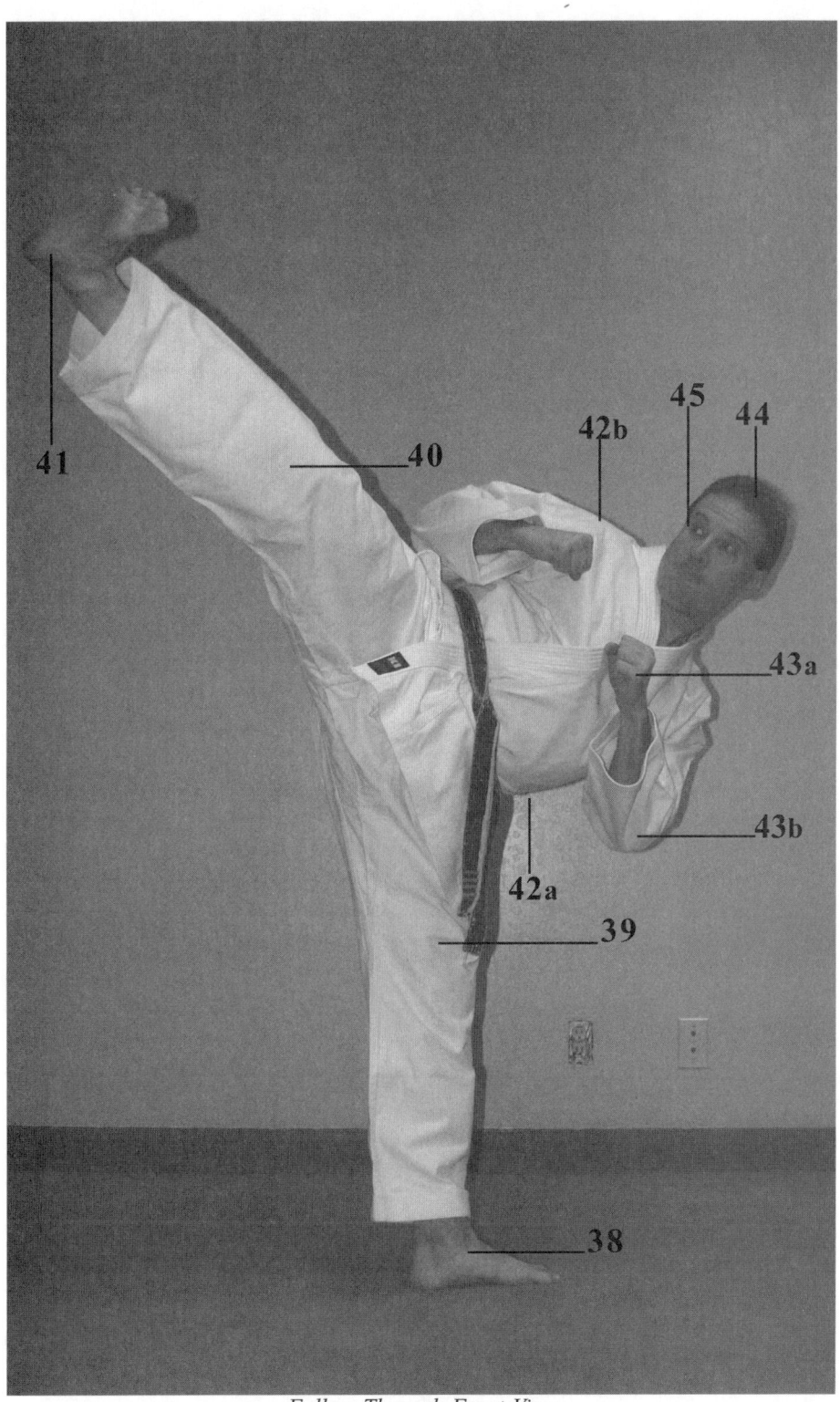

Follow Through Front View

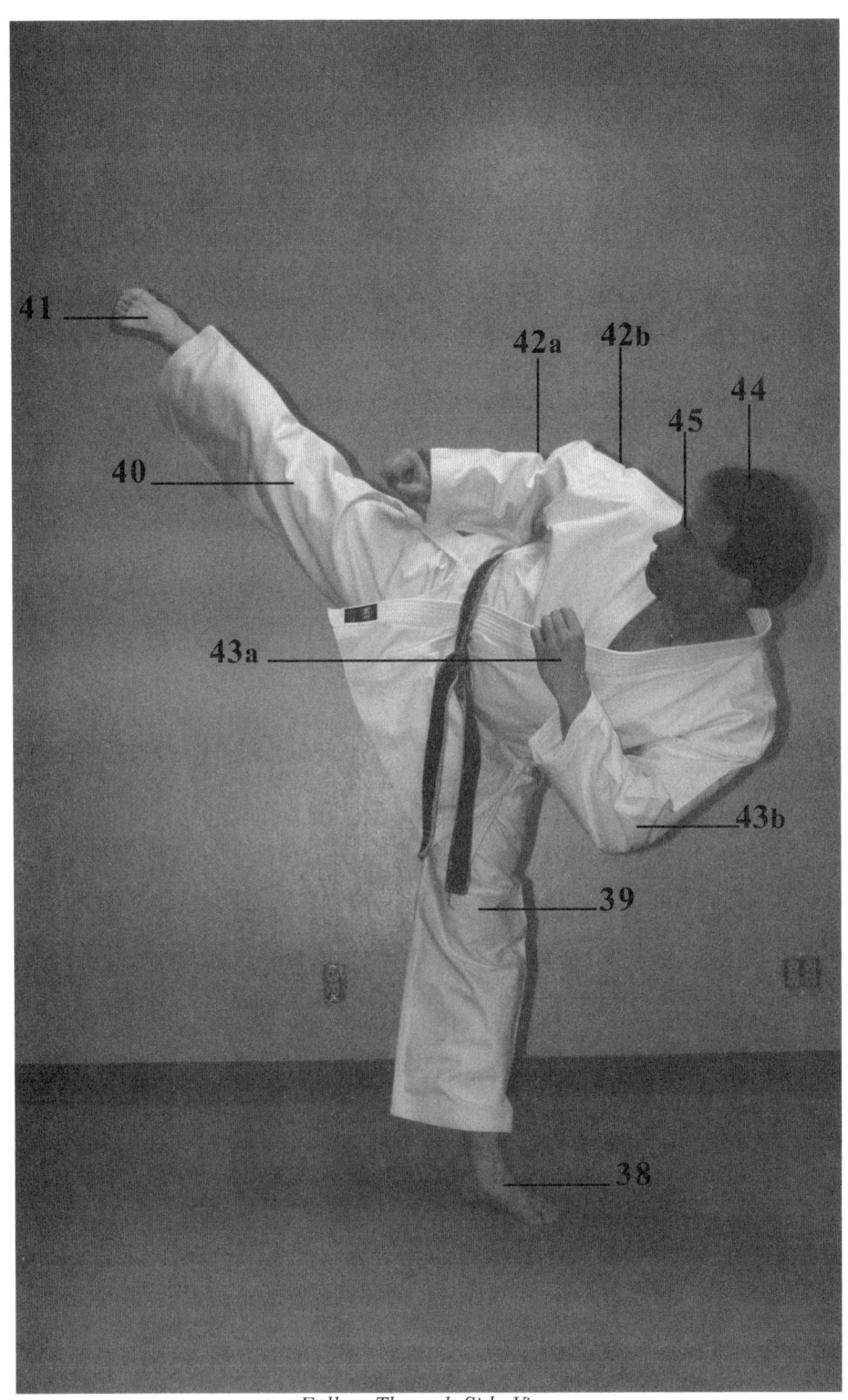

Follow Through Side View

54

End of Trajectory:

Continue pivoting clockwise on the ball of your base leg foot (46) approximately 45-degrees from the previous position to the 6 o'clock position. The toes of your base leg foot should now be pointing directly at your opponent. The base leg knee (47) remains slightly bent, while your base leg continues to bear your entire weight until the kicking leg returns to your original fighting position. The kicking leg foot (49), should momentarily be slightly in front of you and to your right at approximately the height of your base leg knee (at roughly midway between the 2 and 3 o'clock position), as it continues along its circular clockwise path, while decreasing in elevation as it returns to its original starting position. Your kicking leg remains straight with the kicking leg knee (48) slightly bent.

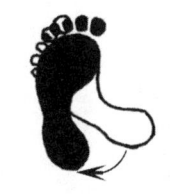

End of Trajectory Foot Position

Often times, a martial artist will tend to slow down his/her kick after striking their target. This results in your kicking foot staying in the air much longer than necessary while continuing to balance on your base leg. This makes it much harder for you to follow up with another kick or technique, and it leaves you much more vulnerable to attack from your opponent. **Remember,** your kicking foot should travel from the target back to its original starting position just as fast, if not faster, than it did from its initial fighting position to the target.

Your back (50a) and (50b), which has continued to move in a clockwise direction, is now facing at the 6 o'clock position, with your chest and abdomen facing directly toward your opponent. Your upper body, which is straight but not rigid, should start returning to the upright position from the 75-degree bent over position.

Your hands (51a) and elbows (51b), are also in relatively the same position as they were in (4a) and (4b).

Your head (52) should return to the same position as in (6). Your eyes (53) should still be on your opponent, although they may not be focused on your opponent's chest if you have knocked him backward or down. **Never take your eyes off of your opponent!**

Note: As you continue to pivot on the ball of your base leg foot in a clockwise motion, the toes of your base leg foot are now pointing at the 12 o'clock position. After reaching the "Follow Through" position (6), your kicking leg will decrease in elevation while continuing its circular motion. This is called the "End of Trajectory," and is located at approximately the 4 o'clock position. Your kicking leg completes its circular path by returning to its original starting position (1).

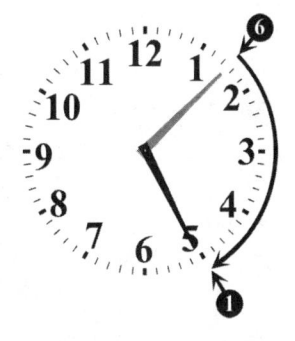

Overhead View

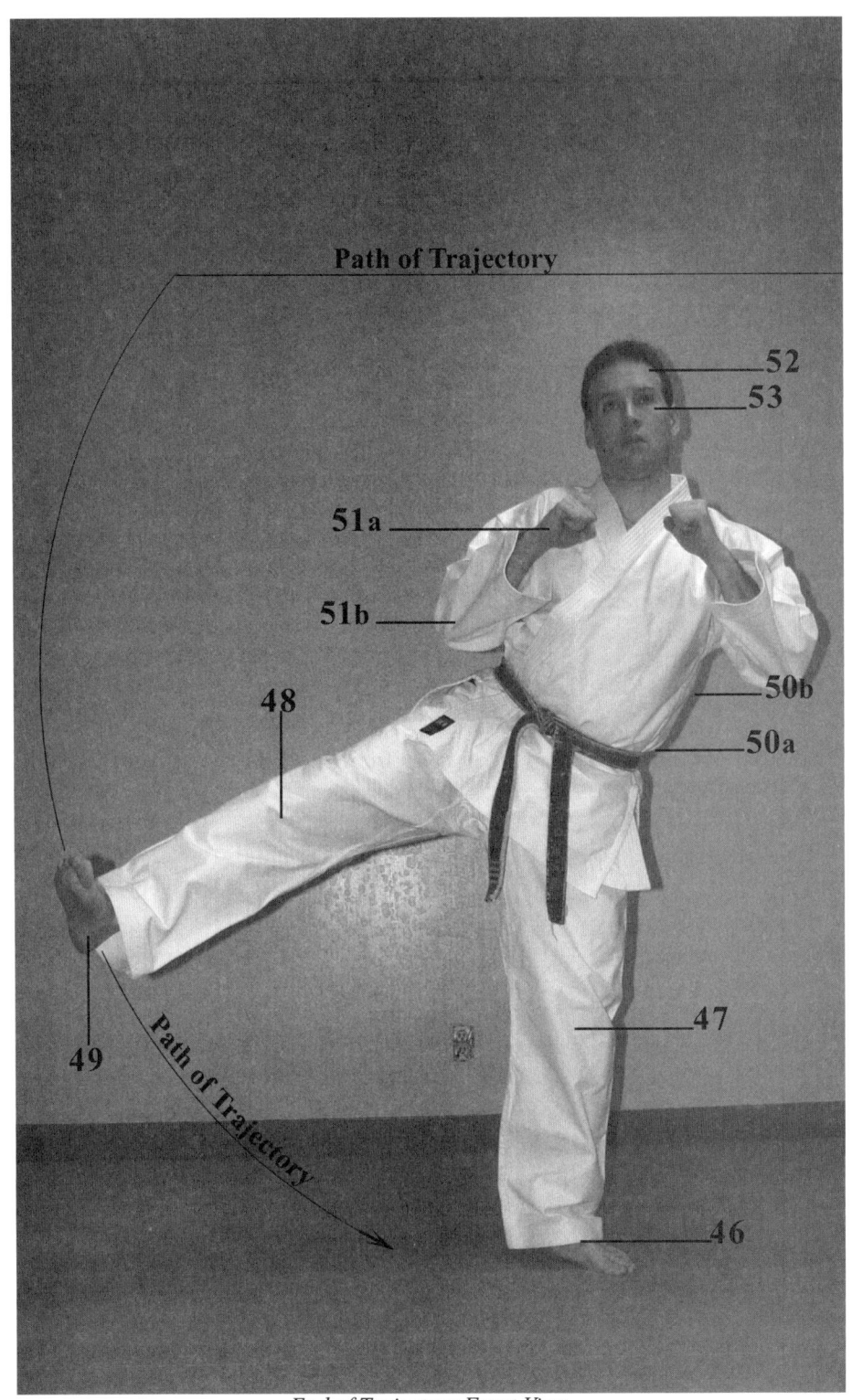

End of Trajectory Front View

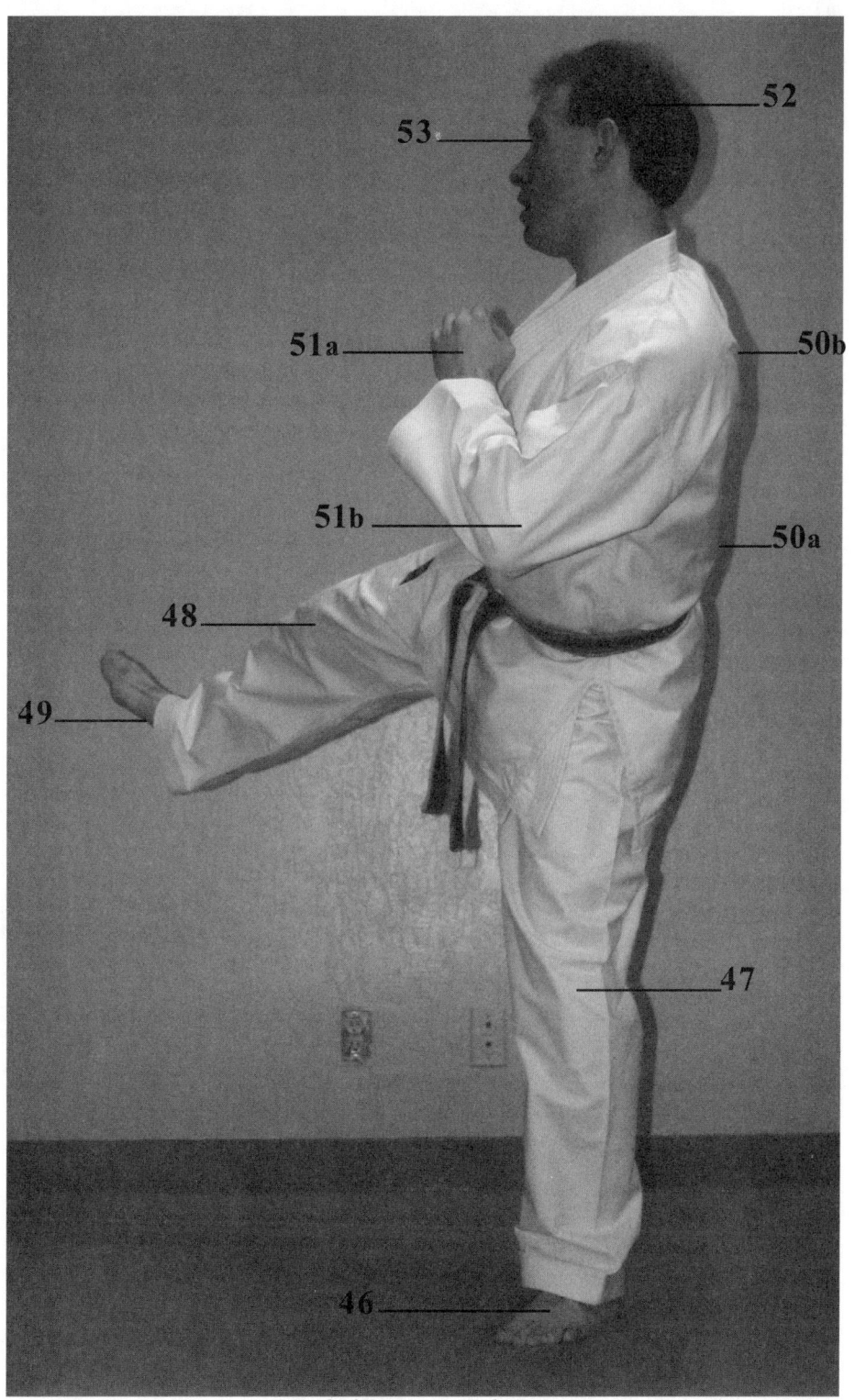

End of Trajectory Side View

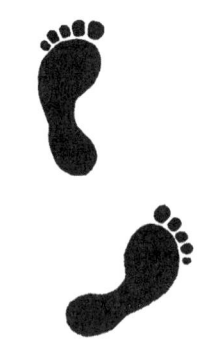

Return to Fighting Position:

Continue turning clockwise (if kicking with the right leg, counterclockwise if you are kicking with the left leg) by pivoting on the ball of your base leg foot, and returning your kicking foot to its original starting position. Your head, shoulders and hips will all come back around to your original fighting position before your kicking leg foot touches the ground. Your entire body should be upright and straight although not rigid throughout the entire return to your original fighting position.

Once you return to Fighting Position, your fighting stance should once again be approximately shoulder width apart with the toes of your front or lead foot (54a) pointed directly at your opponent. The heel of your lead foot (54a) should be in a direct line with the heel of your rear foot (54b). The toes of your back or rear foot (54b) should be pointed away from your body at a 45-degree angle. For example, if your right foot were in the rear position, then the toes of that foot would be pointed to the right at a 45-degree angle. If the left foot were in the rear position, then the toes of your left foot would be pointed to the left at a 45-degree angle.

Return to Fighting Position

Your weight should once again be distributed over the balls of both feet and not over the entire surface area of the feet. The weight distribution over your feet should be approximately 55% over the lead leg and 45% over the rear leg.

Your knees (55) should be slightly but not noticeably bent. The lead leg knee should be slightly bent over the lead leg foot in the direction of the toes. The same also holds true for the rear knee in the fact that it too should be slightly bent over the rear foot in the direction of the rear toes. The bending of the knees contributes to faster movement with the legs as they are not locked straight or rigid and have better mobility when slightly bent rather than straight.

Your body (56) is facing at a 45-degree angle to your opponent. Your hands (57a) and elbows (57b), should still be held up like a boxer's, that is with the lead hand held up at head level and away from your face about 8 to 12 inches (toward your opponent). Your lead elbow should be tucked in along your side in order to protect your ribs and stomach area. Your rear hand is held up alongside your cheek with the palm of that hand facing toward your cheek. Your rear elbow is also tucked in along your side in order to protect your ribs and stomach area.

Your back (58) should be straight but not rigid and your lead shoulder should be raised up slightly in order to protect your chin.

Your head (59) is facing toward your opponent with the chin tucked down behind your upraised lead shoulder. Your eyes (60) should focus like a flashlight on the chest or center of your opponent whether he is still standing or not. At the same time, allow your peripheral vision to scan the rest of your opponent's body and therefore any movements he will make. I cannot stress this enough, **<u>do not</u>** become fixated on a particular spot or point of focus on your opponent. This becomes more of a hindrance than an asset when fighting.

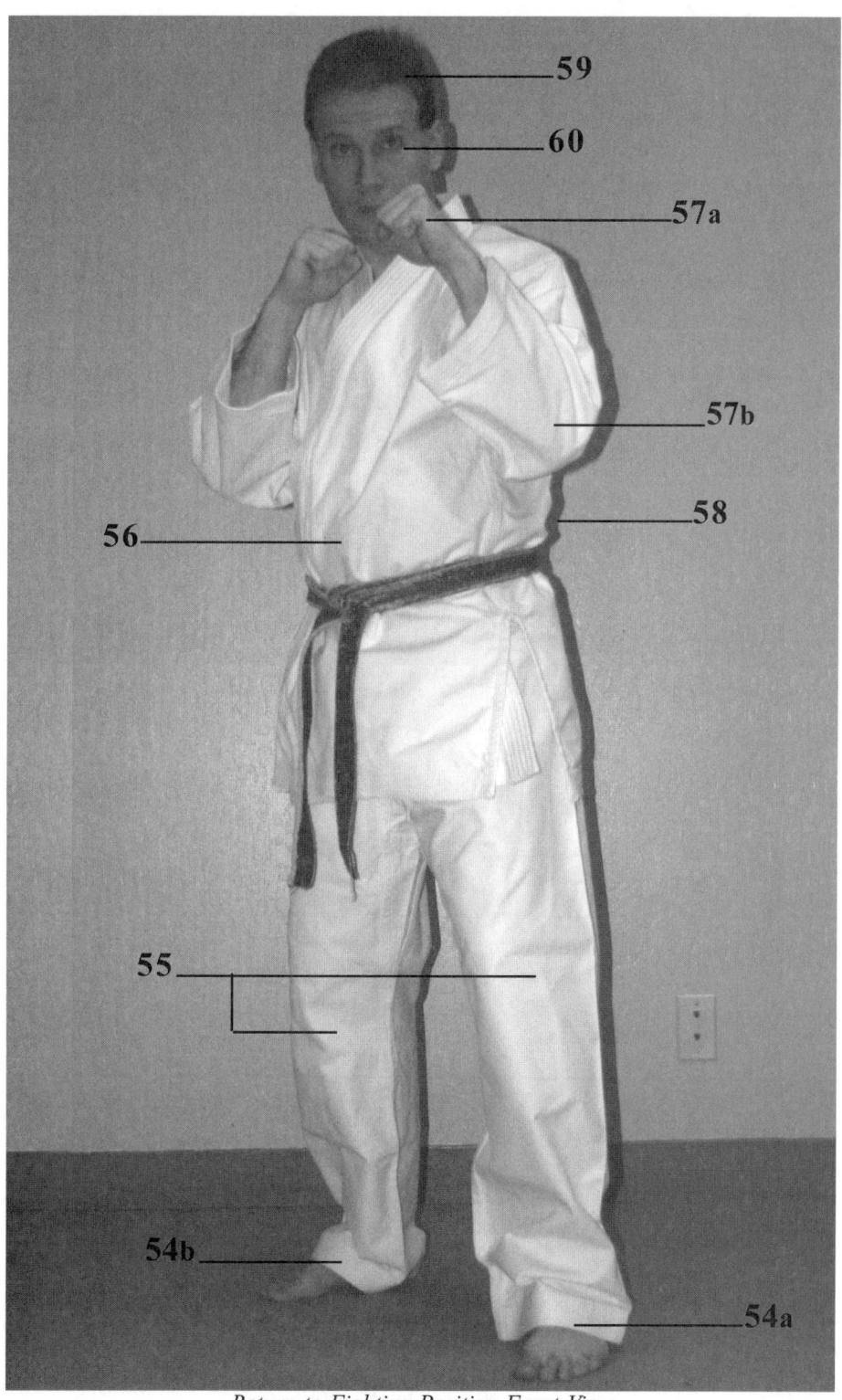

Return to Fighting Position Front View

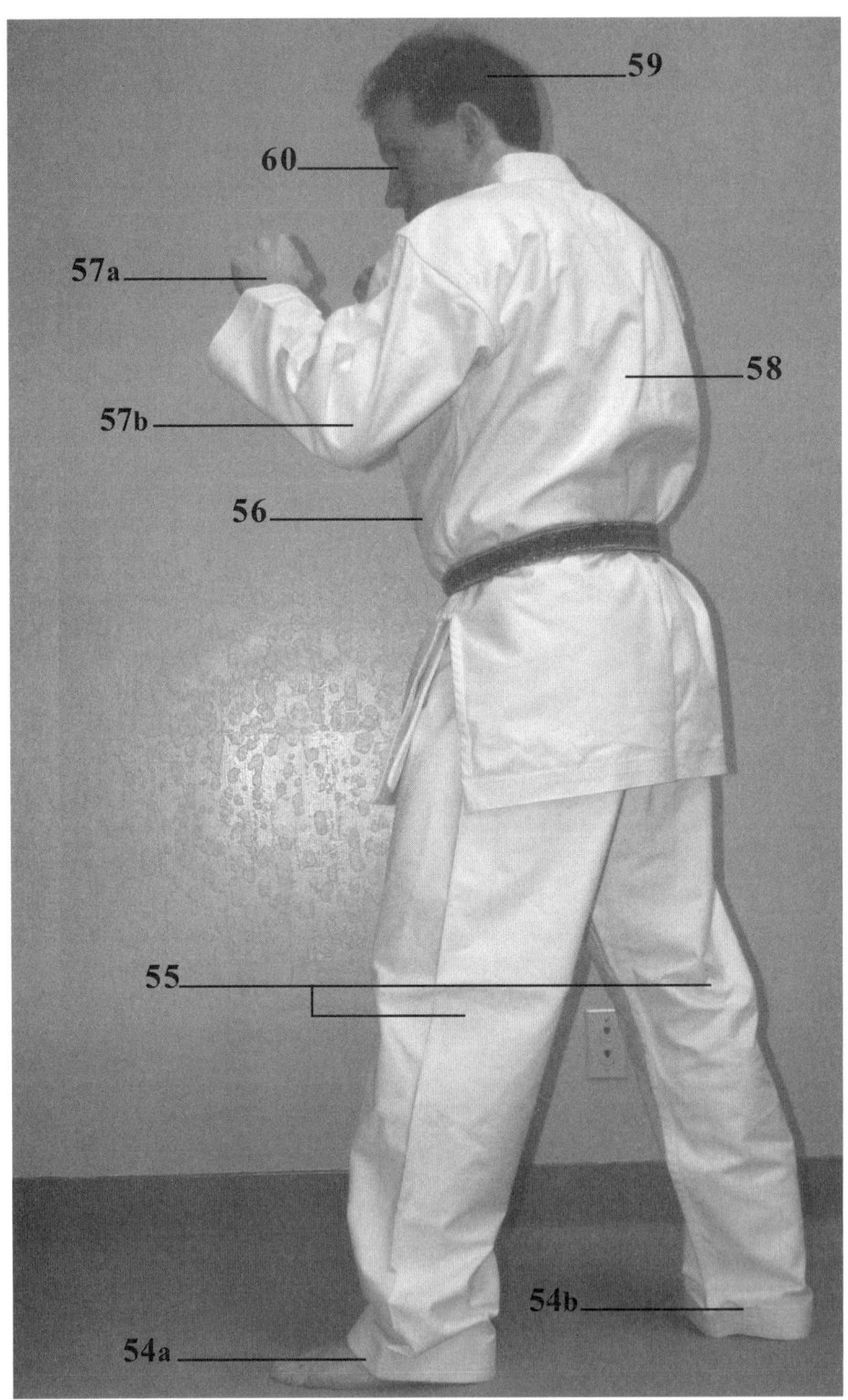

Return to Fighting Position Side View

60

Note: The following illustration, is a visual overview of the "Wheel Kick" clock, showing the sequence of events for the correct execution of a Turning Wheel Kick. The center of the clock (pivot point for the minute hand) represents the ball of your base leg foot, while the minute hand represents your kicking leg.

(1) Fighting Position, (2) Turn & Begin Trajectory, (3) Peak of Trajectory, (4) Initial Impact, (5) Strike Through, (6) Follow Through, and finally, back to (1) End of Trajectory and Return to Fighting Position.

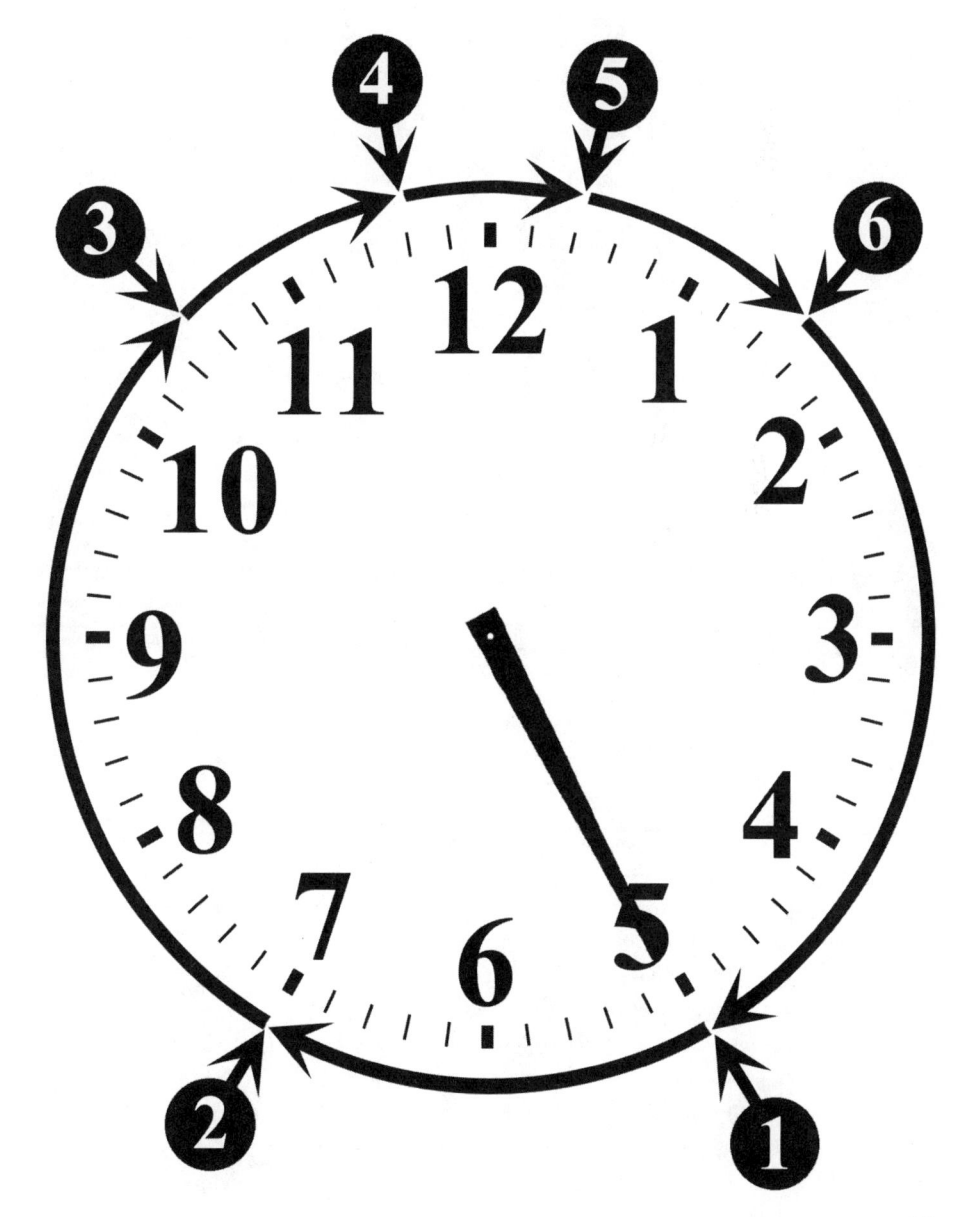

Pictorial Overview:

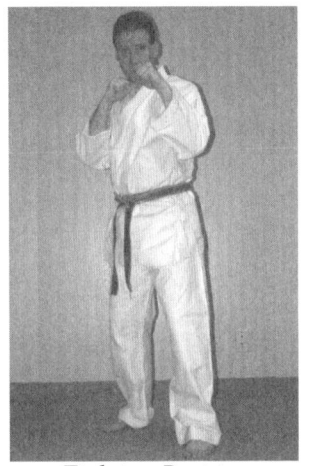

Fighting Position

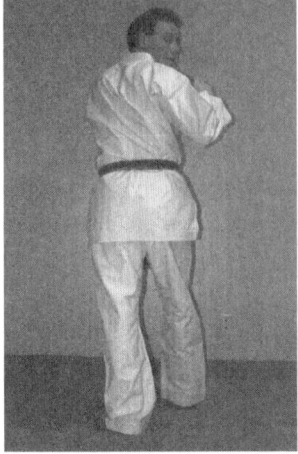

Turn

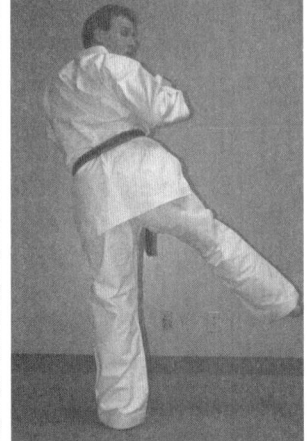

Begin Trajectory

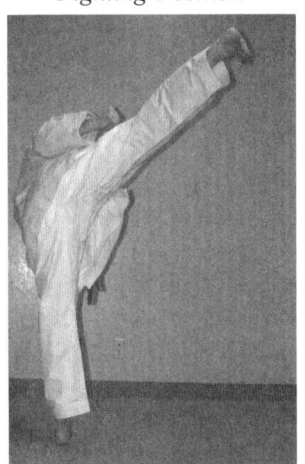

Peak of Trajectory

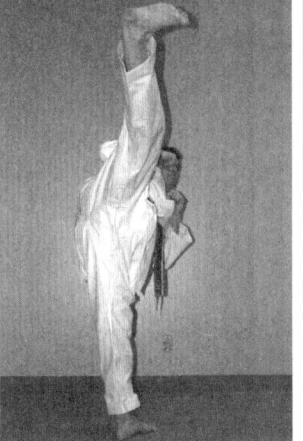

Impact

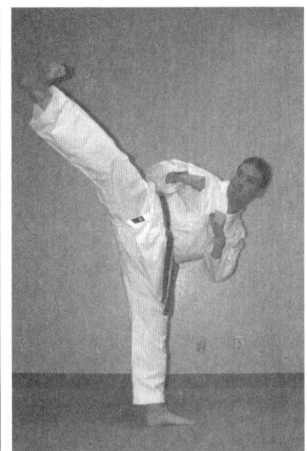

Follow Through

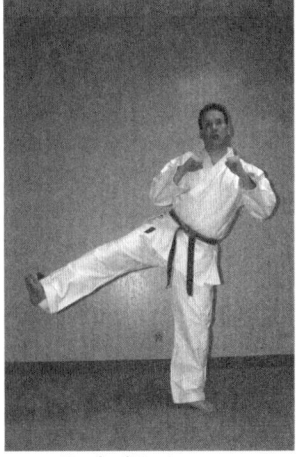

End of Trajectory

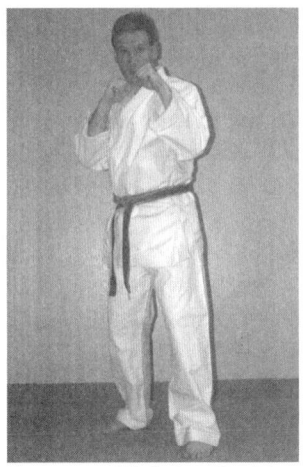

Return to Fighting Position

Variations of the Turning Wheel Kick

This chapter will explain in detail how to properly execute ten variations of the Turning Wheel Kick. Remember that all of these variations are derived from the primary kick, Turning Wheel Kick. Therefore, it is essential that you learn Turning Wheel Kick first before attempting any of these other variations.

To perhaps give you a better understanding of what I mean, let me use the comparison of building a house. Before you start building your house you are first going to need a set of blueprints, this would be the equivalent of the material presented in this book. Next you are going to need the proper materials to begin building with, this would be the equivalent of properly warming-up and stretching before you attempt to practice these kicks.

Next comes the hardest part for students to understand, now in order for your house to be stable, sturdy, and secure, you must first have a very well built and strong foundation. The foundation of your house is made out of concrete, while the foundation of this particular type of kick is, the Turning Wheel Kick. Once you have a strong and proficient Turning Wheel Kick, then you can begin to build upon that with the many different variations of that kick. Just like you would build your frame, walls, ceilings, floors and roof of your house.

If you don't take the time to first build a strong and stable foundation, your kicking skills along with your house, will not last and will collapse when the first strong storm or self-defense situation comes along.

As a general rule of thumb, every time you practice one of the variations of Turning Wheel Kick, you should practice Turning Wheel Kick itself at least ten times. I promise you that if you do this, all of your Wheel Kicks will steadily improve and become stronger.

Step-Back Wheel Kick

The Step-Back Wheel Kick is identical in execution to the Turning Wheel Kick, with one notable exception. A stepping backward motion is performed immediately prior to executing the kick. This step is used to draw your opponent in toward you. The starting or fighting position for this kick begins with your kicking leg in the forward position rather than in the rearward position. The actual stepping back motion of the forward foot prior to the execution of the kick is performed by simply stepping back with the forward foot into another fighting position. Only now the kicking leg is in the rearward rather than the forward position. When executing the stepping back motion, be sure and move your forward foot without initially moving your hips and upper body in order to avoid telegraphing the movement to your opponent. Your hips and upper body will begin to move as your foot begins to set down after stepping back.

Fighting Position:
1. Your fighting position for this kick is exactly the same as it will be for Spinning Wheel Kick. With your kicking leg in the forward position to begin with rather than in the rearward position.
2. This stance is approximately shoulder width apart with the heel of your rear foot in a direct line with the heel of your front foot.
3. Your front or lead foot should be pointing directly at your opponent.
4. Your rear foot is angled toward the left at approximately a 45-degree angle. Your weight should be distributed evenly over the balls of both feet.
5. Your knees are slightly, but not noticeably bent. They should not be locked straight or rigid.
6. Your body should be facing at a 45-degree angle toward your opponent. This presents a smaller target area and also facilitates a faster step-and-turn when utilizing this kick.
7. Your hands should be held up (like a boxers), with the elbows tucked in to protect the ribs and your hands up to protect your head. Your hands should remain as close to this position as possible throughout the entire kick.
8. Your head should be facing your opponent with your chin tucked down and protected by your lead shoulder.
9. Your eyes should be centered on your opponent's chest.

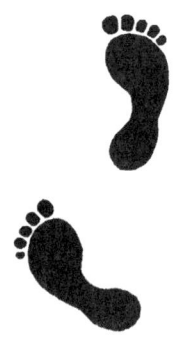

Fighting Position Foot Position

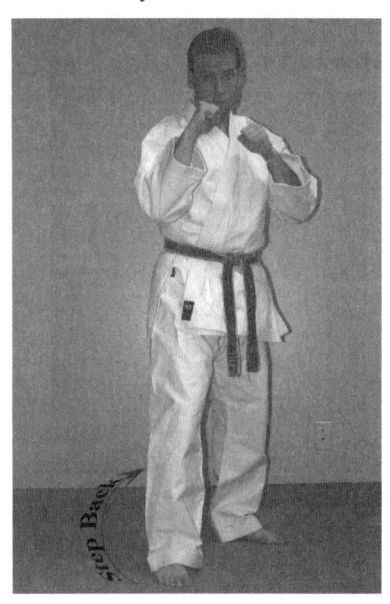

Fighting Position Front View

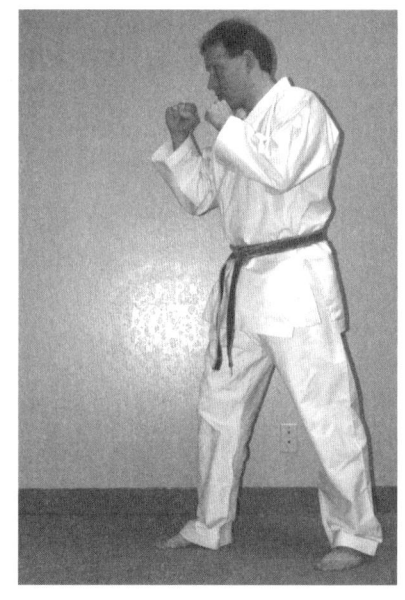

Fighting Position Side View

Step-Back & Turn Back:
10. Take a step backward with your front foot. And...
11. As you step backward with your front foot, pivot on the ball of your base leg. This will have the effect of turning your back towards your opponent.
12. While you are stepping back, and as you begin to turn, you should be turning your head and looking over your kicking leg shoulder at your opponent. Your eyes should be centered on your opponent's chest.
13. When you set your front foot down, only the ball of your kicking leg foot should be touching the ground. However, when initially learning this kick, make sure you have your entire kicking foot in contact with the ground. Your kicking foot should not only be behind you, but should also be approximately 8 inches to the side. This allows for better balance and a more accurate kick. Your back should now be toward your opponent, and the heel of your now-base leg foot should also be pointed toward your opponent.

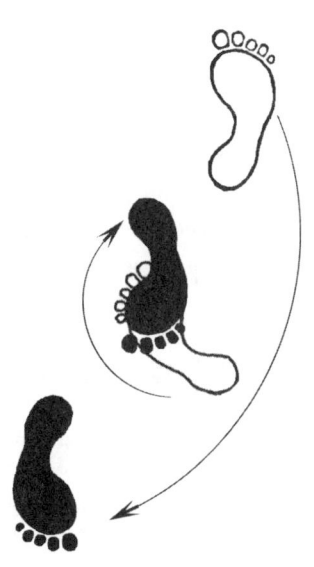

Step Back & Turn Back Foot Position

Note: Your head should always turn first when executing any turning kick, so that you can maintain constant eye contact with your opponent.

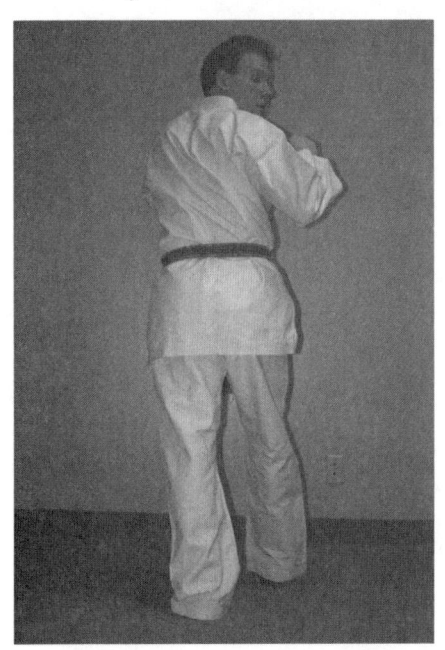

Step Back & Turn Front View

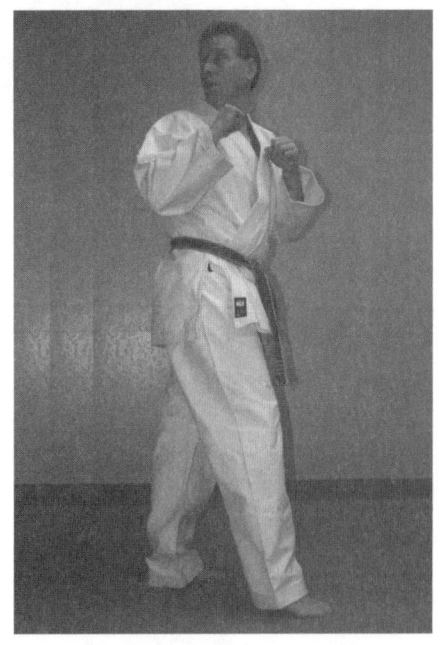

Step Back & Turn Side View

Begin Trajectory:

14. Using the toes of your kicking foot, push off the floor and bring your kicking leg up at a 45-degree angle between the direction your body is facing and your right hand side. Your leg should be straight, with a slight bend in the knee. In this position, your kicking foot should already be in the correct position to strike your opponent.
15. As you bring your kicking leg up, your upper body should start bending over slightly, from the waist, to the left. Your back will remain straight.
16. Your head is still up and turned over your kicking shoulder, your eyes should always remain in contact with your opponent throughout the entire kick.
17. Your back should no longer be facing directly towards your opponent, but should start turning, along with your shoulders, in the direction of the kick.

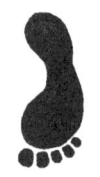

Begin Trajectory Foot Position

Note: Your kicking foot will make a complete 360-degree circle throughout the entire execution of a Wheel Kick, from your initial "Fighting Position" to "Return to Fighting Position." This is done while simultaneously increasing the elevation of the kicking foot to the correct target height by the time it reaches the "Peak of Trajectory" position, and decreasing the elevation from the "Follow Through" position, until the foot returns to its original starting position.

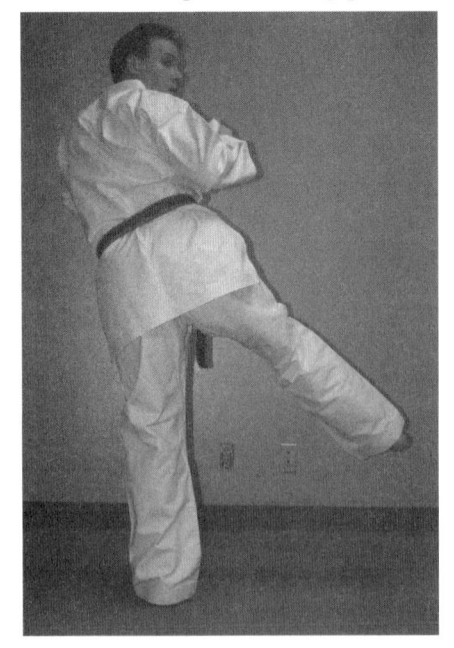

Begin Trajectory Front View

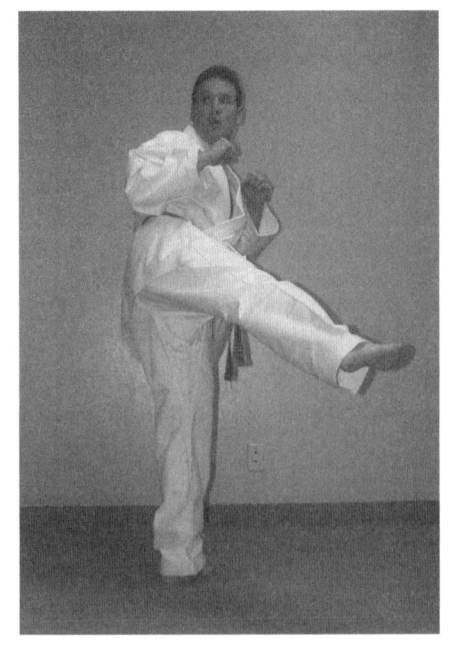

Begin Trajectory Side View

Peak of Trajectory:

18. Your base leg foot should now have moved approximately 45-degrees (clockwise) by pivoting on the ball of your foot. While your kicking leg, with the knee slightly bent, has now moved up to the correct height to strike your target.
19. The heel of the kicking foot should follow a straight line of trajectory from the "Peak of Trajectory" through the target (Impact), to the "Follow Through" position.
20. Your upper body should now be leaning to your left at almost a 75-degree angle in relation to your bodys upright position, and almost parallel with the ground.
21. Although your body is now in the above position, your head should still be looking over your kicking leg shoulder at your opponent.
22. Your back is no longer facing toward your opponent. It should now be facing at a 45-degree angle to your opponent's left in approximately the same direction that your kicking leg will be in, when it is in the "Follow Through" position.

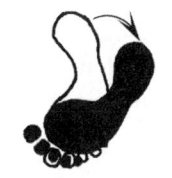

Peak of Trajectory Foot Position

Note: One of the most important factors needed for the correct execution of a Wheel Kick, or any kick for that matter, is the proper pivoting on the ball of the base leg foot throughout the entire execution of the kick.

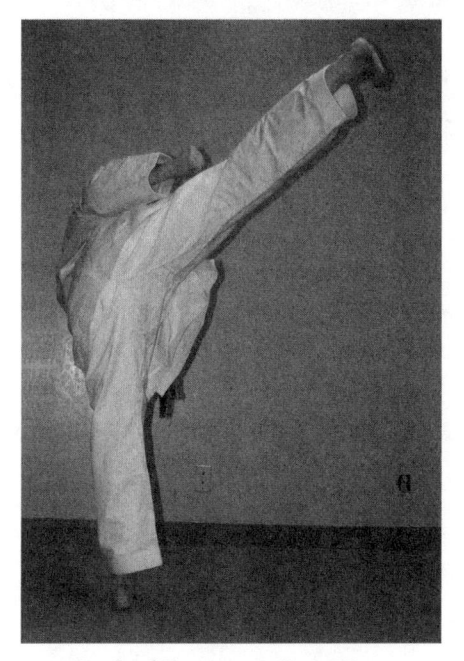

Peak of Trajectory Front View   *Peak of Trajectory Side View*

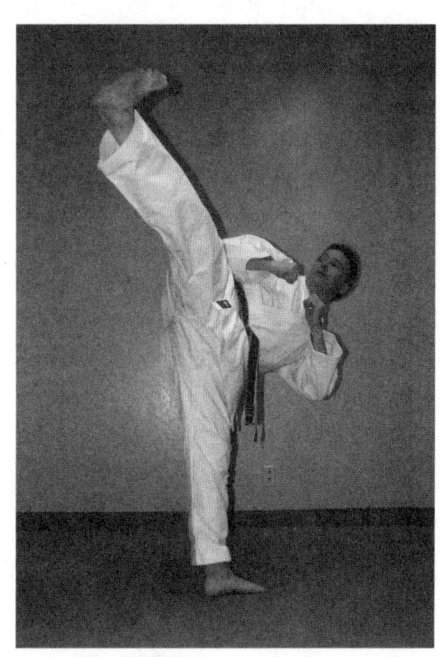

67

Impact:

23. Your base leg foot has now moved another 45-degrees (clockwise), by pivoting on the ball of the foot, with the arch of your foot now facing towards your opponent.
24. Your upper body should still be leaning to your left at almost a 75-degree angle in relation to your bodys upright position, and almost parallel with the ground. Although it has moved clockwise prior to the movement of your kicking leg and foot. At the moment of impact, your entire body should tighten to add power to the kick, as your foot continues to travel through the target.
25. Notice how your kicking foot, kicking leg (with knee slightly bent), hips, back, shoulders and head are all in a straight line at the initial moment of "Impact". Also, notice how the toes of the kicking foot are pulled back towards your body and pointed. This helps insure that contact with the target is made with the back of the heel.
26. Your head should still be up and looking over the kicking leg shoulder. Eye contact with your opponent is maintained at all times.

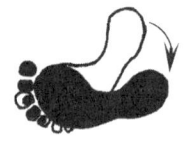

Impact Foot Position

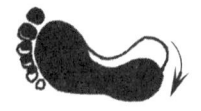

Impact (ADVANCED) Foot Position

Note: As you can clearly see in the photographs on pages, 67, 68, 69, and 70, I have not pivoted correctly on the ball of my base leg foot throughout...

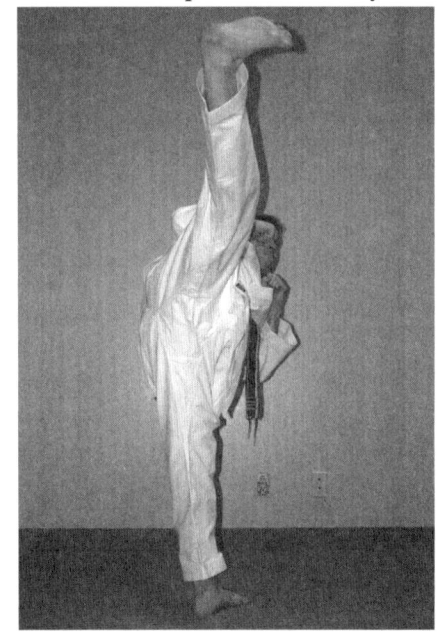

Impact Front View

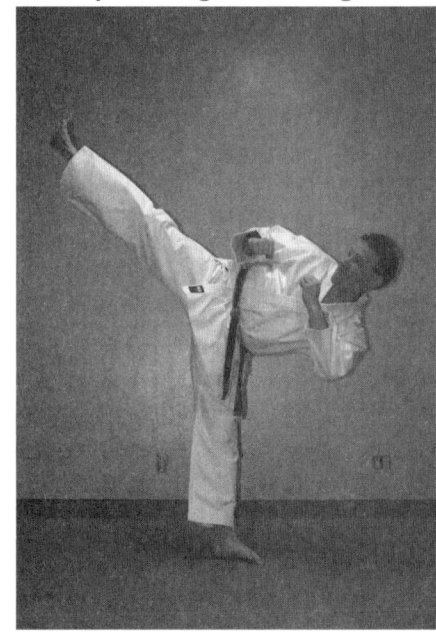

Impact Side View

Follow Through:

27. Your base leg foot should have moved another 45-degrees (clockwise) by pivoting on the ball of the foot.
28. Your upper body should still be leaning to your left at almost a 75-degree angle in relation to your bodys upright position, and almost parallel with the ground. Although it has once again moved clockwise prior to the movement of your kicking leg and foot. Your back is straight and the front of your body is now at approximately a 45-degree angle to the front of your opponent.
29. Your kicking leg foot should continue along exactly the same path it followed from the "Peak of Trajectory" to "Impact." Your foot should be approximately 45-degrees past your target.
30. Your head should no longer be looking over your kicking leg shoulder. However, your eyes are still looking at your opponent.

Follow Through Foot Position

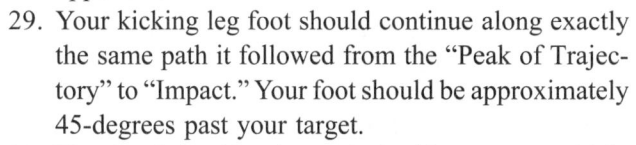

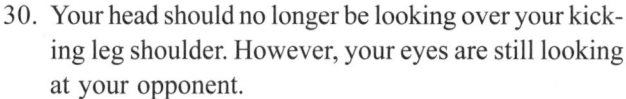

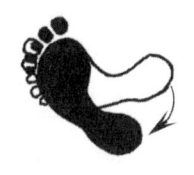

Note: ...the entire sequence, from "Peak of Trajectory" through "End of Trajectory." I have intentionally done this in order to make you aware of the single most common mistake made when executing a Wheel Kick, improper pivoting on the ball of the base leg foot. As you can see in the series of photographs mentioned on the previous page, my hips,...

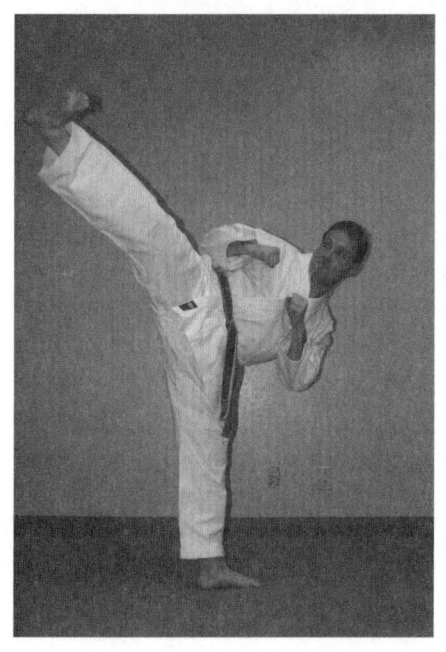

Follow Through Front View   *Follow Through Side View*

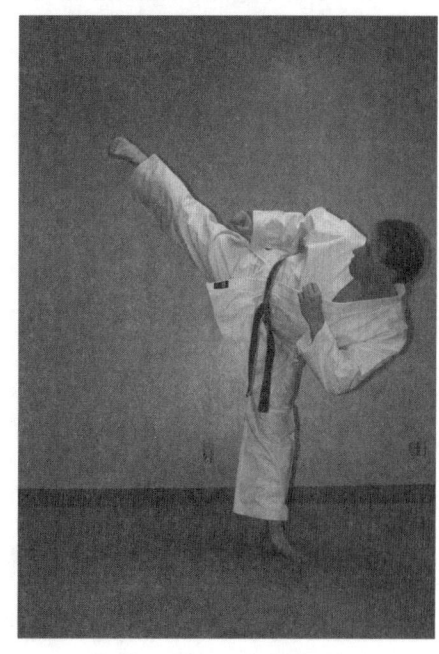

69

End of Trajectory:

31. Your base leg foot should have moved another 45-degrees (clockwise) by pivoting on the ball of the foot. The toes of your base leg foot should now be pointing directly at your opponent.
32. Your kicking leg remains straight with the knee slightly bent. Your kicking foot is now slightly in front of you and to your right at approximately the height of your base leg knee.
33. Your upper body will straighten up from the approximately 75-degree bent over position you were in when kicking. Your back remains straight and your upper body is now facing directly toward your opponent.
34. Your head should still be up and looking directly over the center of your chest. Your eyes are still in contact with your opponent, whether he is still standing, or lying on the ground.

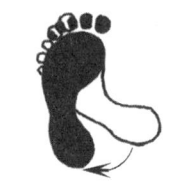

End of Trajectory Foot Position

Note: ...kicking leg, and upper body, are all moving before I am pivoting on the ball of my base leg foot. This not only makes your Wheel Kick far less effective, but it can also lead to serious damage to your base leg knee. Remember that pivoting on the ball of your base leg foot should precede all other movement.

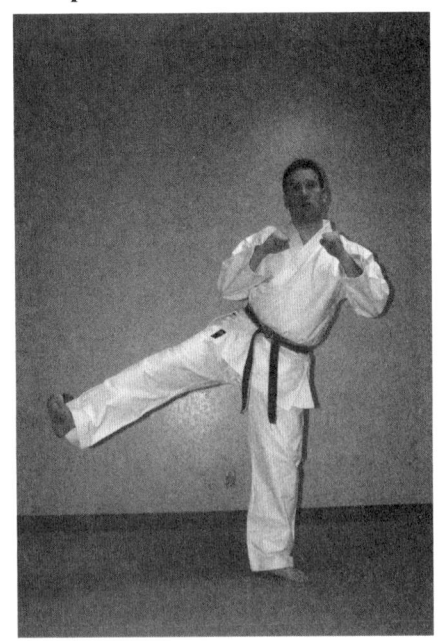

End of Trajectory Front View   *End of Trajectory Side View*

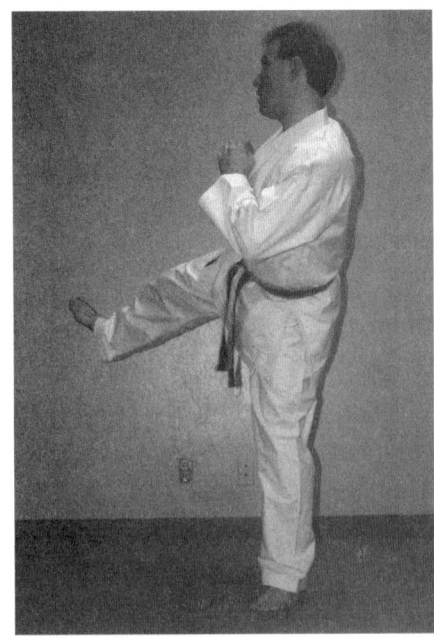

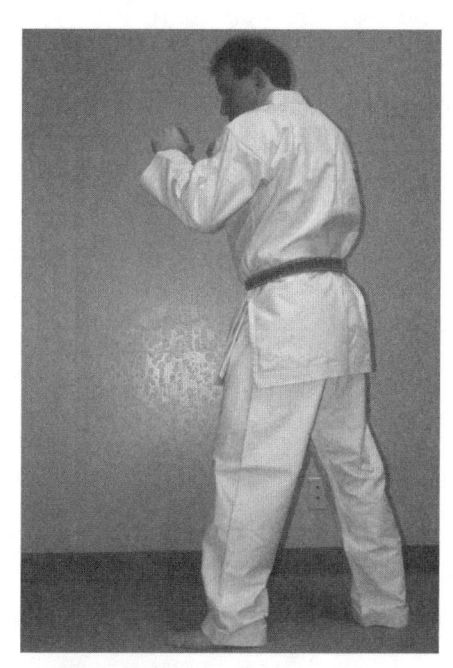

Return to Fighting Position:

35. Your entire body from your head to your toes, should be in exactly the same fighting position that you would be in if you were going to execute a Turning Wheel Kick with your right leg. Although, you won't be in exactly the same location.
36. Your kicking leg foot continues the 360-degree motion and returns to its original starting position. Although your kicking leg knee will remain slightly bent as it returns to the starting position.
37. Your hands, which should have remained as close to this position as possible throughout the entire kick, are held up (like a boxer's), with the elbows tucked in to protect the ribs and your hands up to protect your head.
38. Your head should now be looking over your lead leg shoulder with your eyes in contact with your opponent.

Return to Fighting Position Foot Position

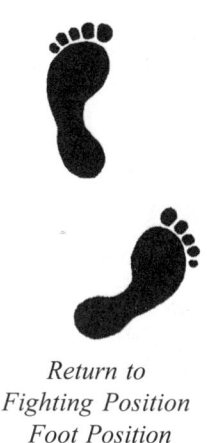

Note: The only time your entire base leg foot is in contact with the ground, is in the initial "Fighting Position," during the "Impact" phase of the kick, and in the "Return to Fighting Position."

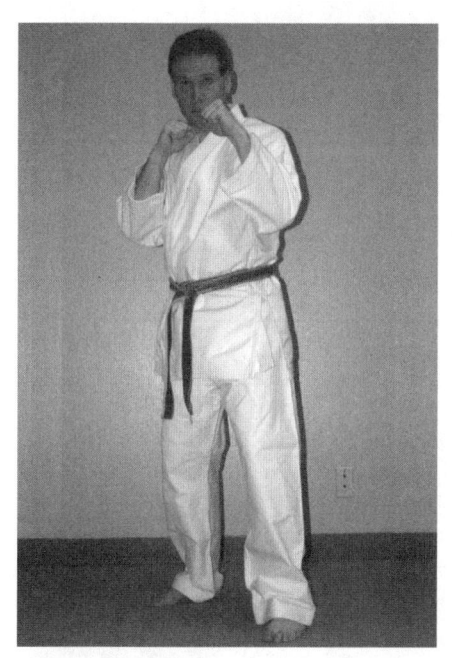

Return to Fighting Position Front View   *Return to Fighting Position Side View*

Pictorial Overview:

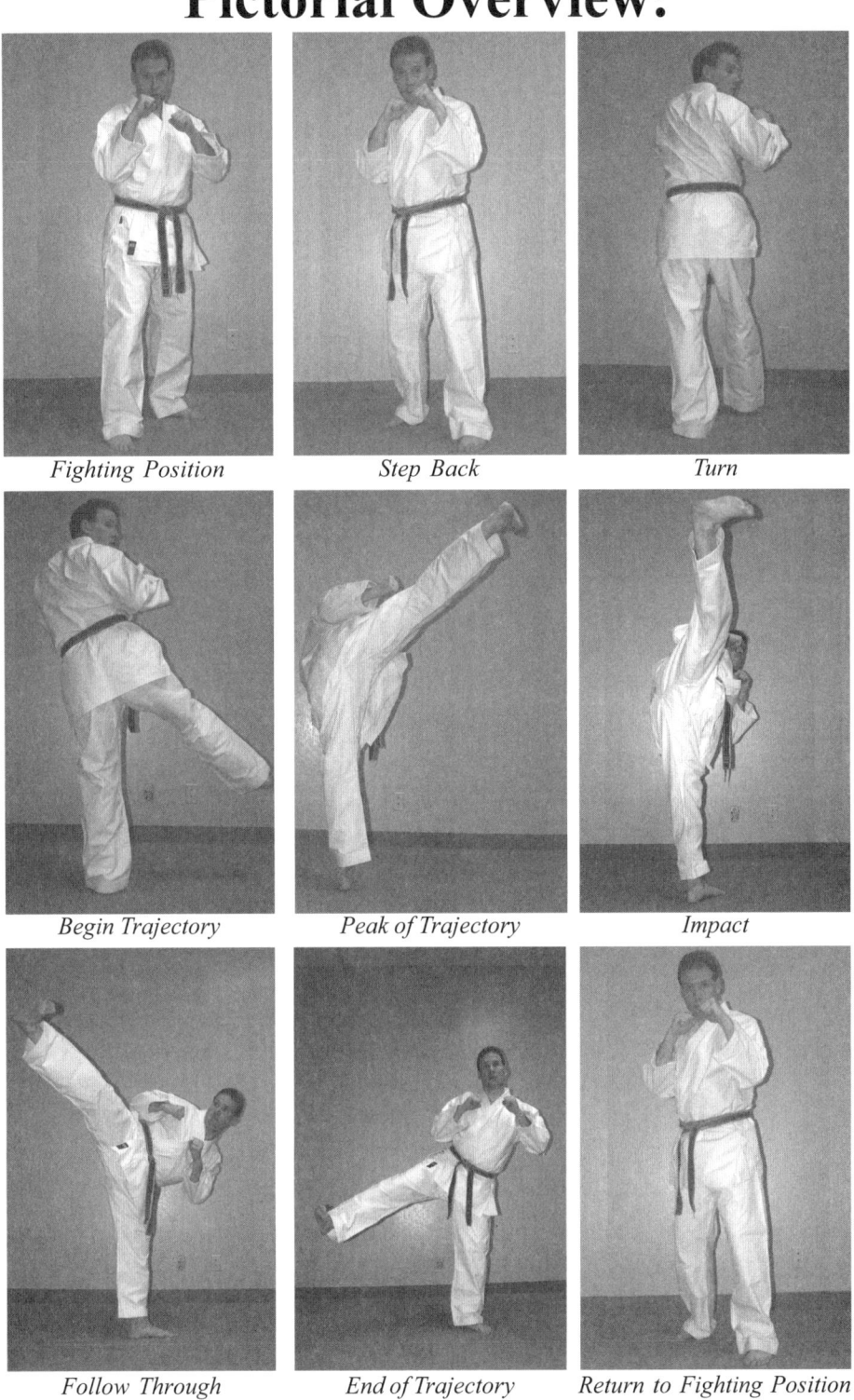

Fighting Position

Step Back

Turn

Begin Trajectory

Peak of Trajectory

Impact

Follow Through

End of Trajectory

Return to Fighting Position

Spinning Wheel Kick

The Spinning Wheel Kick is identical in execution to the Turning Wheel Kick, with one notable exception. A stepping forward motion, which is performed before executing the kick. This step is used to close the distance with ones opponent and can also increase the power in this kick due to the added momentum obtained from stepping forward. The actual spinning motion of the rearward foot prior to execution of the kick is performed by simply stepping forward with the rearward foot into another fighting position. Only now the kicking leg is in the rearward rather than the forward position. When executing the step forward/spinning motion, be sure and move your rearward foot without initially moving your hips and upper body in order to avoid telegraphing the movement to your opponent. Your hips and upper body will begin to move as you set your foot back down on the ground.

Fighting Position:
1. Your fighting position for this kick is exactly the same as it was for Step-Back Wheel Kick, with your kicking leg in the forward position to begin with rather than in the rear.
2. This stance is approximately shoulder width apart with the heel of your rear foot directly in line with the heel of your front foot.
3. Your front or lead foot should be pointed directly at your opponent.
4. Your rear foot is angled toward the left at approximately a 45-degree angle. Your weight should be distributed evenly over the balls of both feet.

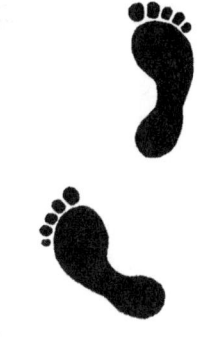

Fighting Position Foot Position

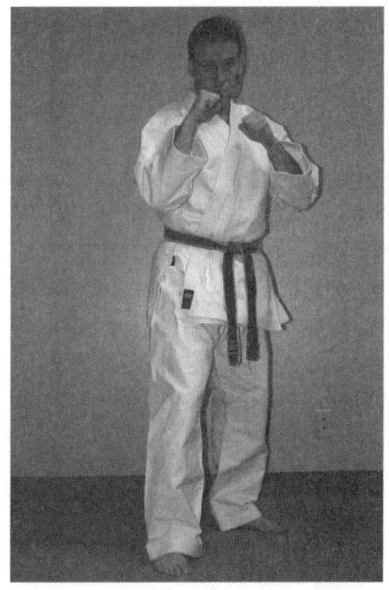

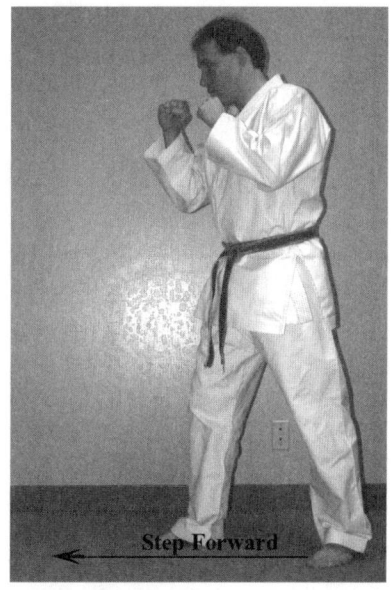

Fighting Position Front View

Fighting Position Side View

5. Your knees are slightly, but not noticeably bent. They should not be locked straight or rigid.
6. Your body should be facing at a 45-degree angle towards your opponent. This presents a smaller target area and also facilitates a faster step-and-turn when utilizing this kick.
7. Your hands should be held up (like a boxer's), with the elbows tucked in to protect the ribs and your hands up to protect your head. Your hands should remain as close to this position as possible throughout the entire kick.
8. Your head should be facing your opponent with your chin tucked down and protected by your lead shoulder.
9. Your eyes should be centered on your opponent's chest.

Step Forward & Turn Back:

10. Take a step forward with your rear foot. And...
11. As you step forward with your rear leg, pivot on the ball of your base leg foot. This will have the effect of turning your back toward your opponent.
12. Your eyes should still be centered on your opponent's chest
13. When you set your rear foot down, it should be not only in front of you, but also approximately 8 inches to the side. This allows for better balance and a more accurate kick. Your back should now be toward your opponent, and the heel of your now-base leg foot should also be pointed toward your opponent.

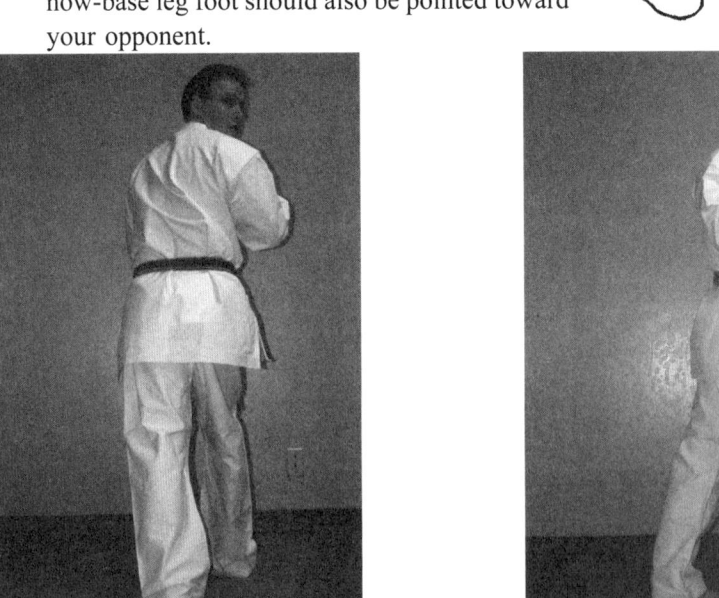

Step Forward & Turn Back Foot Position

Step Forward & Turn Front View

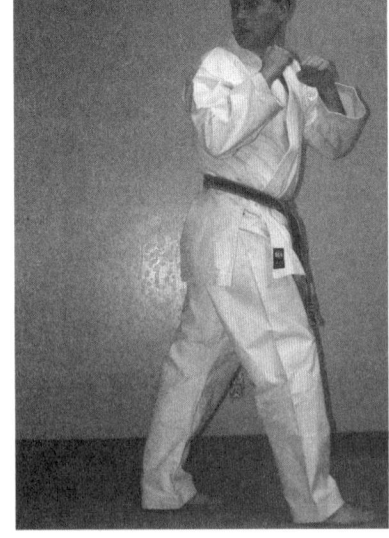

Step Forward & Turn Side View

Begin Trajectory:

14. Using the toes of your kicking foot, push off the floor and bring your kicking leg up at a 45-degree angle between the direction your body is facing and your right hand side. Your leg should be straight, with a slight bend in the knee. In this position, your kicking foot should already be in the correct position to strike your opponent.
15. As you bring your kicking leg up, your upper body should start bending over slightly, from the waist, to the left. Your back will remain straight.
16. Your head is still up and turned over your kicking shoulder, your eyes should always remain in contact with your opponent throughout the entire kick.
17. Your back should no longer be facing directly towards your opponent, but should start turning, along with your shoulders, in the direction of the kick.

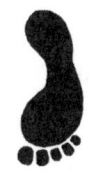

Begin Trajectory Foot Position

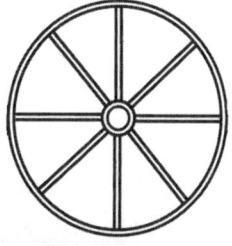

Note: The overhead view of a Wheel Kick can also be compared to a wagon wheel, which is shown here on the right. The hub or center or the wagon wheel is representative of your entire body, with the exception of your kicking leg, which is represented by the spokes in the wagon wheel, while your kicking foot is represented by the outer rim.

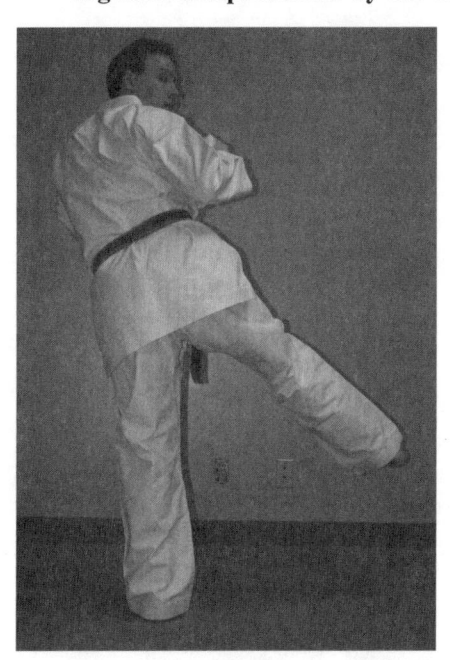

Begin Trajectory Front View   *Begin Trajectory Side View*

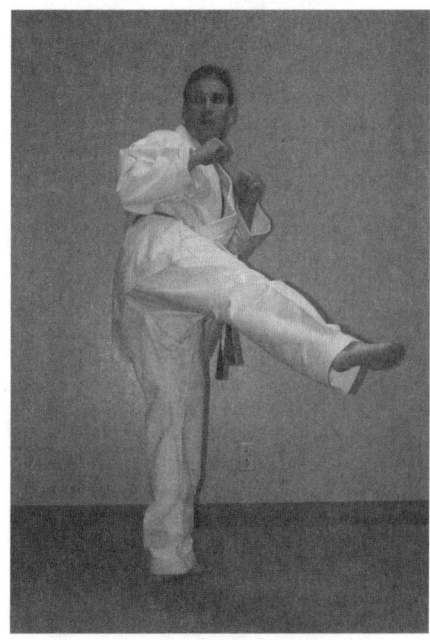

75

Peak of Trajectory:

18. Your base leg foot should now have moved approximately 45-degrees (clockwise) by pivoting on the ball of your foot. While your kicking leg, with the knee slightly bent, has now moved up to the correct height to strike your target.
19. The heel of the kicking foot should follow a straight line of trajectory from the "Peak of Trajectory" through the target (Impact), to the "Follow Through" position.
20. Your upper body should now be leaning to your left at almost a 75-degree angle in relation to your bodys upright position, and almost parallel with the ground.
21. Although your body is now in the above position, your head should still be looking over your kicking leg shoulder at your opponent.
22. Your back is no longer facing toward your opponent. It should now be facing at a 45-degree angle to your opponent's left in approximately the same direction that your kicking leg will be in, when it is in the "Follow Through" position.

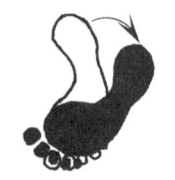

Peak of Trajectory Foot Position

Note: Your "Peak of Trajectory" should be at the exact same height as your intended target, and should travel along a straight path from the "Peak of Trajectory" through "Impact" to the "Follow Through" position.

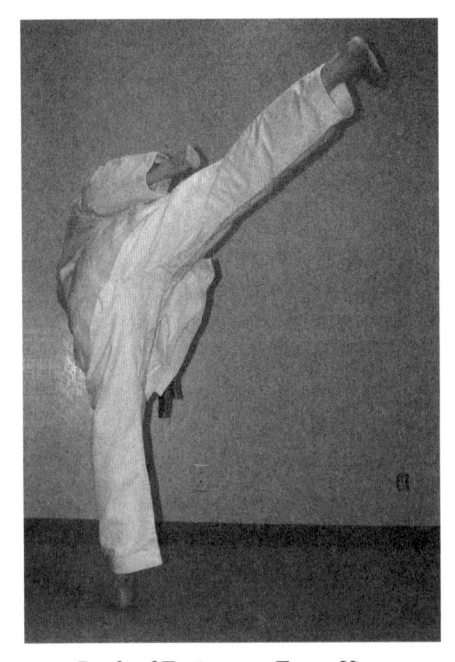

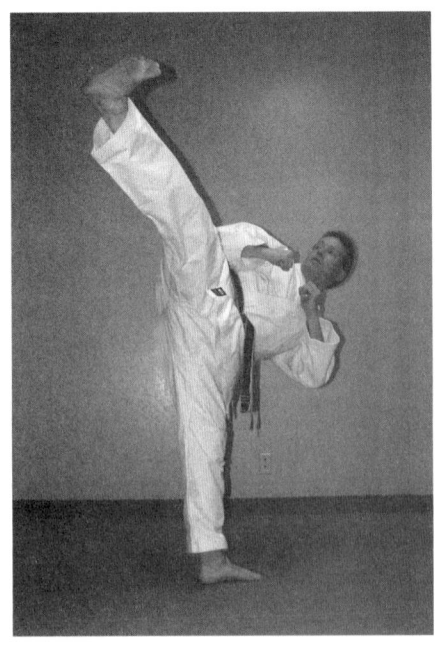

Peak of Trajectory Front View   *Peak of Trajectory Side View*

Impact:

23. Your base leg foot has now moved another 45-degrees (clockwise), by pivoting on the ball of the foot, with the arch of your foot now facing towards your opponent.
24. Your upper body should still be leaning to your left at almost a 75-degree angle in relation to your bodys upright position, and almost parallel with the ground. Although it has moved clockwise prior to the movement of your kicking leg and foot. At the moment of impact, your entire body should tighten to add power to the kick, as your foot continues to travel through the target.
25. Notice how your kicking foot, kicking leg (with knee slightly bent), hips, back, shoulders and head are all in a straight line at the initial moment of "Impact". Also, notice how the toes of the kicking foot are pulled back towards your body and pointed. This helps insure that contact with the target is made with the back of the heel.
26. Your head should still be up and looking over the kicking leg shoulder. Eye contact with your opponent is maintained at all times.

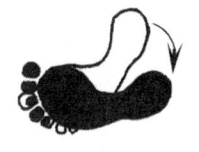

Impact Foot Position

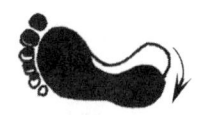

Impact (ADVANCED) Foot Position

Note: For optimum results upon impact, you must use a combination of proper technique, along with an explosive combination of speed and strength.

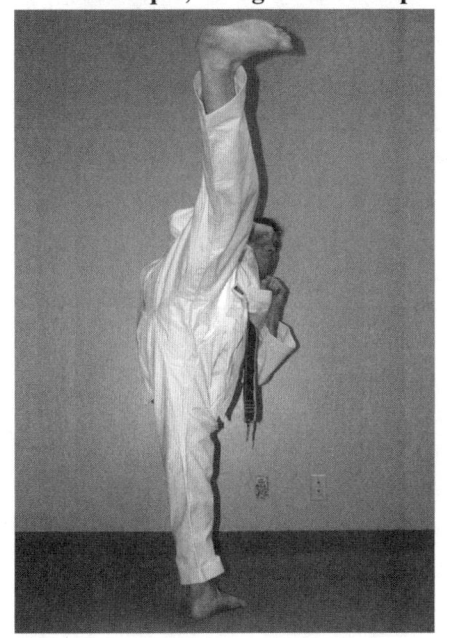

Impact Front View   *Impact Side View*

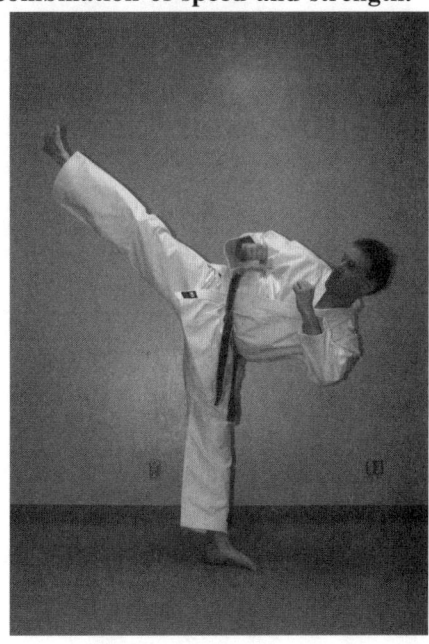

Follow Through:

27. Your base leg foot should have moved another 45-degrees (clockwise) by pivoting on the ball of the foot.
28. Your upper body should still be leaning to your left at almost a 75-degree angle in relation to your bodys upright position, and almost parallel with the ground. Although it has once again moved clockwise prior to the movement of your kicking leg and foot. Your back is straight and the front of your body is now at approximately a 45-degree angle to the front of your opponent.
29. Your kicking leg foot should continue along exactly the same path it followed from the "Peak of Trajectory" to "Impact." Your foot should be approximately 45-degrees past your target.
30. Your head should no longer be looking over your kicking leg shoulder. However, your eyes are still looking at your opponent.

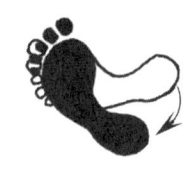

Follow Through Foot Position

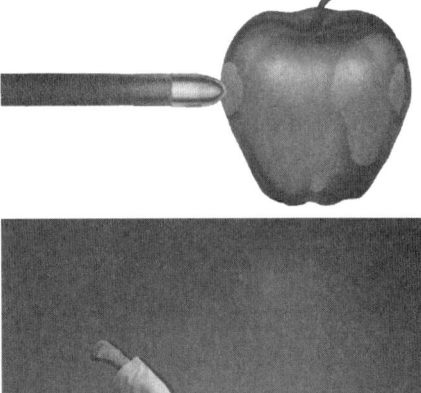

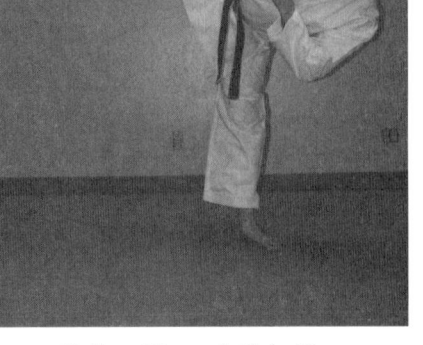

Note: In the illustration on the right, and on pages; 88, 96, 104, 112, and 122, your kicking foot and your "Path of Trajectory" are represented by the bullet and the bullets trajectory, while the apple...

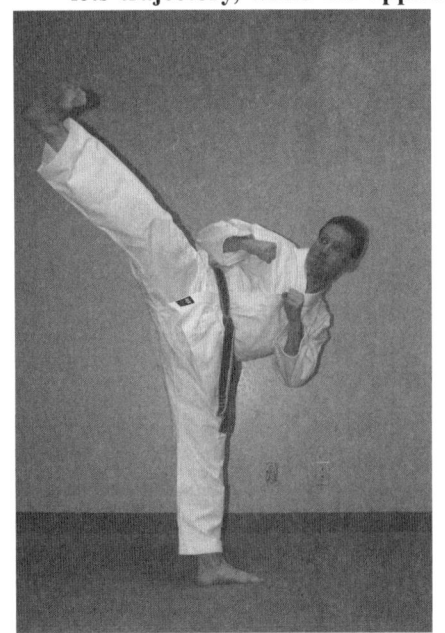

Follow Through Front View *Follow Through Side View*

End of Trajectory:
31. Your base leg foot should have moved another 45-degrees (clockwise) by pivoting on the ball of the foot. The toes of your base leg foot should now be pointing directly at your opponent.
32. Your kicking leg remains straight with the knee slightly bent. Your kicking foot is now slightly in front of you and to your right at approximately the height of your base leg knee.
33. Your upper body will straighten up from the approximately 75-degree bent over position you were in when kicking. Your back remains straight and your upper body is now facing directly toward your opponent.
34. Your head should still be up and looking directly over the center of your chest. Your eyes are still in contact with your opponent, whether he is still standing, or lying on the ground..

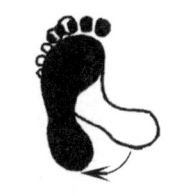

End of Trajectory Foot Position

Note: ...represents the head of your opponent. As you can see in the illustration presented on the previous page, if you merely strike the target surface without applying all of the proper principles outlined in this book, you will end up with a much less effective "surface strike."

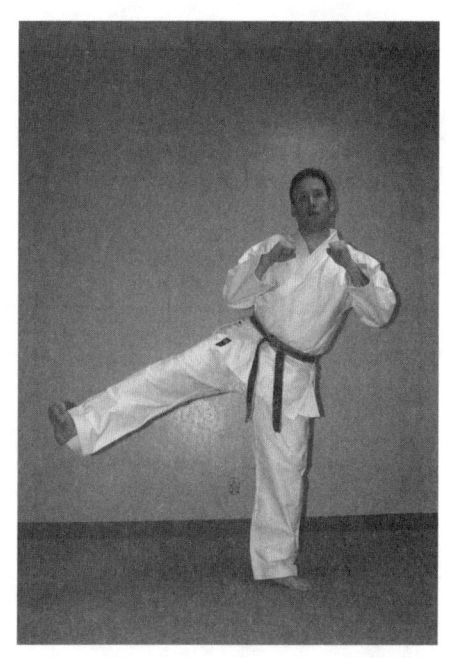

End of Trajectory Front View   *End of Trajectory Side View*

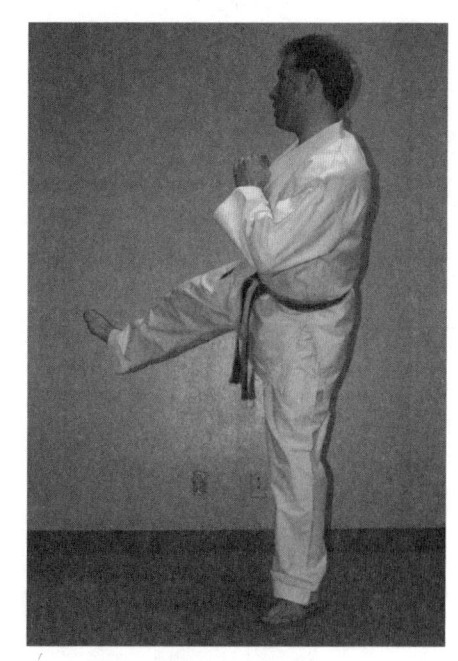

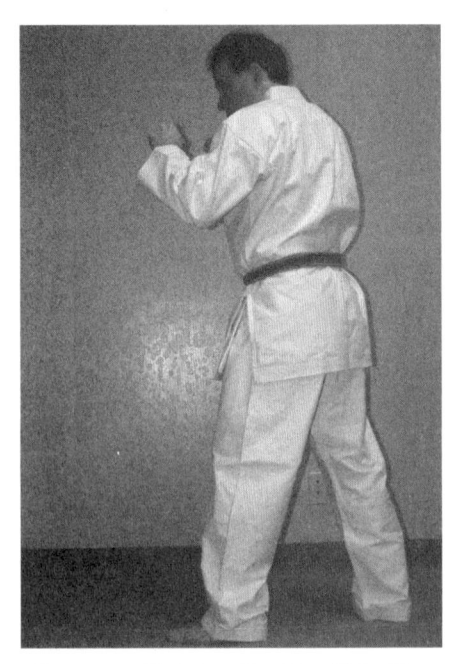

Return to Fighting Position:

35. Your entire body from your head to your toes, should be in exactly the same fighting position that you would be in if you were going to execute a Turning Wheel Kick with your right leg. Although, you won't be in exactly the same location.
36. Your kicking leg foot continues the 360-degree motion and returns to its original starting position. Although your kicking leg knee will remain slightly bent as it returns to the starting position.
37. Your hands, which should have remained as close to this position as possible throughout the entire kick, are held up (like a boxer's), with the elbows tucked in to protect the ribs and your hands up to protect your head.
38. Your head should now be looking over your lead leg shoulder with your eyes in contact with your opponent.

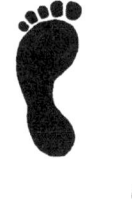

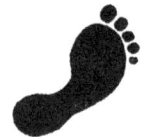

Return to Fighting Position Foot Position

Note: Your kicking leg should be just as fast, if not faster, traveling from "Impact" to "Return to Fighting Position," than it is traveling from "Fighting Position" to "Impact."

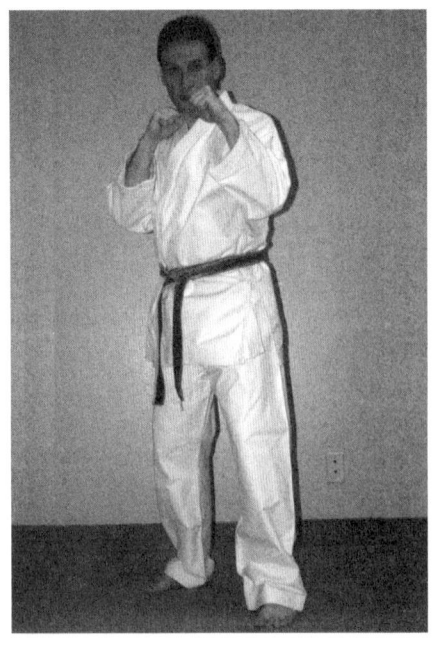

Return to Fighting Position Front View   *Return to Fighting Position Side View*

Pictorial Overview:

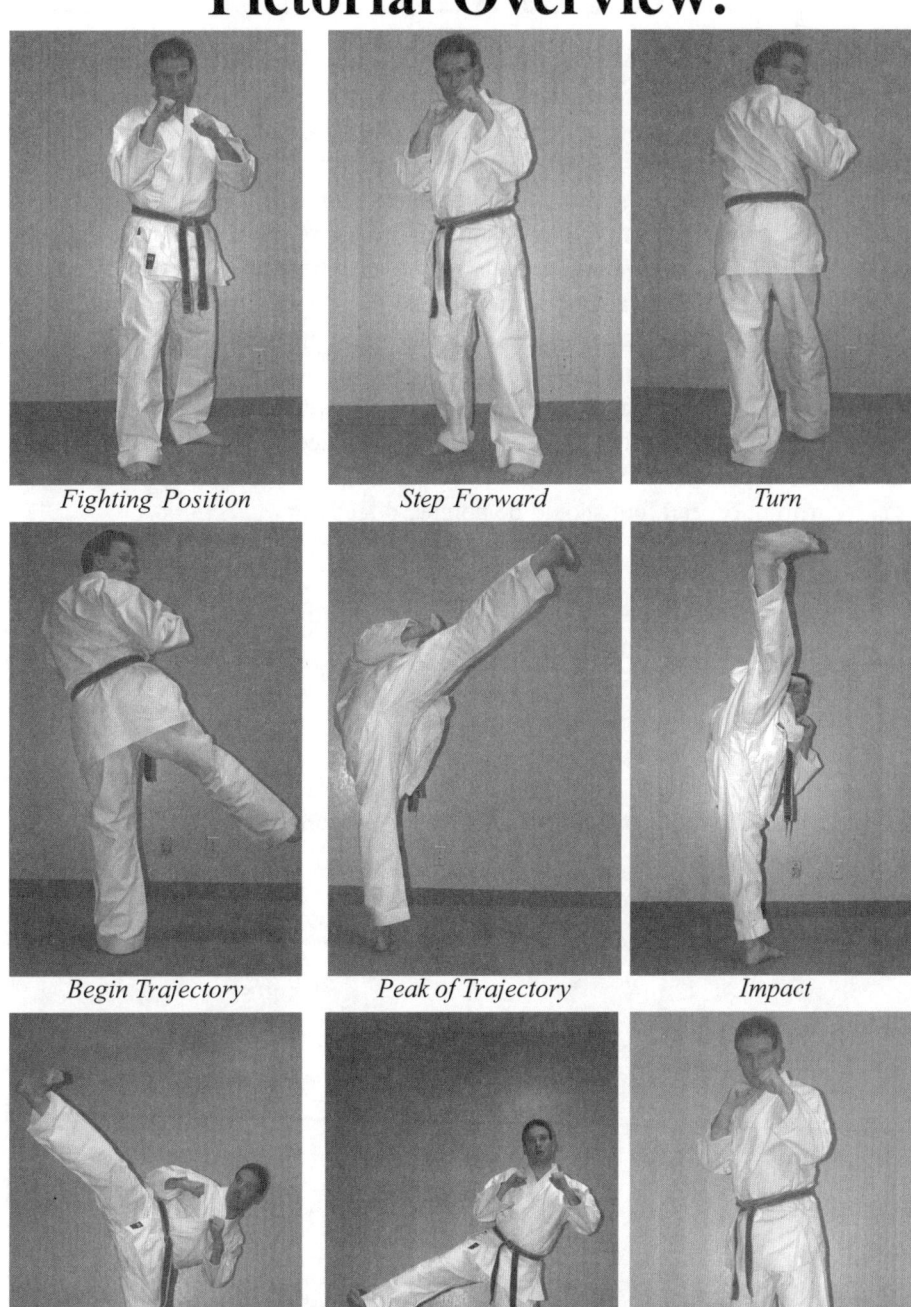

Fighting Position	*Step Forward*	*Turn*
Begin Trajectory	*Peak of Trajectory*	*Impact*
Follow Through	*End of Trajectory*	*Return to Fighting Position*

Hop/Slide Forward Wheel Kick

The Hopping/Sliding Forward Wheel Kick is identical in execution to the Turning Wheel Kick, with one notable exception. A hopping/sliding forward motion, which is performed immediately prior to executing the kick. This motion is used to close the distance between yourself and your opponent. It can also increase the power in this kick due to the added momentum of hopping/sliding forward. The actual hop or slide motion is performed by both feet simultaneously moving forward keeping the same distance between them. The hop or slide can be anywhere from a few inches up to 18 inches. Keep your hips and upper body as still as possible throughout the hop or slide in order to avoid telegraphing the move to your opponent.

Fighting Position:
1. This stance is approximately shoulder width apart with the heel of your rear foot directly in line with the heel of your front foot.
2. Your front or lead foot should be pointed directly at your opponent.
3. Your rear foot is angled toward the right at approximately a 45-degree angle. Your weight should be distributed evenly over the balls of both feet.
4. Your knees are slightly, but not noticeably bent. They should not be locked straight or rigid.
5. Your body should be facing at a 45-degree angle toward your opponent. This presents a smaller target area and also facilitates a faster turn when utilizing this kick.

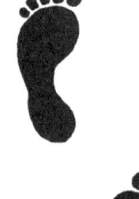

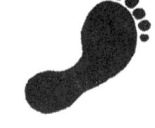

Fighting Position Foot Position

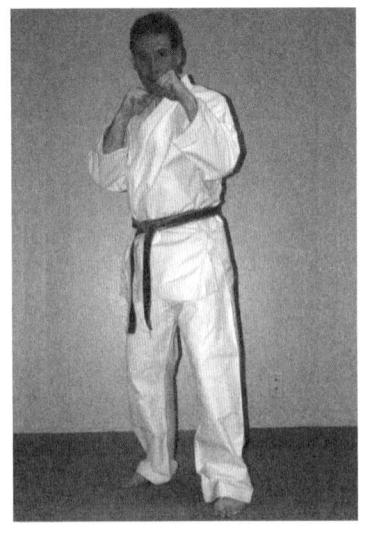

Fighting Position Front View

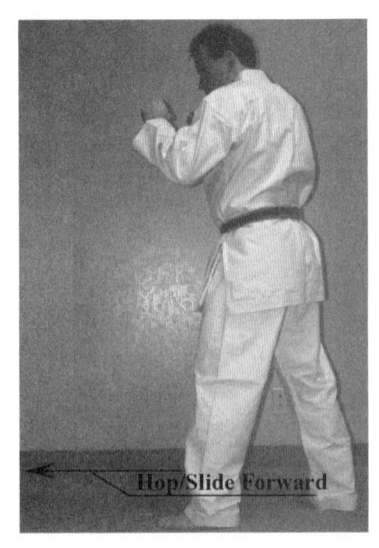

Fighting Position Side View

6. Your hands should be held up (like a boxer's), with the elbows tucked in to protect the ribs and your hands up to protect your head. Your hands should remain as close to this position as possible throughout the entire kick.
7. Your head should be facing your opponent with your chin tucked down and protected by your lead shoulder.
8. Your eyes should be centered on your opponent's chest.

Hop/Slide Forward & Turn Back:
9. Moving on the balls of your feet, move both feet forward approximately 3 to 18 inches, utilizing a hopping/sliding motion. Simultaneously pivot on the balls of both feet and point the heels of both feet at your opponent. Your rear foot will slide out approximately 8 inches to your right. This allows for better balance and a more accurate kick.
10. While you are hopping/sliding forward, and as you begin to turn, you should be turning your head and looking over your kicking leg shoulder at your opponent.
11. Your back should be facing directly toward your opponent.

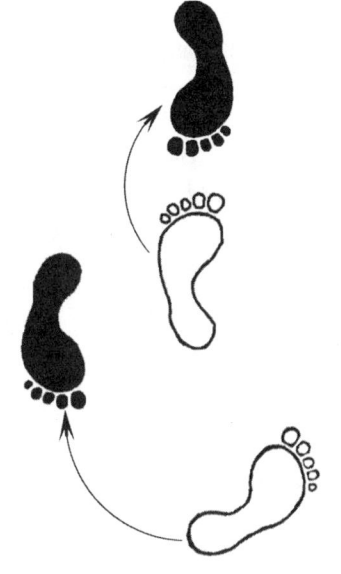

Hop/Slide Forward & Turn Back Foot Position

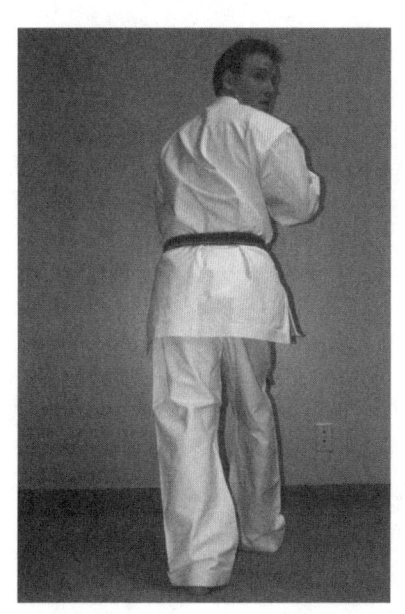

Hop/Slide Forward &... Front View

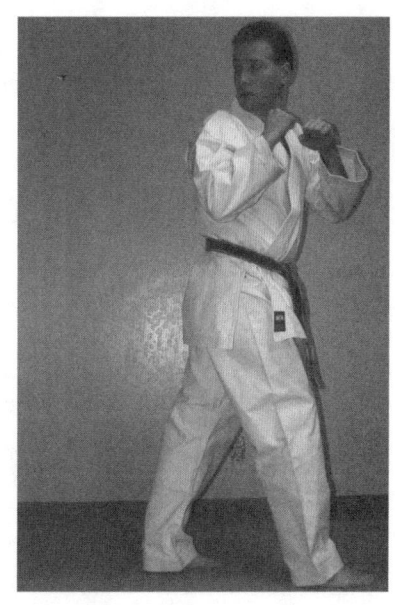

Hop/Slide Forward &... Side View

Begin Trajectory:

12. Using the toes of your kicking foot, push off the floor and bring your kicking leg up at a 45-degree angle between the direction your body is facing and your right hand side. Your leg should be straight, with a slight bend in the knee. In this position, your kicking foot should already be in the correct position to strike your opponent.
13. As you bring your kicking leg up, your upper body should start bending over slightly, from the waist, to the left. Your back will remain straight.
14. Your head is still up and turned over your kicking shoulder, your eyes should always remain in contact with your opponent throughout the entire kick.
15. Your back should no longer be facing directly towards your opponent, but should start turning, along with your shoulders, in the direction of the kick.

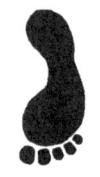

Begin Trajectory Foot Position

Note: After you have become sufficiently proficient executing the kicks described in this book wearing gi pants and being barefoot, you will want to also start practicing them wearing your normal everyday clothes and shoes. There is a big difference between kicking in gi pants and barefoot, and kicking in everyday clothes and shoes.

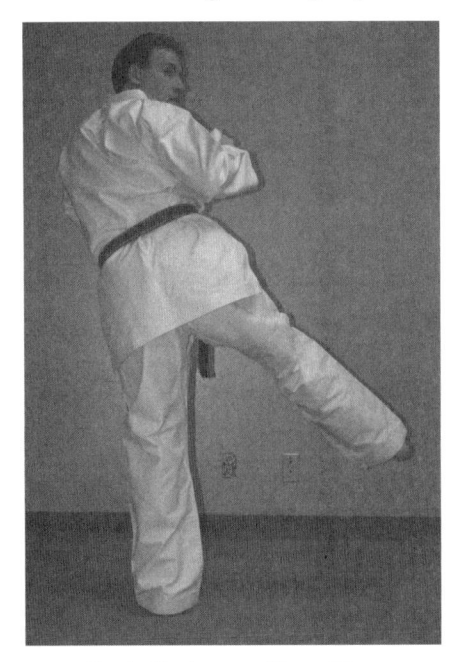

Begin Trajectory Front View   *Begin Trajectory Side View*

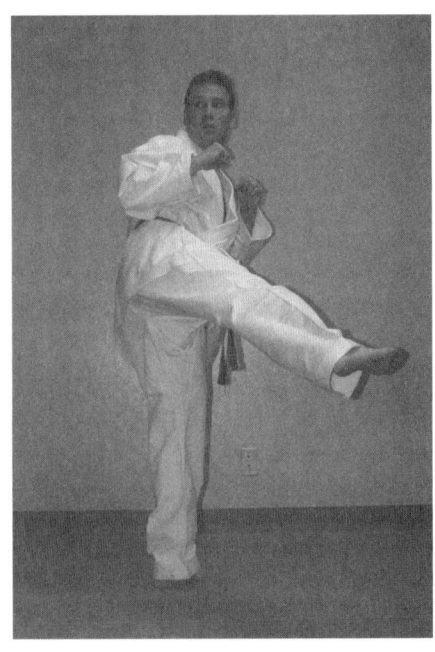

Peak of Trajectory:

16. Your base leg foot should now have moved approximately 45-degrees (clockwise) by pivoting on the ball of your foot. While your kicking leg, with the knee slightly bent, has now moved up to the correct height to strike your target.
17. The heel of the kicking foot should follow a straight line of trajectory from the "Peak of Trajectory" through the target (Impact), to the "Follow Through" position.
18. Your upper body should now be leaning to your left at almost a 75-degree angle in relation to your bodys upright position, and almost parallel with the ground.
19. Although your body is now in the above position, your head should still be looking over your kicking leg shoulder at your opponent.
20. Your back is no longer facing toward your opponent. It should now be facing at a 45-degree angle to your opponent's left in approximately the same direction that your kicking leg will be in, when it is in the "Follow Through" position.

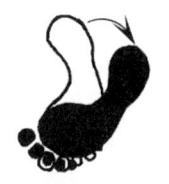

Peak of Trajectory Foot Position

Note: If you are too slow in bringing your kicking leg from the "Peak of Trajectory" position through "Impact" to the "Follow Through" position, I guarantee you that your opponent will not be slow in grabbing it.

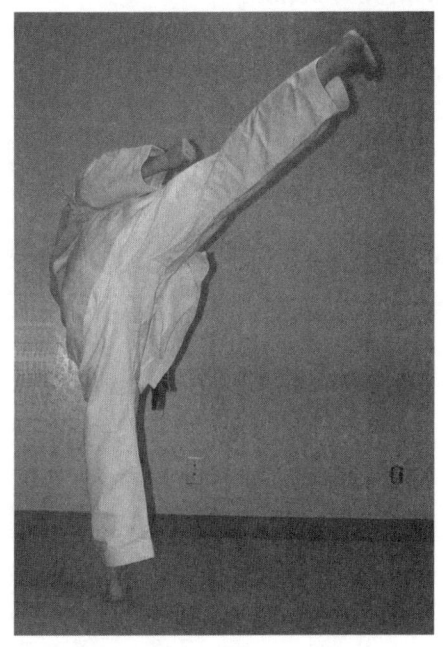

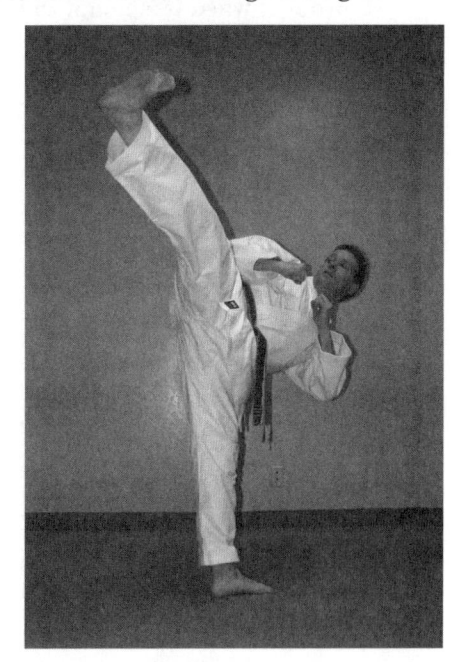

Peak of Trajectory Front View *Peak of Trajectory Side View*

85

Impact:

21. Your base leg foot has now moved another 45-degrees (clockwise), by pivoting on the ball of the foot, with the arch of your foot now facing towards your opponent.
22. Your upper body should still be leaning to your left at almost a 75-degree angle in relation to your bodys upright position, and almost parallel with the ground. Although it has moved clockwise prior to the movement of your kicking leg and foot. At the moment of impact, your entire body should tighten to add power to the kick, as your foot continues to travel through the target.
23. Notice how your kicking foot, kicking leg (with knee slightly bent), hips, back, shoulders and head are all in a straight line at the initial moment of "Impact". Also, notice how the toes of the kicking foot are pulled back towards your body and pointed. This helps insure that contact with the target is made with the back of the heel.
24. Your head should still be up and looking over the kicking leg shoulder. Eye contact with your opponent is maintained at all times.

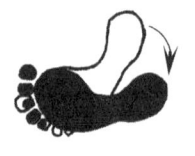

Impact Foot Position

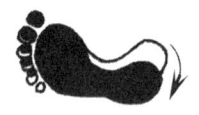

Impact (ADVANCED) Foot Position

Note: You must learn to control the body's innate response to pull back or slow down when it is about to impact with something.

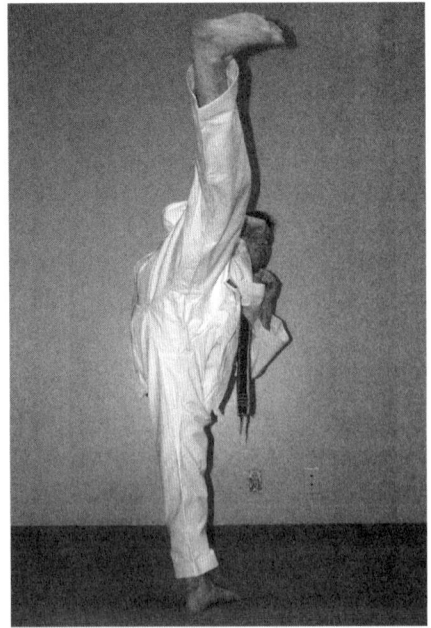

Impact Front View   *Impact Side View*

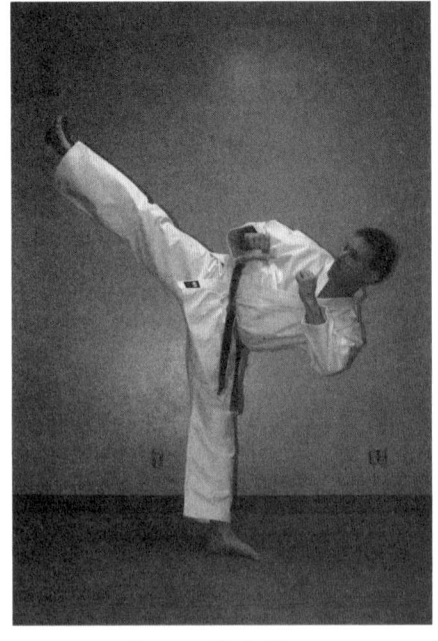

Follow Through:

25. Your base leg foot should have moved another 45-degrees (clockwise) by pivoting on the ball of the foot.
26. Your upper body should still be leaning to your left at almost a 75-degree angle in relation to your bodys upright position, and almost parallel with the ground. Although it has once again moved clockwise prior to the movement of your kicking leg and foot. Your back is straight and the front of your body is now at approximately a 45-degree angle to the front of your opponent.
27. Your kicking leg foot should continue along exactly the same path it followed from the "Peak of Trajectory" to "Impact." Your foot should be approximately 45-degrees past your target.
28. Your head should no longer be looking over your kicking leg shoulder. However, your eyes are still looking at your opponent.

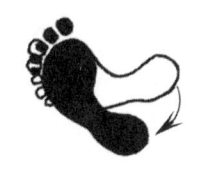

Follow Through Foot Position

Note: Your first line of defense should be your kicks, as they are your longest and most powerful weapons in your arsenal. Kicking falls into the "Long Range" category, while punching and hand strikes fall into the "Mid Range" category. Knee and elbow strikes fall into the "Short Range" category, while joint techniques fall into your final range, Grappling."

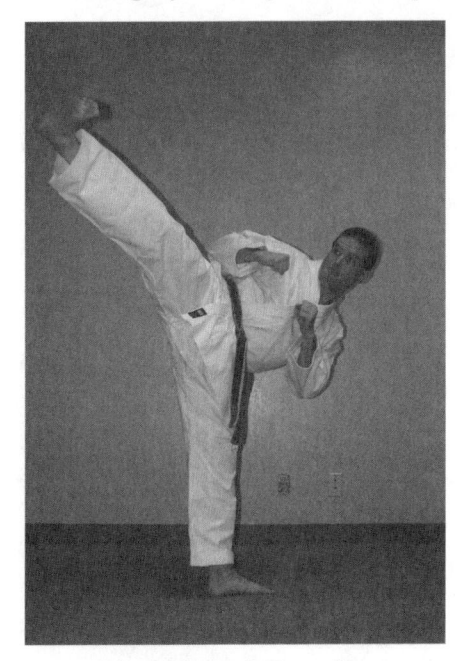

Follow Through Front View   *Follow Through Side View*

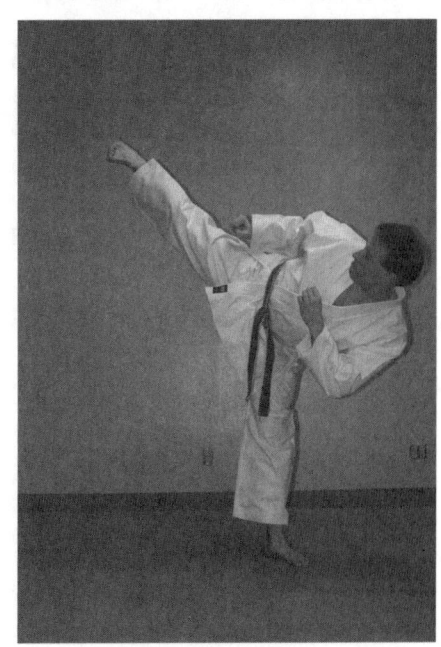

End of Trajectory:

29. Your base leg foot should have moved another 45-degrees (clockwise) by pivoting on the ball of the foot. The toes of your base leg foot should now be pointing directly at your opponent.
30. Your kicking leg remains straight with the knee slightly bent. Your kicking foot is now slightly in front of you and to your right at approximately the height of your base leg knee.
31. Your upper body will straighten up from the approximately 75-degree bent over position you were in when kicking. Your back remains straight and your upper body is now facing directly toward your opponent.
32. Your head should still be up and looking directly over the center of your chest. Your eyes are still in contact with your opponent, whether he is still standing, or lying on the ground..

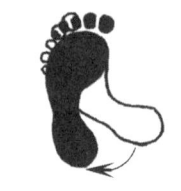

End of Trajectory Foot Position

Note: In the illustration on the right, the mushroomed bullet represents the tightening of the kicking foot upon impact with the selected target area. In this example, if you merely strike the target surface applying...

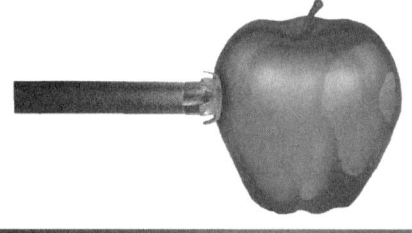

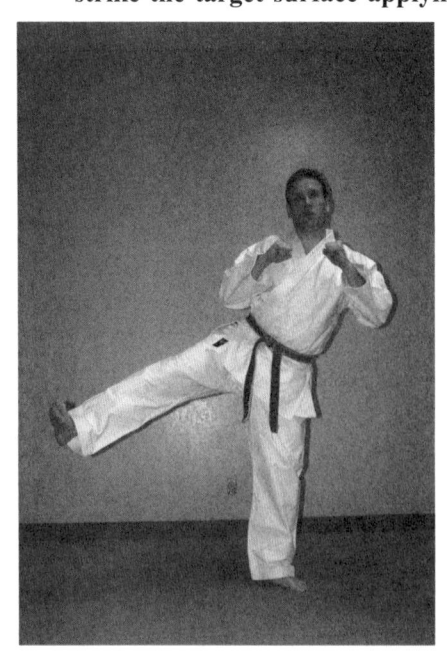

End of Trajectory Front View *End of Trajectory Side View*

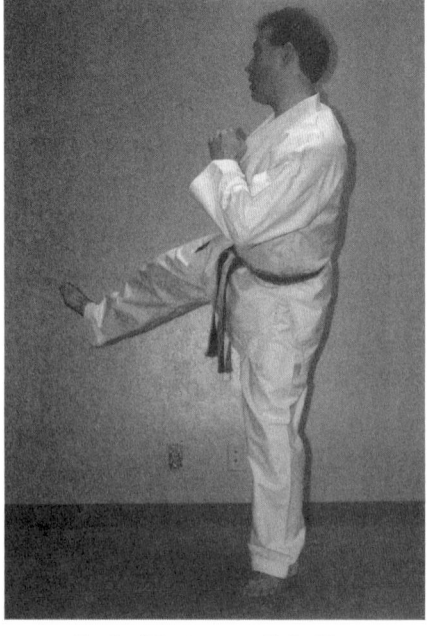

Return to Fighting Position:

33. Your entire body from your head to your toes, should be in exactly the same position that you initially started in (refer to the Fighting Position section of this kick), prior to executing this kick. Although, you won't be in exactly the same location.
34. Your kicking leg foot continues the 360-degree motion and returns to its original starting position. Although your kicking leg knee will remain slightly bent as it returns to the starting position.
35. Your hands, which should have remained as close to this position as possible throughout the entire kick, are once again in the same position they were in prior to executing the kick.
36. Your head should now be looking over your lead leg shoulder with your eyes in contact with your opponent.

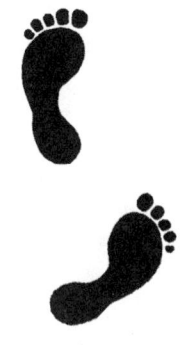

Return to Fighting Position Foot Position

Note: ...only the tightening of the kicking foot upon impact, you will end up with a slightly harder "surface strike" than what was demonstrated on page 78. In order to maximize the effectiveness of your kicks, you must, correctly, apply all of the proper principles outlined in this book.

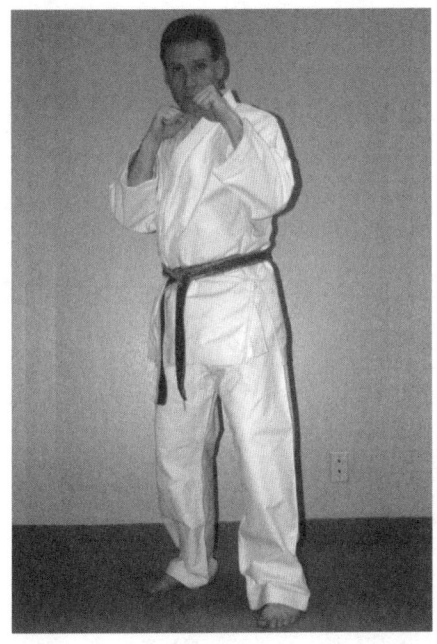

Return to Fighting Position Front View

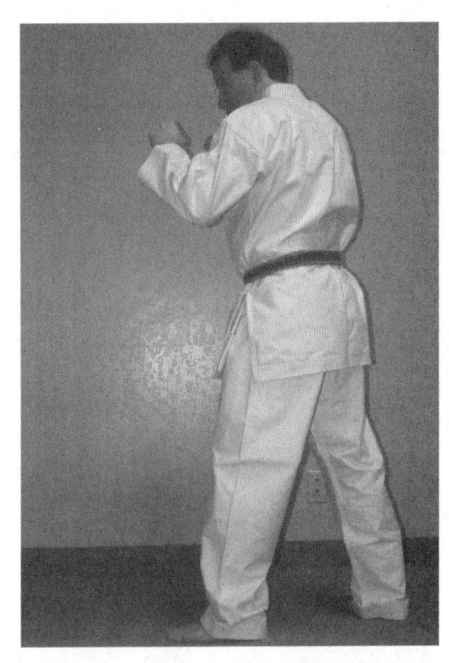

Return to Fighting Position Side View

Pictorial Overview:

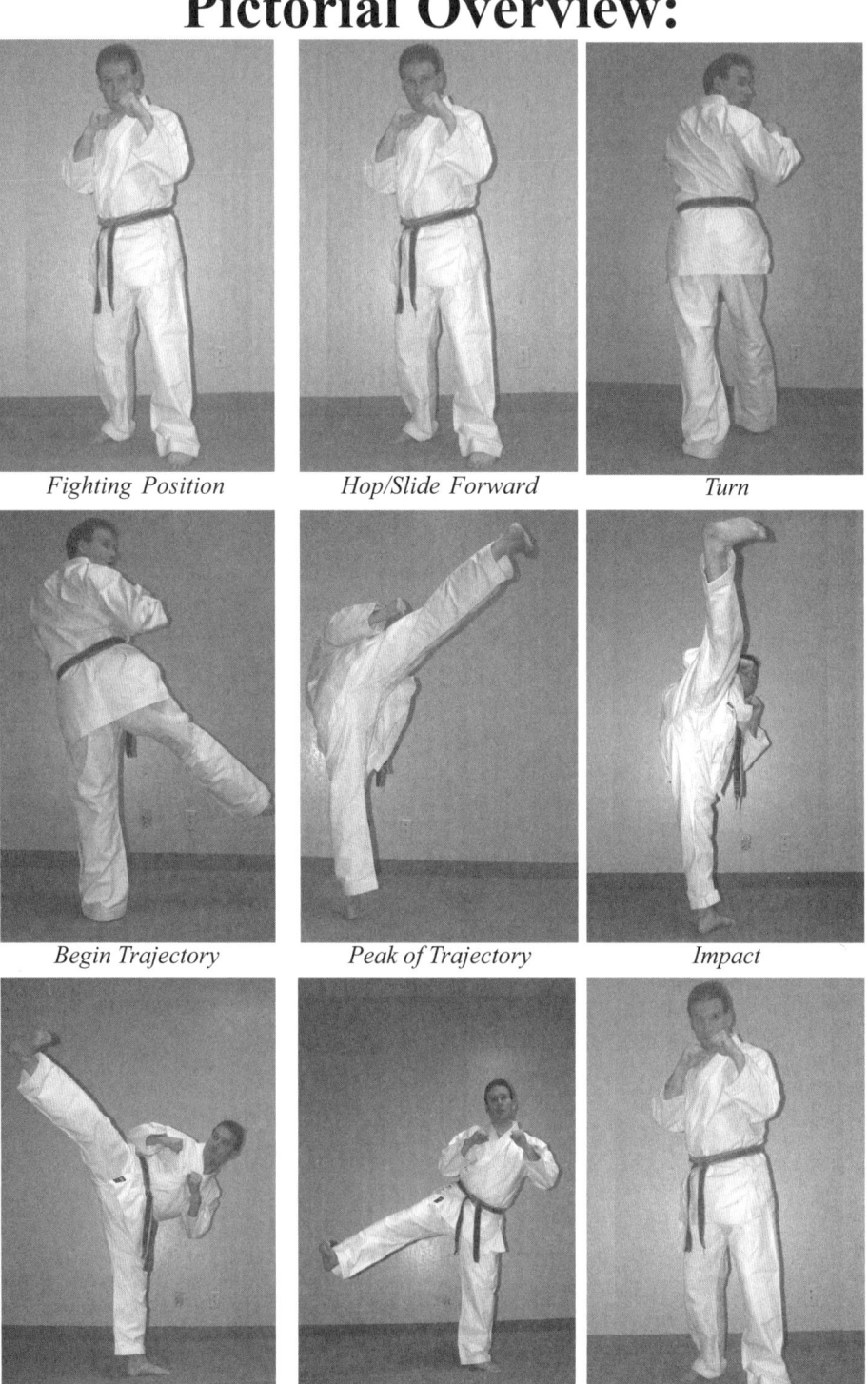

Fighting Position	*Hop/Slide Forward*	*Turn*
Begin Trajectory	*Peak of Trajectory*	*Impact*
Follow Through	*End of Trajectory*	*Return to Fighting Position*

Hop/Slide Backward Wheel Kick

The Hopping/Sliding Backward Wheel Kick is identical in execution to the Turning Wheel Kick, with one notable exception. A hopping/sliding backward motion, which is performed immediately prior to executing the kick. This hopping/sliding backward motion is used to draw your opponent into you, or to avoid an attack. It can also increase the power in this kick due to the added momentum of hopping/sliding backward. The actual hop or slide motion is performed by both feet simultaneously moving backward keeping the same distance between them. The hop or slide can be anywhere from a few inches up to 18 inches. Keep your hips and upper body as still as possible throughout the hop or slide in order to avoid telegraphing the move to your opponent.

Fighting Position:
1. This stance is approximately shoulder width apart with the heel of your rear foot directly in line with the heel of your front foot.
2. Your front of lead foot should be pointed directly at your opponent.
3. Your rear foot is angled towards the right at approximately a 45-degree angle. Your weight should be distributed evenly over the balls of both feet.
4. Your knees are slightly, but not noticeably bent. They should not be locked straight or rigid.
5. Your body should be facing at a 45-degree angle toward your opponent. This presents a smaller target area and also facilitates a faster turn when utilizing this kick.

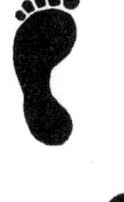

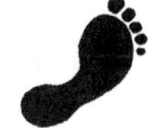

Fighting Position Foot Position

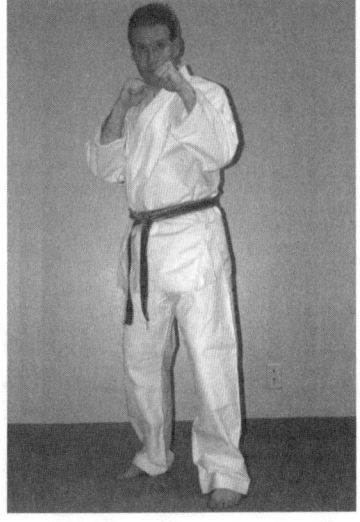

Fighting Position Front View

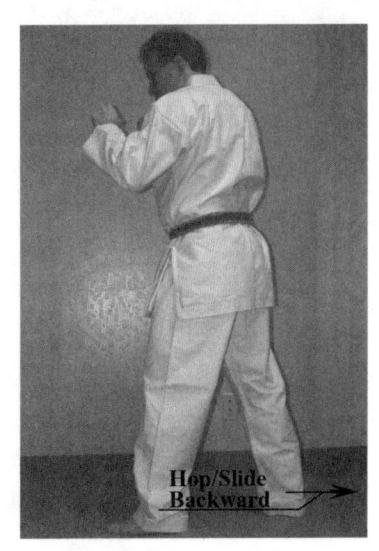

Fighting Position Side View

6. Your hands should be held up (like a boxer's), with the elbows tucked in to protect the ribs and your hands up to protect your head. Your hands should remain as close to this position as possible throughout the entire kick.
7. Your head should be facing your opponent with your chin tucked down and protected by your lead shoulder.
8. Your eyes should be centered on your opponent's chest.

Hop/Slide Backward & Turn Back:
9. Moving on the balls of your feet, move both feet forward approximately 3 to 18 inches, utilizing a hopping/sliding motion. Simultaneously pivot on the balls of both feet and point the heels of both feet at your opponent. Your rear foot will slide out approximately 8 inches to your right. This helps maintain your balance while giving you a direct line of trajectory to your target.
10. While you are hopping/sliding forward, and as you begin to turn, you should be turning your head and looking over your kicking leg shoulder at your opponent.
11. Your back should be facing directly toward your opponent.

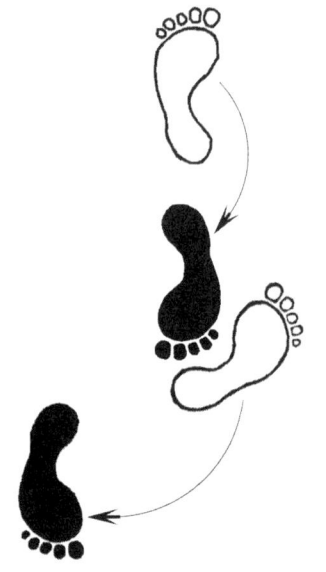

*Hop/Slide Backward
& Turn Back
Foot Position*

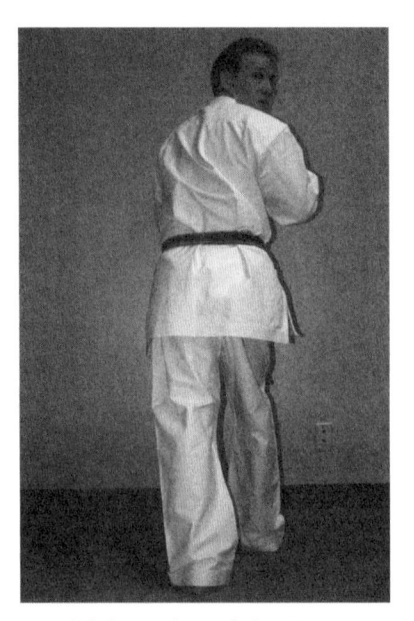

Hop/Slide Backward &... Front View

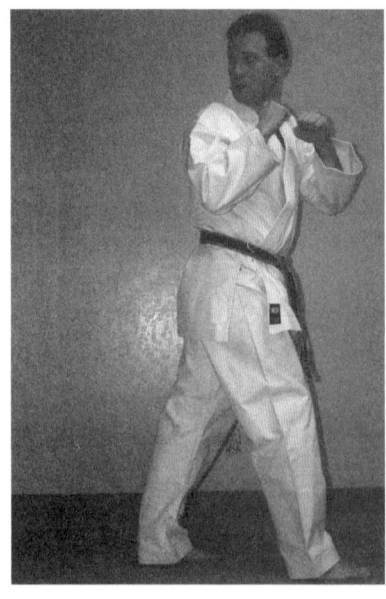

Hop/Slide Backward &... Side View

Begin Trajectory:

12. Using the toes of your kicking foot, push off the floor and bring your kicking leg up at a 45-degree angle between the direction your body is facing and your right hand side. Your leg should be straight, with a slight bend in the knee. In this position, your kicking foot should already be in the correct position to strike your opponent.
13. As you bring your kicking leg up, your upper body should start bending over slightly, from the waist, to the left. Your back will remain straight.
14. Your head is still up and turned over your kicking shoulder, your eyes should always remain in contact with your opponent throughout the entire kick.
15. Your back should no longer be facing directly towards your opponent, but should start turning, along with your shoulders, in the direction of the kick.

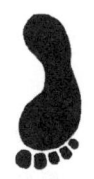

Begin Trajectory Foot Position

Note: Although you have been confronted by an opponent, the decision to execute a technique, whether it is a kick, punch, throw or joint technique, should be determined by you and you alone, not the actions, or inactions of your opponent.

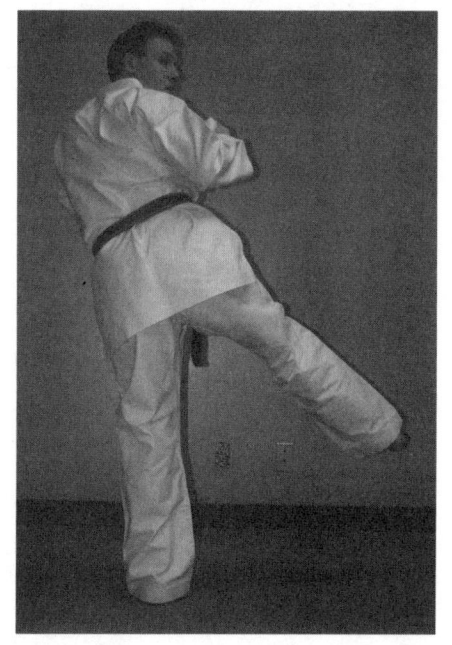

Begin Trajectory Front View   *Begin Trajectory Side View*

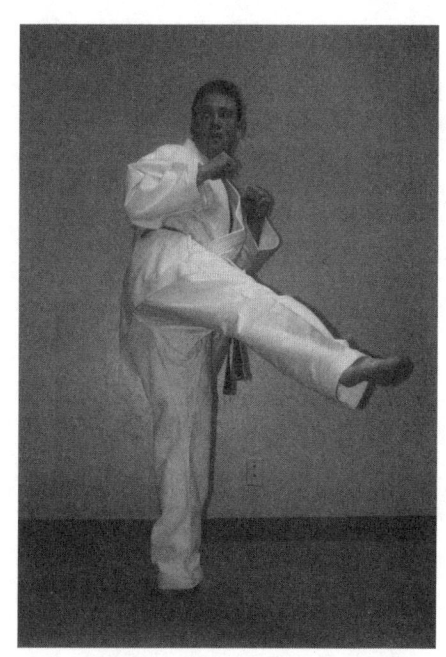

93

Peak of Trajectory:

16. Your base leg foot should now have moved approximately 45-degrees (clockwise) by pivoting on the ball of your foot. While your kicking leg, with the knee slightly bent, has now moved up to the correct height to strike your target.
17. The heel of the kicking foot should follow a straight line of trajectory from the "Peak of Trajectory" through the target (Impact), to the "Follow Through" position.
18. Your upper body should now be leaning to your left at almost a 75-degree angle in relation to your bodys upright position, and almost parallel with the ground.
19. Although your body is now in the above position, your head should still be looking over your kicking leg shoulder at your opponent.
20. Your back is no longer facing toward your opponent. It should now be facing at a 45-degree angle to your opponent's left in approximately the same direction that your kicking leg will be in, when it is in the "Follow Through" position.

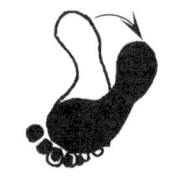

Peak of Trajectory Foot Position

Note: Although the Wheel Kick is used primarily to strike the head of an opponent at a high section level, you should also practice the Wheel Kick at a midsection (stomach) level, and low section (knee) level.

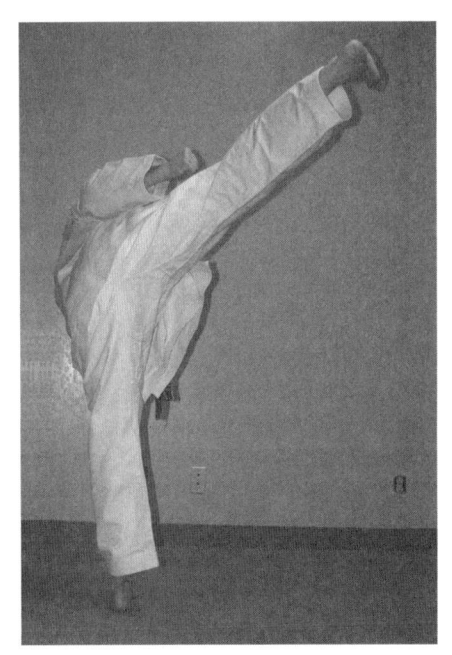

Peak of Trajectory Front View   *Peak of Trajectory Side View*

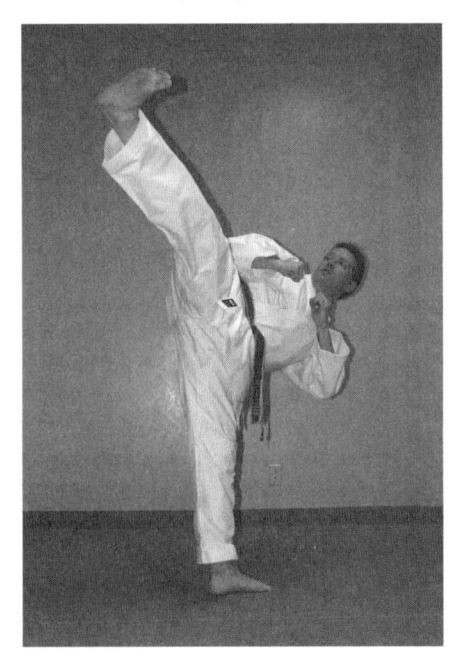

Impact:
21. Your base leg foot has now moved another 45-degrees (clockwise), by pivoting on the ball of the foot, with the arch of your foot now facing towards your opponent.
22. Your upper body should still be leaning to your left at almost a 75-degree angle in relation to your bodys upright position, and almost parallel with the ground. Although it has moved clockwise prior to the movement of your kicking leg and foot. At the moment of impact, your entire body should tighten to add power to the kick, as your foot continues to travel through the target.
23. Notice how your kicking foot, kicking leg (with knee slightly bent), hips, back, shoulders and head are all in a straight line at the initial moment of "Impact". Also, notice how the toes of the kicking foot are pulled back towards your body and pointed. This helps insure that contact with the target is made with the back of the heel.
24. Your head should still be up and looking over the kicking leg shoulder. Eye contact with your opponent is maintained at all times.

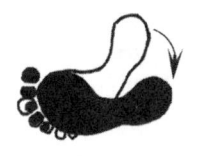

Impact Foot Position

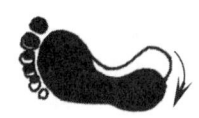

Impact (ADVANCED) Foot Position

Note: Don't over-extend your technique by "reaching" for your opponent. Create the proper distance using footwork before executing your kick.

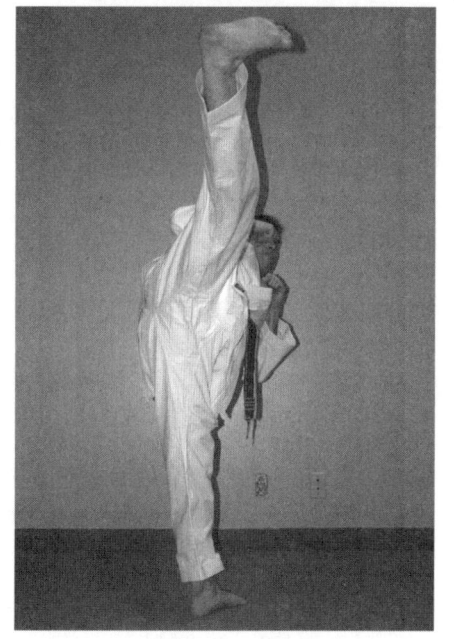

Impact Front View   *Impact Side View*

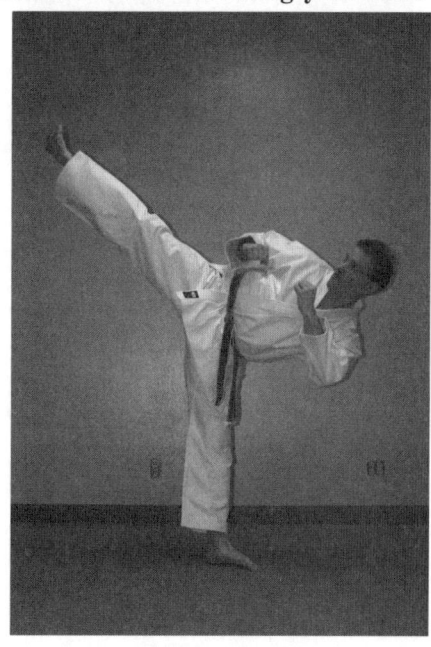

Follow Through:

25. Your base leg foot should have moved another 45-degrees (clockwise) by pivoting on the ball of the foot.
26. Your upper body should still be leaning to your left at almost a 75-degree angle in relation to your bodys upright position, and almost parallel with the ground. Although it has once again moved clockwise prior to the movement of your kicking leg and foot. Your back is straight and the front of your body is now at approximately a 45-degree angle to the front of your opponent.
27. Your kicking leg foot should continue along exactly the same path it followed from the "Peak of Trajectory" to "Impact." Your foot should be approximately 45-degrees past your target.
28. Your head should no longer be looking over your kicking leg shoulder. However, your eyes are still looking at your opponent.

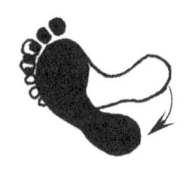

Note: In the illustration on the right, the bullet, which represents your kicking foot, has penetrated through the target area and into the target. However, in this example, if you merely "strike into" the target, rather...

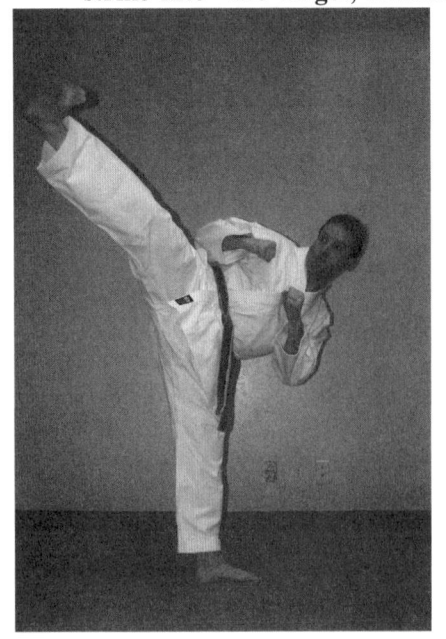

Follow Through Foot Position

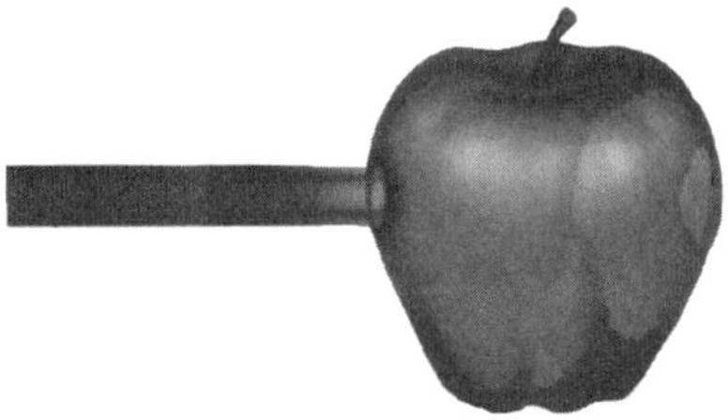

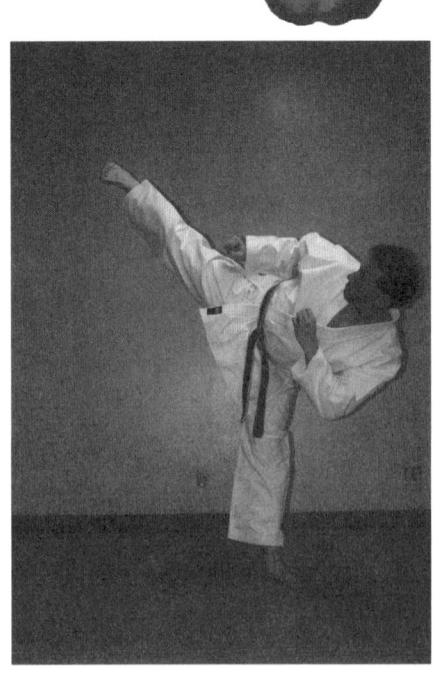

Follow Through Front View

Follow Through Side View

End of Trajectory:

29. Your base leg foot should have moved another 45-degrees (clockwise) by pivoting on the ball of the foot. The toes of your base leg foot should now be pointing directly at your opponent.
30. Your kicking leg remains straight with the knee slightly bent. Your kicking foot is now slightly in front of you and to your right at approximately the height of your base leg knee.
31. Your upper body will straighten up from the approximately 75-degree bent over position you were in when kicking. Your back remains straight and your upper body is now facing directly toward your opponent.
32. Your head should still be up and looking directly over the center of your chest. Your eyes are still in contact with your opponent, whether he is still standing, or lying on the ground.

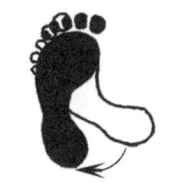

End of Trajectory Foot Position

Note: ...than "striking through" the target, you will end up with a slightly more effective "penetrating strike," rather than the two distinctively separate "surface strikes" that were demonstrated on pages 78 and 88. Once again, in order to maximize the effectiveness of your kicks, you must, correctly, apply all of the proper principles outlined in this book.

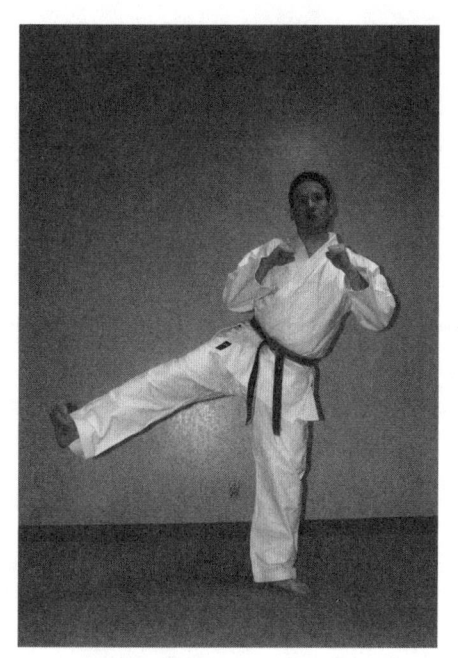

End of Trajectory Front View   *End of Trajectory Side View*

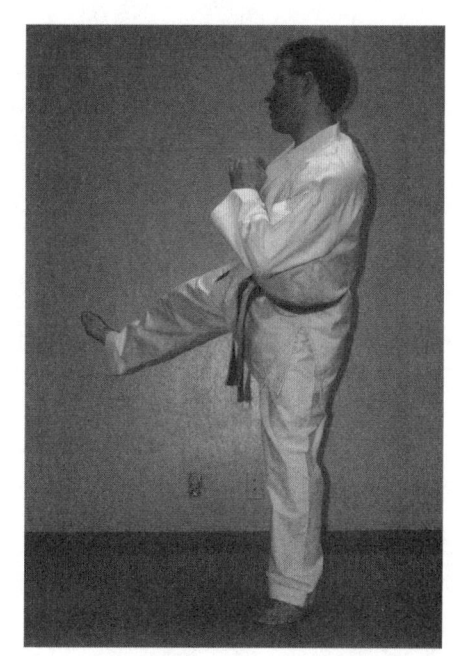

Return to Fighting Position:

33. Your entire body from your head to your toes, should be in exactly the same position that you initially started in (refer to the Fighting Position section of this kick), prior to executing this kick. Although, you won't be in exactly the same location.
34. Your kicking leg foot continues the 360-degree motion and returns to its original starting position. Although your kicking leg knee will remain slightly bent as it returns to the starting position.
35. Your hands, which should have remained as close to this position as possible throughout the entire kick, are once again in the same position they were in prior to executing the kick.
36. Your head should now be looking over your lead leg shoulder with your eyes in contact with your opponent.

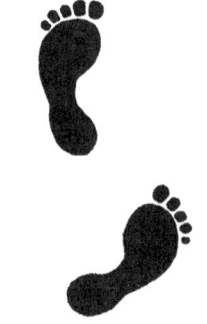

Return to Fighting Position Foot Position

Note: **The principles and techniques described within this book are not specific to any particular style. The information supplied within this book is intended to be used by any martial artist, practicing any style, anywhere in the world.**

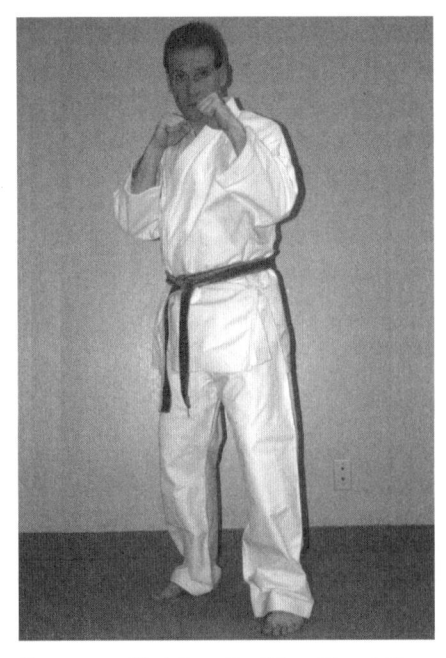

Return to Fighting Position Front View

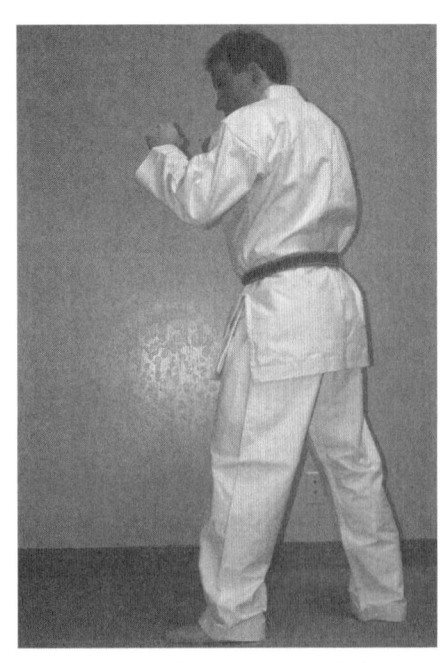

Return to Fighting Position Side View

Pictorial Overview:

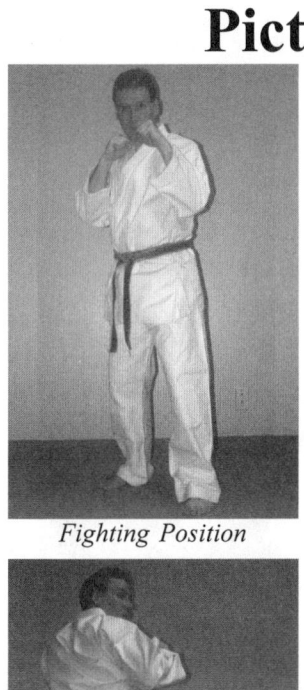

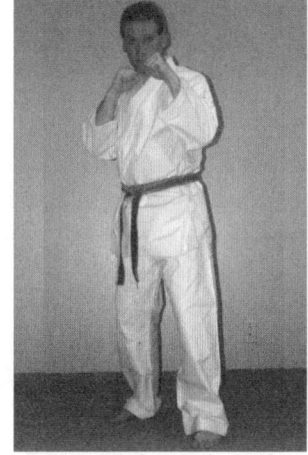

Fighting Position

Hop/Slide Backward

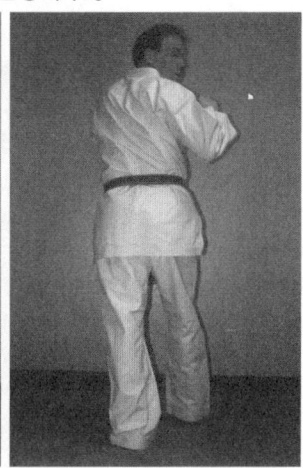

Turn

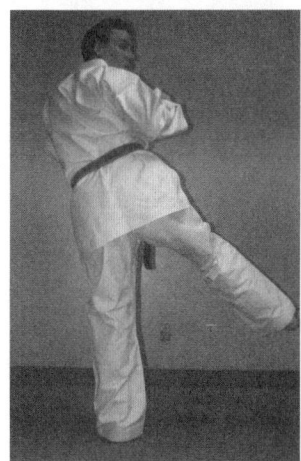

Begin Trajectory

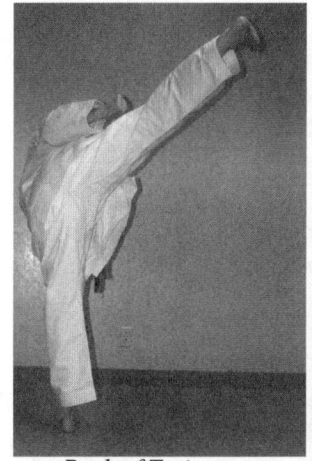

Peak of Trajectory

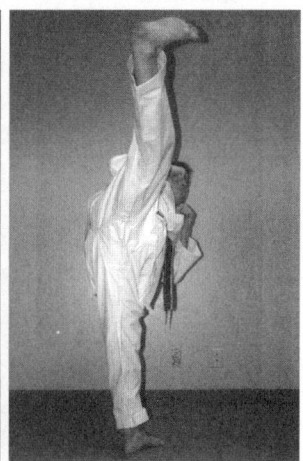

Impact

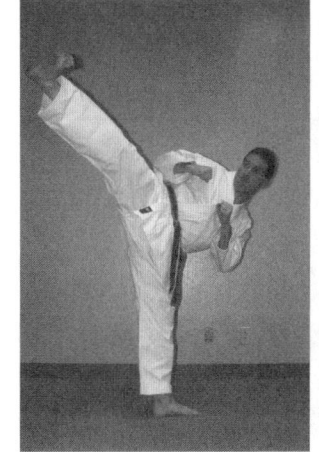

Follow Through

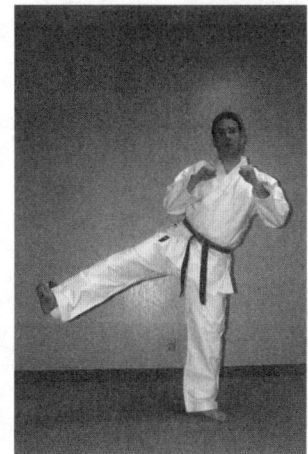

End of Trajectory

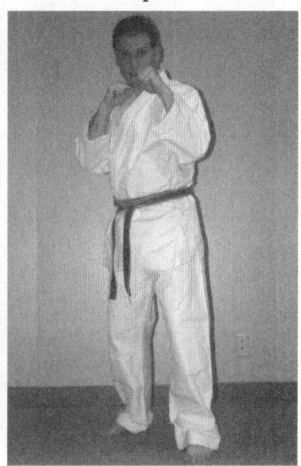

Return to Fighting Position

Front Leg Wheel Kick

The Front Leg Wheel Kick is unique in the fact that it does not utilize a 360-degree turning motion during the execution of the kick. As a matter of fact, at no time during the execution of this kick do you turn your back towards your opponent. This kick is executed by shifting your weight onto your rear leg while bringing your front leg up and across your body into the "Begin Trajectory" phase of the kick. Although this is perhaps the weakest of all the Wheel Kicks in this book, it is still a necessary and very effective kick. With practice, this can be one of the fastest Wheel Kicks in your kicking arsenal.

Fighting Position:
1. This stance is approximately shoulder width apart with the heel of your rear foot directly in line with the heel of your front foot.
2. Your front of lead foot should be pointed directly at your opponent.
3. Your rear foot is angled towards the right at approximately a 45-degree angle. Your weight should be distributed evenly over the balls of both feet.
4. Your knees are slightly, but not noticeably bent. They should not be locked straight or rigid.
5. Your body should be facing at a 45-degree angle toward your opponent. This presents a smaller target area and also facilitates a faster turn when utilizing this kick.

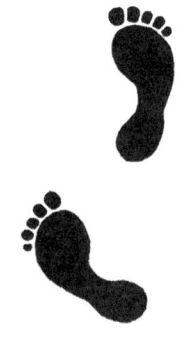

Fighting Position Foot Position

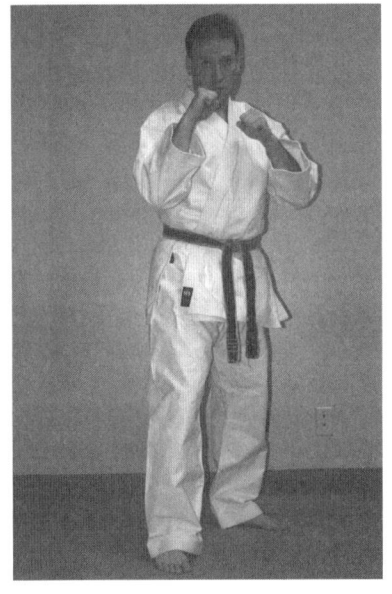

Fighting Position Front View

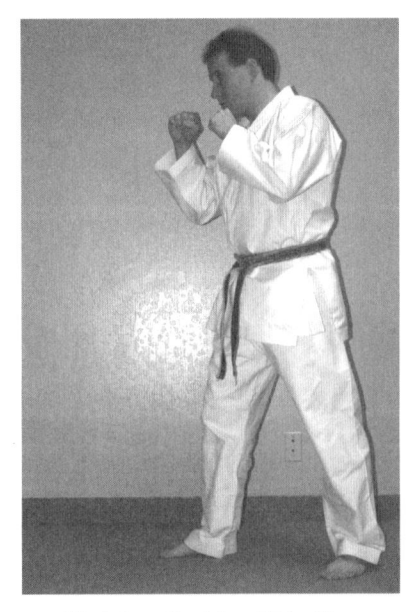

Fighting Position Side View

6. Your hands should be held up (like a boxer's), with the elbows tucked in to protect the ribs and your hands up to protect your head. Your hands should remain as close to this position as possible throughout the entire kick.
7. Your head should be facing your opponent with your chin tucked down and protected by your lead shoulder.
8. Your eyes should be centered on your opponent's chest.

Begin Trajectory:
9. Using the toes of your kicking foot, push off the floor and bring your kicking leg up at a 45-degree angle between the direction your body is facing and your right hand side. Your leg should be straight, with a slight bend in the knee. In this position, your kicking foot should already be in the correct position to strike your opponent.
10. As you bring your kicking leg up, your upper body should start bending over slightly, from the waist, to the left. Your back will remain straight.
11. Your head is still up and turned over your kicking shoulder, your eyes should always remain in contact with your opponent throughout the entire kick.
12. Your right hand side should now be facing directly towards your opponent, while your back is at a 90-degree angle to your opponent's left.

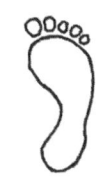

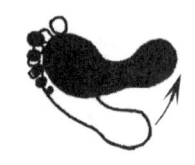

Begin Trajectory Foot Position

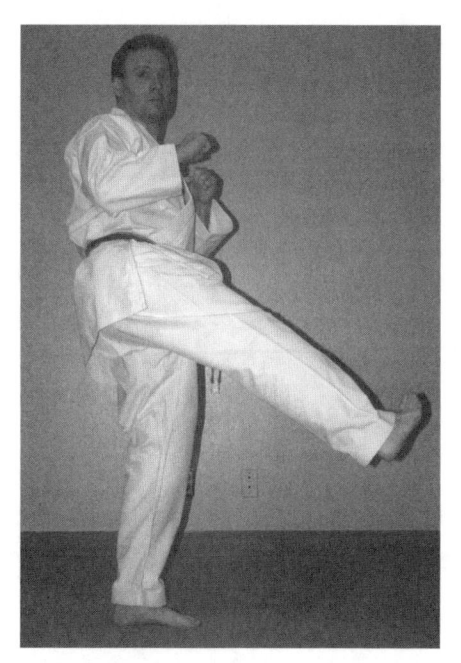

Begin Trajectory Front View   *Begin Trajectory Side View*

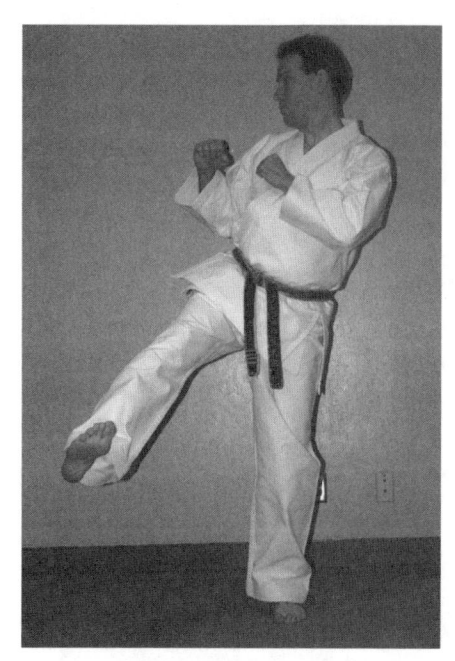

101

Peak of Trajectory:

13. Your base leg foot should now have moved approximately 45-degrees (clockwise) by pivoting on the ball of your foot. While your kicking leg, with the knee slightly bent, has now moved up to the correct height to strike your target.
14. The heel of the kicking foot should follow a straight line of trajectory from the "Peak of Trajectory" through the target (Impact), to the "Follow Through" position.
15. Your upper body should now be leaning to your left at almost a 75-degree angle in relation to your bodys upright position, and almost parallel with the ground.
16. Although your body is now in the above position, your head should still be looking over your kicking leg shoulder at your opponent.
17. Your back is now be facing at a 45-degree angle to your opponent's left in approximately the same direction that your kicking leg will be in, when it is in the "Follow Through" position.

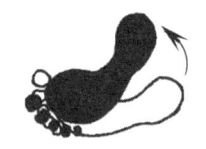

Peak of Trajectory Foot Position

Note: The head, which can easily be compared to the ever popular "bobblehead" dolls, makes for a difficult target with a kick due to the ease in which the head can "bob and weave" like a boxer in order to avoid being hit.

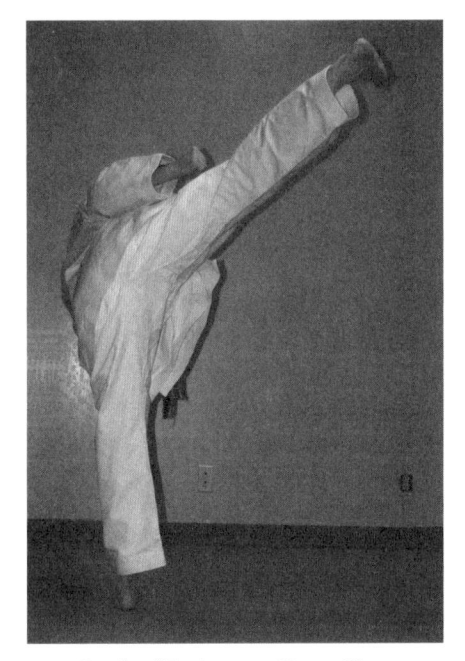

Peak of Trajectory Front View   *Peak of Trajectory Side View*

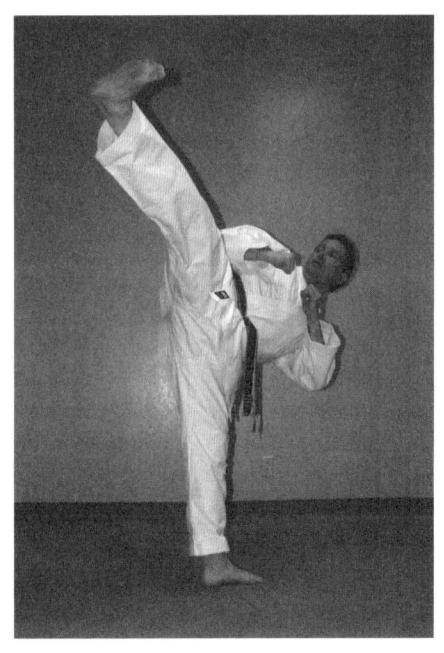

Impact:
18. Your base leg foot has now moved another 45-degrees (clockwise), by pivoting on the ball of the foot, with the arch of your foot now facing towards your opponent.
19. Your upper body should still be leaning to your left at almost a 75-degree angle in relation to your bodys upright position, and almost parallel with the ground. Although it has moved clockwise prior to the movement of your kicking leg and foot. At the moment of impact, your entire body should tighten to add power to the kick, as your foot continues to travel through the target.
20. Notice how your kicking foot, kicking leg (with knee slightly bent), hips, back, shoulders and head are all in a straight line at the initial moment of "Impact". Also, notice how the toes of the kicking foot are pulled back towards your body and pointed. This helps insure that contact with the target is made with the back of the heel.
21. Your head should still be up and looking over the kicking leg shoulder. Eye contact with your opponent is maintained at all times.

Note: Look closely at the photographs below, see how vulnerable you are in this position? Constantly strive to kick faster than you can blink!

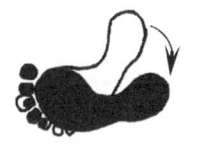

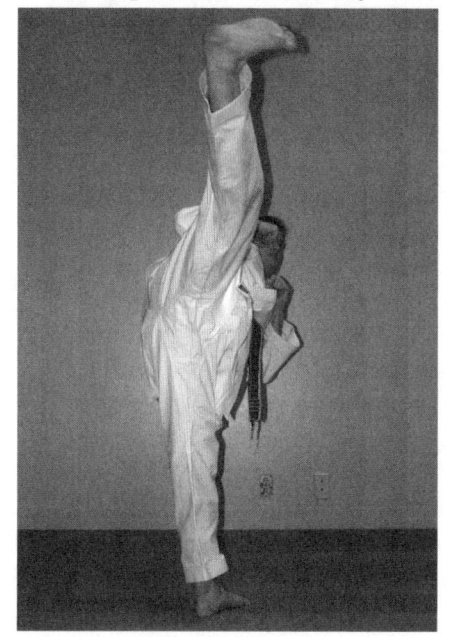

Impact Foot Position

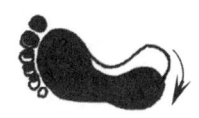

Impact (ADVANCED) Foot Position

Impact Front View

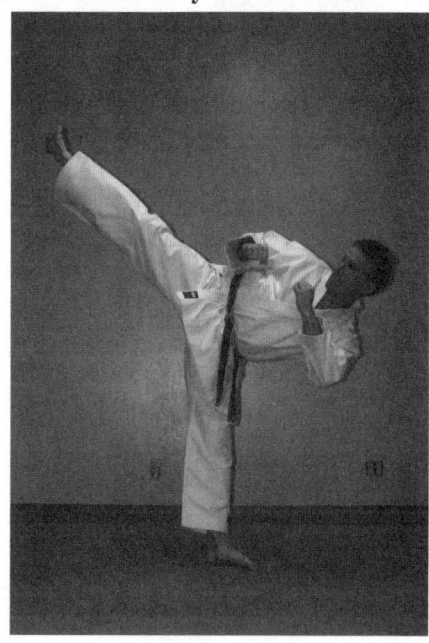

Impact Side View

Follow Through:

22. Your base leg foot should have moved another 45-degrees (clockwise) by pivoting on the ball of the foot.
23. Your upper body should still be leaning to your left at almost a 75-degree angle in relation to your bodys upright position, and almost parallel with the ground. Although it has once again moved clockwise prior to the movement of your kicking leg and foot. Your back is straight and the front of your body is now at approximately a 45-degree angle to the front of your opponent.
24. Your kicking leg foot should continue along exactly the same path it followed from the "Peak of Trajectory" to "Impact." Your foot should be approximately 45-degrees past your target.
25. Your head should no longer be looking over your kicking leg shoulder. However, your eyes are still looking at your opponent.

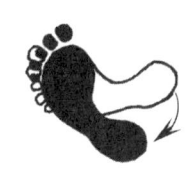

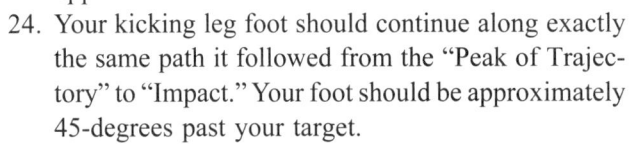

Follow Through Foot Position

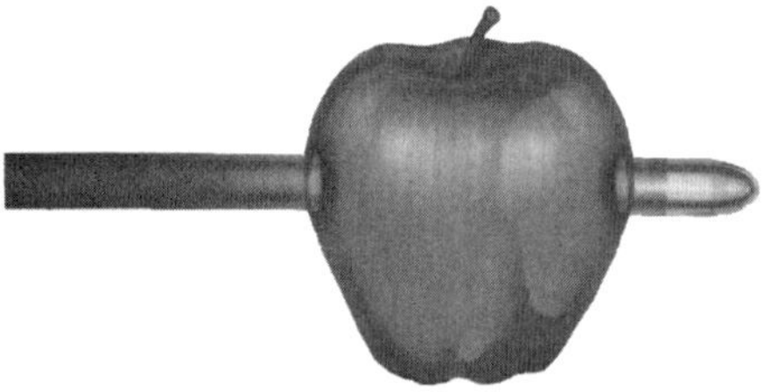

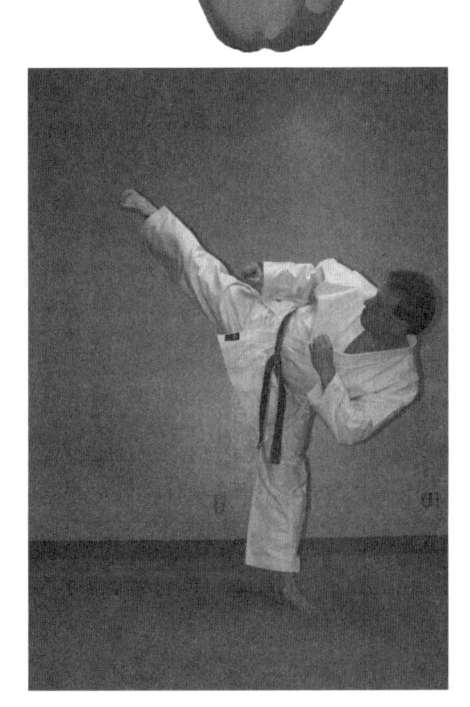

Note: In the illustration on the right, the bullet, which represents your kicking foot, has penetrated into and completely through the target. However, in this example, if you merely "strike through" the...

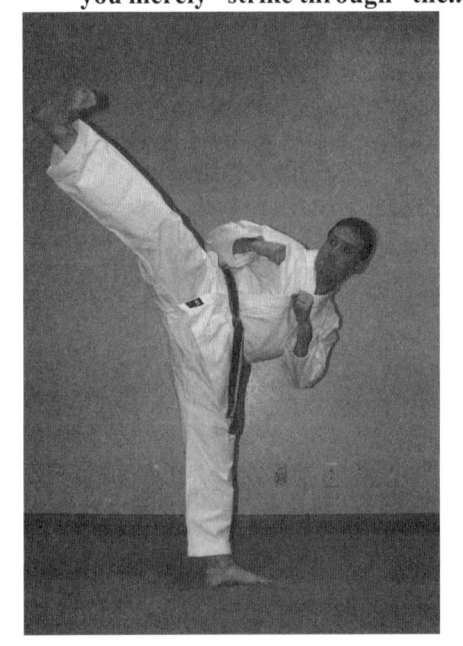

Follow Through Front View   *Follow Through Side View*

104

End of Trajectory:
26. Your base leg foot should have moved another 45-degrees (clockwise) by pivoting on the ball of the foot. The toes of your base leg foot should now be pointing directly at your opponent.
27. Your kicking leg remains straight with the knee slightly bent. Your kicking foot is now slightly in front of you and to your right at approximately the height of your base leg knee.
28. Your upper body will straighten up from the approximately 75-degree bent over position you were in when kicking. Your back remains straight and your upper body is now facing directly toward your opponent.
29. Your head should still be up and looking directly over the center of your chest. Your eyes are still in contact with your opponent, whether he is still standing, or lying on the ground.

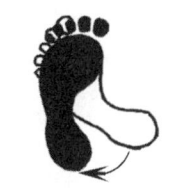

End of Trajectory Foot Position

Note: ...target without adding the tightening of the entire body upon impact, you will end up with a slightly more effective kick that the three previous examples which were demonstrated on pages, 78, 88 and 96. However, you still will not have reached the maximum effectiveness of your kick, because you still have not correctly applied all of the proper principles which I have outlined for you in this book.

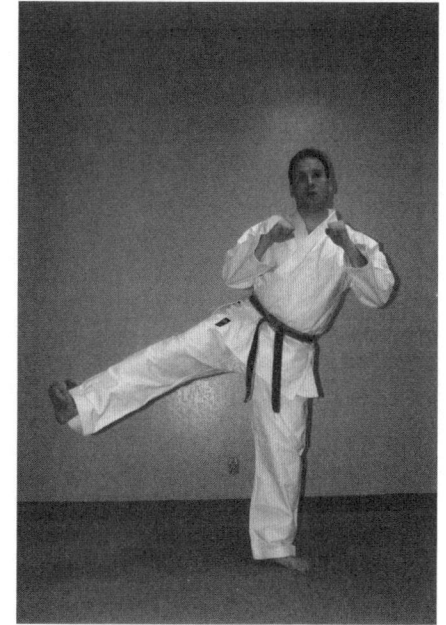

End of Trajectory Front View *End of Trajectory Side View*

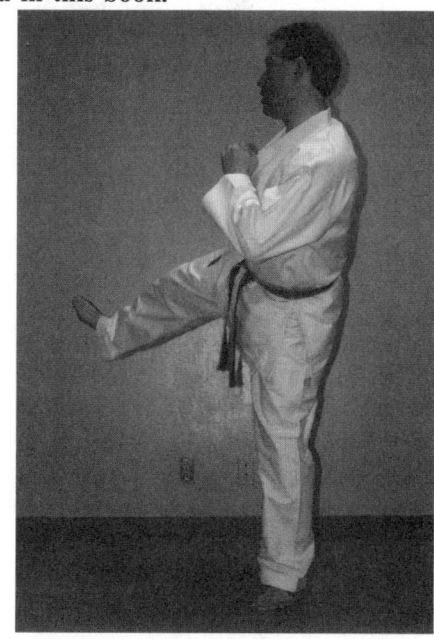

Return to Fighting Position:

30. Your entire body from your head to your toes, should be in exactly the same position that you initially started in (refer to the Fighting Position section of this kick), prior to executing this kick.
31. Your kicking leg foot continues the 360-degree motion and returns to its original starting position. Although your kicking leg knee will remain slightly bent as it returns to the starting position.
32. Your hands, which should have remained as close to this position as possible throughout the entire kick, are once again in the same position they were in prior to executing the kick.
33. Your head should now be looking over your lead leg shoulder with your eyes in contact with your opponent.

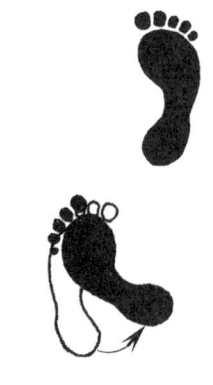

Return to Fighting Position Foot Position

Note: Would you hammer a nail into a piece of wood with a saw? Would you cut a board with a hammer? Remember to use the correct tool for each particular situation. Kicking may be effective in one situation, but ineffective in another. A Wheel Kick may be the correct kick to use in one kicking situation, but totally ineffective in another.

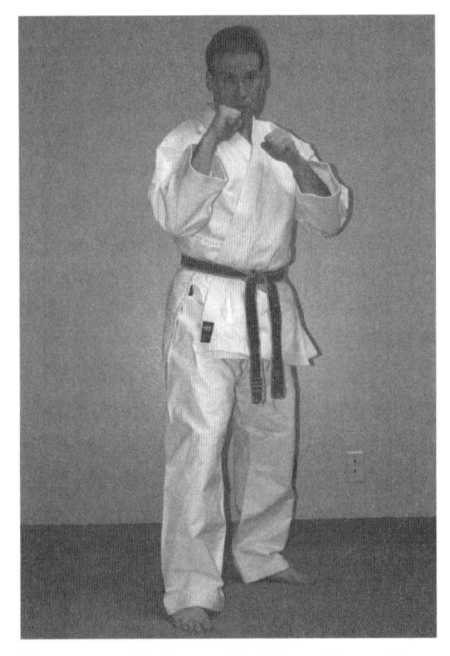

Return to Fighting Position Front View   *Return to Fighting Position Side View*

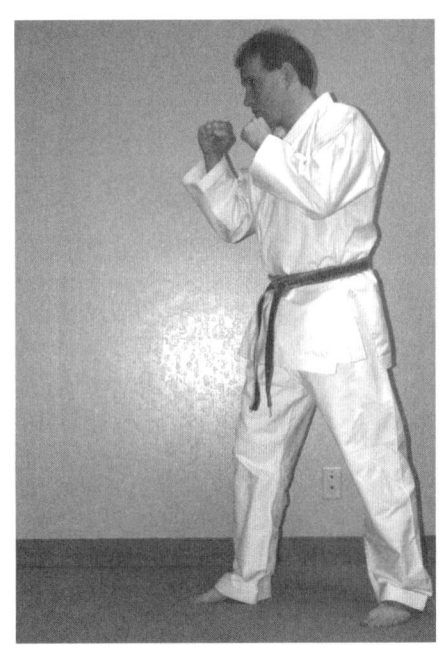

Pictorial Overview:

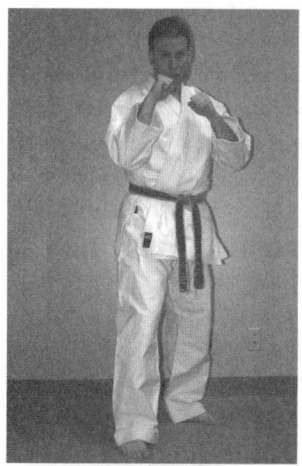

Fighting Position

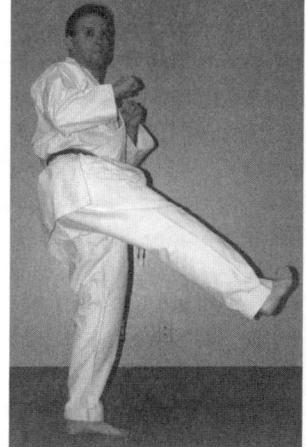

Begin Trajectory

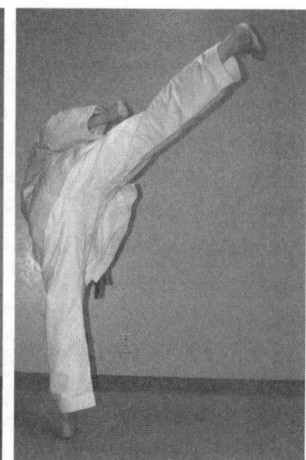

Peak of Trajectory

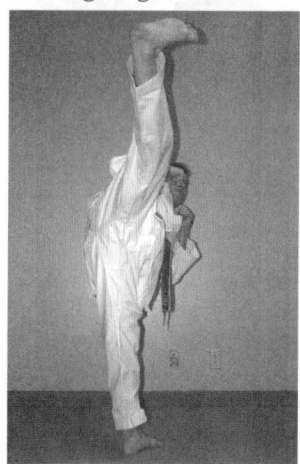

Impact

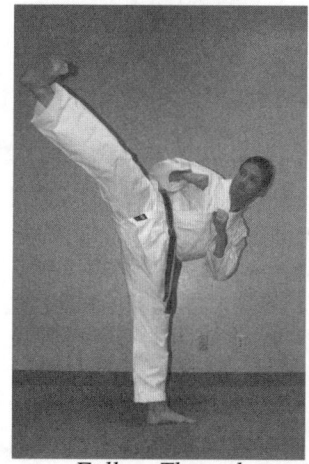

Follow Through

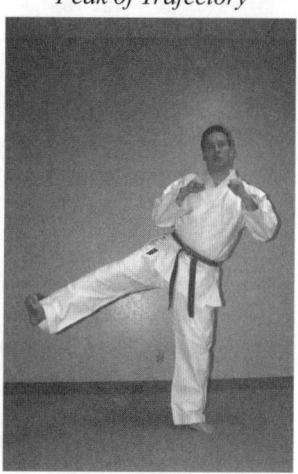

End of Trajectory

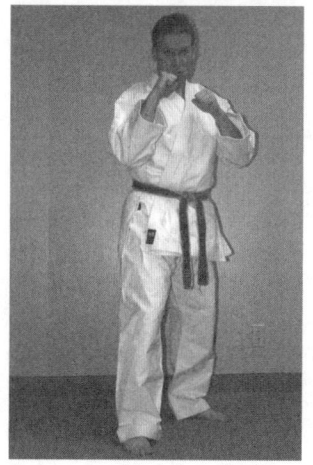

Return to Fighting Position

Back Leg Wheel Kick

    The Back Leg Wheel Kick is identical in execution to the Front Leg Wheel Kick, with one notable exception. Your kicking leg, which was in the forward position on the Front Leg Wheel Kick, is now in the rearward position. As with the Front Leg Wheel Kick, at no time during the execution of this kick do you turn your back towards your opponent. This kick is executed by shifting your weight onto your front leg while bringing your rear leg up and across your body into the "Begin Trajectory" phase of the kick. This kick tends to be a little more powerful than the Front Leg Wheel Kick due to the fact that your are executing the kick off of your rear leg. Although it is not as powerful as a Turning Wheel Kick, it is still a very necessary and effective Wheel Kick to have in your arsenal of kicking techniques.

Fighting Position:

1. This stance is approximately shoulder width apart with the heel of your rear foot directly in line with the heel of your front foot.
2. Your front of lead foot should be pointed directly at your opponent.
3. Your rear foot is angled towards the right at approximately a 45-degree angle. Your weight should be distributed evenly over the balls of both feet.
4. Your knees are slightly, but not noticeably bent. They should not be locked straight or rigid.
5. Your body should be facing at a 45-degree angle toward your opponent. This presents a smaller target area and also facilitates a faster turn when utilizing this kick.

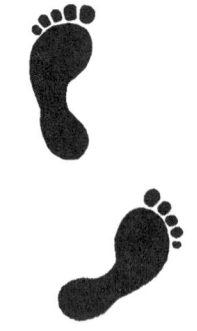

Fighting Position Foot Position

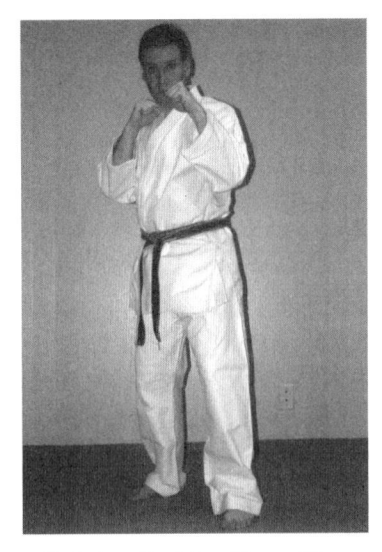

Fighting Position Front View

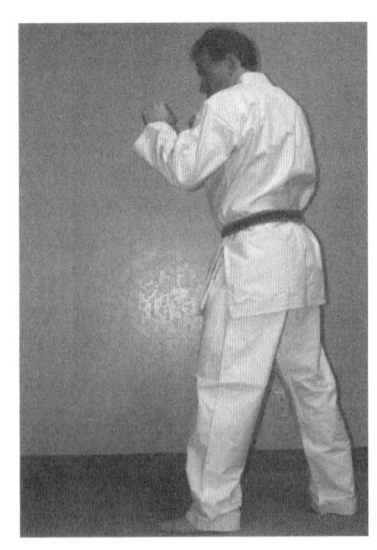

Fighting Position Side View

6. Your hands should be held up (like a boxer's), with the elbows tucked in to protect the ribs and your hands up to protect your head. Your hands should remain as close to this position as possible throughout the entire kick.
7. Your head should be facing your opponent with your chin tucked down and protected by your lead shoulder.
8. Your eyes should be centered on your opponent's chest.

Begin Trajectory:

9. Using the toes of your kicking foot, push off the floor and bring your kicking leg up and across your body at a 45-degree angle between the direction your body is facing and your right hand side. Your leg should be straight, with a slight bend in the knee. In this position, your kicking foot should already be in the correct position to strike your opponent.
10. As you bring your kicking leg up, your upper body should start bending over slightly, from the waist, to the left. Your back will remain straight.
11. Your head is still up and turned over your kicking shoulder, your eyes should always remain in contact with your opponent throughout the entire kick.
12. Your right hand side should now be facing directly towards your opponent, while your back is at a 90-degree angle to your opponent's left.

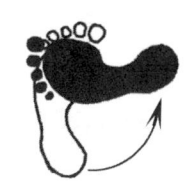

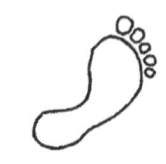

Begin Trajectory Foot Position

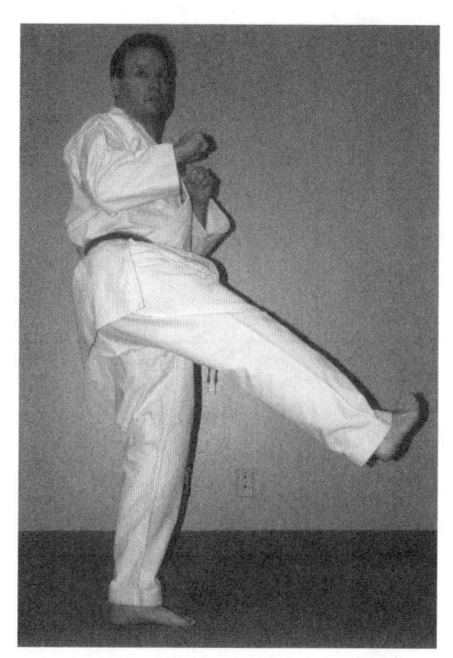

Begin Trajectory Front View   *Begin Trajectory Side View*

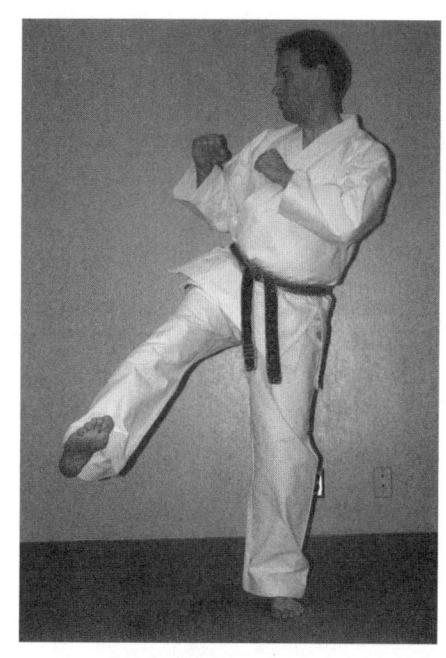

Peak of Trajectory:

13. Your base leg foot should now have moved approximately 45-degrees (clockwise) by pivoting on the ball of your foot. While your kicking leg, with the knee slightly bent, has now moved up to the correct height to strike your target.
14. The heel of the kicking foot should follow a straight line of trajectory from the "Peak of Trajectory" through the target (Impact), to the "Follow Through" position.
15. Your upper body should now be leaning to your left at almost a 75-degree angle in relation to your bodys upright position, and almost parallel with the ground.
16. Although your body is now in the above position, your head should still be looking over your kicking leg shoulder at your opponent.
17. Your back is now be facing at a 45-degree angle to your opponent's left in approximately the same direction that your kicking leg will be in, when it is in the "Follow Through" position.

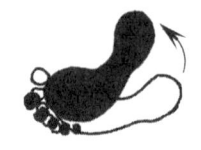

Peak of Trajectory Foot Position

Note: The kicking motion of the Back Leg Wheel Kick is very similar in nature to that of the Reverse Crescent Kick, which is the primary kick discussed in great detail in Volume Five.

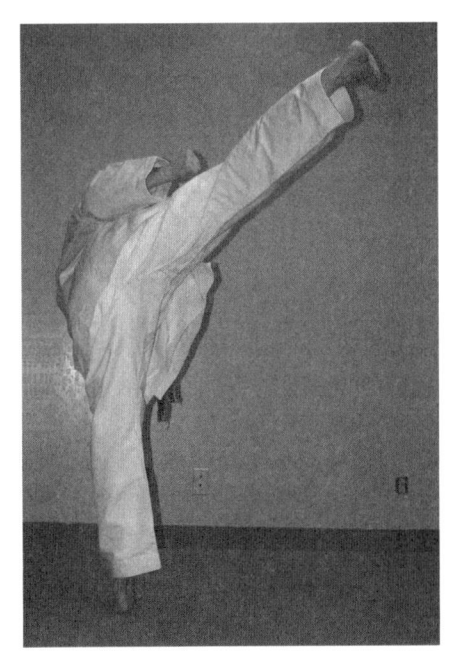

Peak of Trajectory Front View   *Peak of Trajectory Side View*

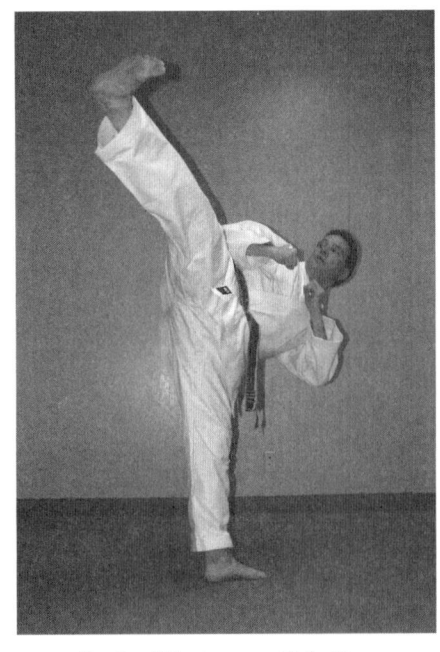

Impact:

18. Your base leg foot has now moved another 45-degrees (clockwise), by pivoting on the ball of the foot, with the arch of your foot now facing towards your opponent.
19. Your upper body should still be leaning to your left at almost a 75-degree angle in relation to your bodys upright position, and almost parallel with the ground. Although it has moved clockwise prior to the movement of your kicking leg and foot. At the moment of impact, your entire body should tighten to add power to the kick, as your foot continues to travel through the target.
20. Notice how your kicking foot, kicking leg (with knee slightly bent), hips, back, shoulders and head are all in a straight line at the initial moment of "Impact". Also, notice how the toes of the kicking foot are pulled back towards your body and pointed. This helps insure that contact with the target is made with the back of the heel.
21. Your head should still be up and looking over the kicking leg shoulder. Eye contact with your opponent is maintained at all times.

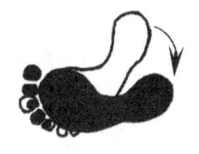

Impact Foot Position

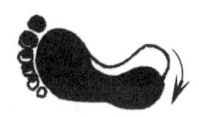

Impact (ADVANCED) Foot Position

Note: A sharp exhalation of air or KIAA!, should be executed at the initial moment of impact to tighten your body and add power to your kick.

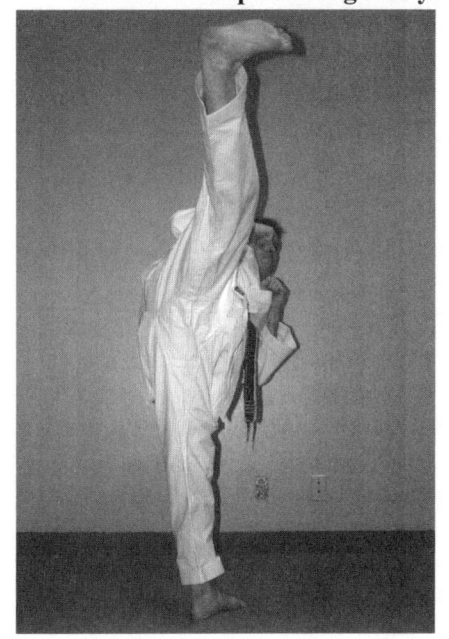

Impact Front View

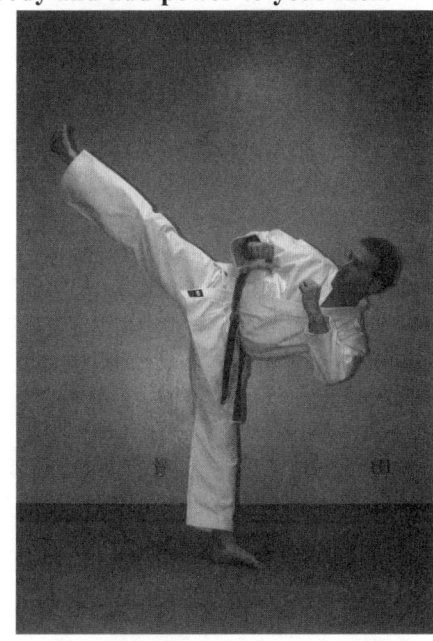

Impact Side View

111

Follow Through:

22. Your base leg foot should have moved another 45-degrees (clockwise) by pivoting on the ball of the foot.
23. Your upper body should still be leaning to your left at almost a 75-degree angle in relation to your bodys upright position, and almost parallel with the ground. Although it has once again moved clockwise prior to the movement of your kicking leg and foot. Your back is straight and the front of your body is now at approximately a 45-degree angle to the front of your opponent.
24. Your kicking leg foot should continue along exactly the same path it followed from the "Peak of Trajectory" to "Impact." Your foot should be approximately 45-degrees past your target.
25. Your head should no longer be looking over your kicking leg shoulder. However, your eyes are still looking at your opponent.

Follow Through Foot Position

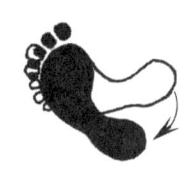

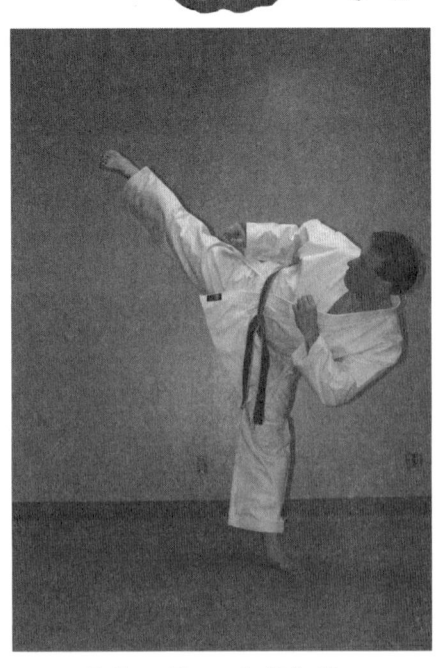

Note: In the illustration on the right, the bullet, which represents your kicking foot, has penetrated through the target area, into the target and through your opponent's...

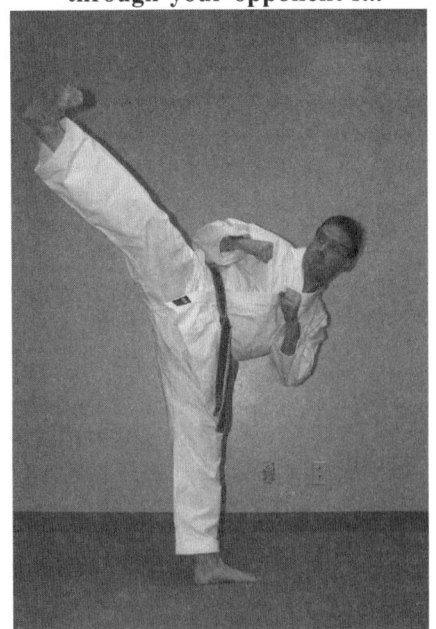

Follow Through Front View   *Follow Through Side View*

End of Trajectory:
26. Your base leg foot should have moved another 45-degrees (clockwise) by pivoting on the ball of the foot. The toes of your base leg foot should now be pointing directly at your opponent.
27. Your kicking leg remains straight with the knee slightly bent. Your kicking foot is now slightly in front of you and to your right at approximately the height of your base leg knee.
28. Your upper body will straighten up from the approximately 75-degree bent over position you were in when kicking. Your back remains straight and your upper body is now facing directly toward your opponent.
29. Your head should still be up and looking directly over the center of your chest. Your eyes are still in contact with your opponent, whether he is still standing, or lying on the ground..

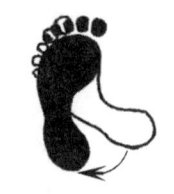

End of Trajectory Foot Position

Note: ...head, which is represented by the apple. However, in this example, your kicking foot has been left hanging in the air after successfully striking through your target, instead of executing the kick correctly by returning to its initial starting position. Always remember, that your kicking foot should be just as fast, if not faster, returning to the "Fighting Position" from just after the initial moment of impact, than from the beginning "Fighting Position" to the initial moment of impact.

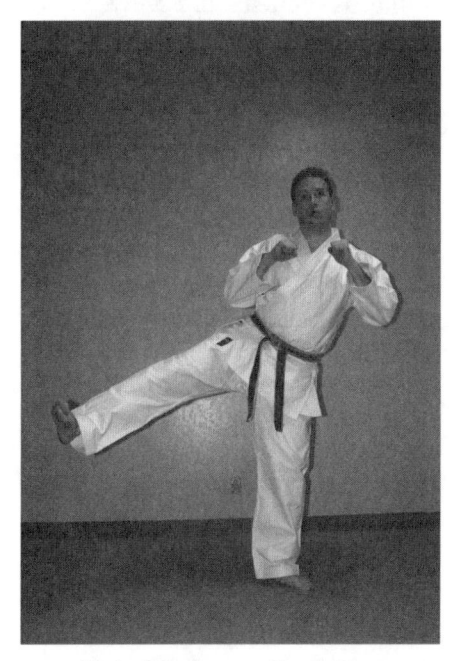

End of Trajectory Front View   *End of Trajectory Side View*

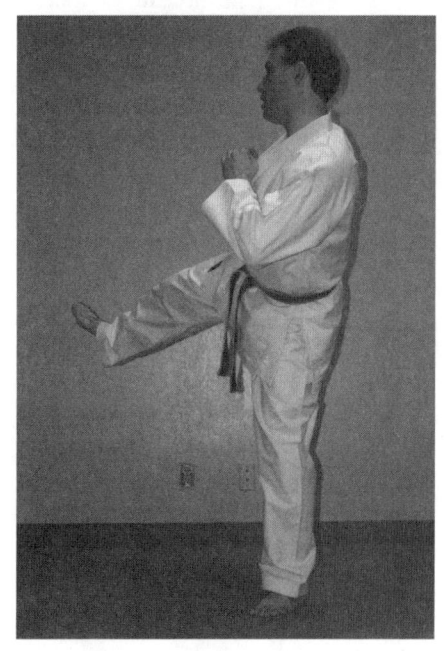

Return to Fighting Position:

30. Your entire body from your head to your toes, should be in exactly the same position that you initially started in (refer to the Fighting Position section of this kick), prior to executing this kick.
31. Your kicking leg foot continues the 360-degree motion and returns to its original starting position. Although your kicking leg knee will remain slightly bent as it returns to the starting position.
32. Your hands, which should have remained as close to this position as possible throughout the entire kick, are once again in the same position they were in prior to executing the kick.
33. Your head should now be looking over your lead leg shoulder with your eyes in contact with your opponent.

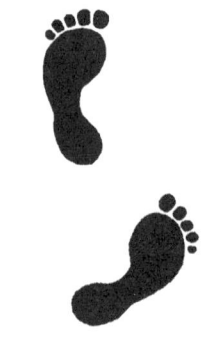

Return to Fighting Position Foot Position

Note: Not pivoting correctly on the ball of your base leg foot, throughout the entire execution of a Wheel Kick, can be likened to the act of "ringing out" a wet hand towel. Each end of the towel is grasped firmly in each hand, then both hands twist the towel in opposite directions, which results in the tightening of the towel in the middle, creating a tremendous amount of pressure on the towel which forces the water out. This is exactly what happens to your knee when you fail to pivot properly on the ball of your base leg foot. However, unlike the towel who's pressure is slow and gradual, the pressure on your knee is sudden and EXPLOSIVE!

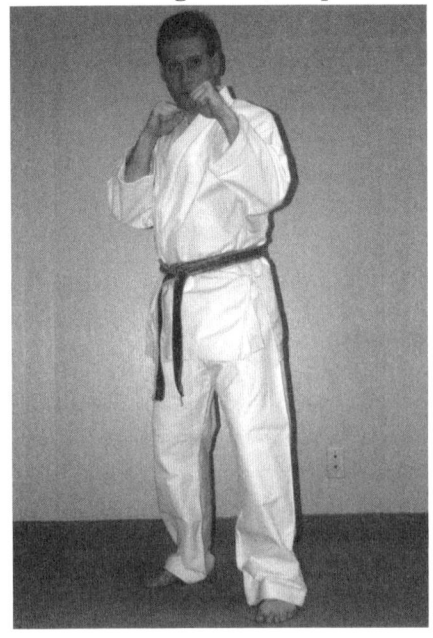

Return to Fighting Position Front View

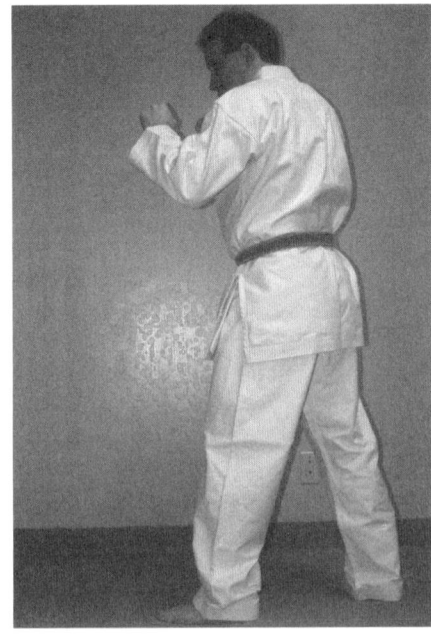

Return to Fighting Position Side View

Pictorial Overview:

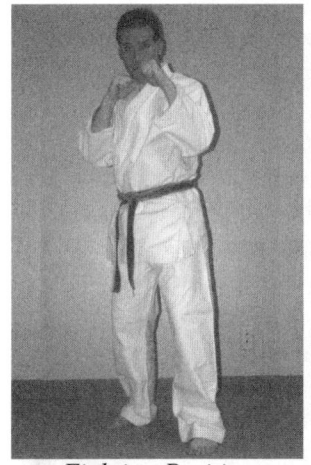

Fighting Position

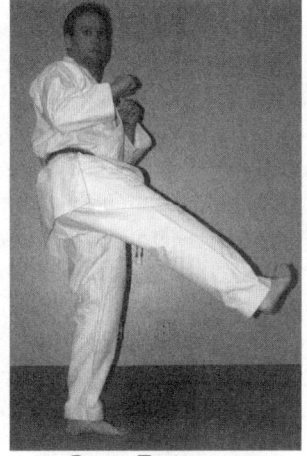

Begin Trajectory

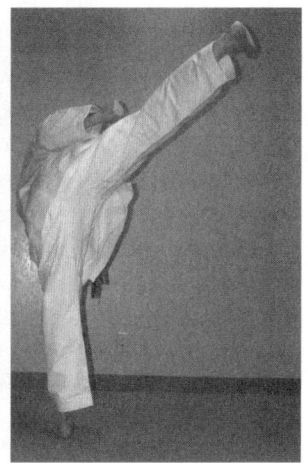

Peak of Trajectory

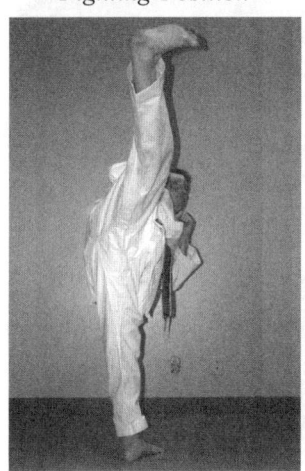

Impact

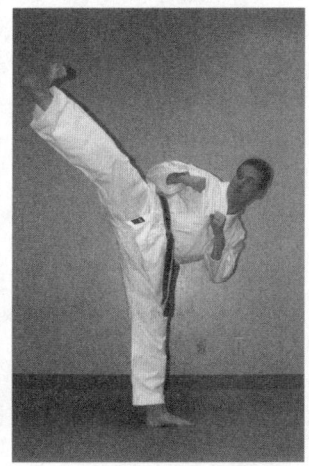

Follow Through

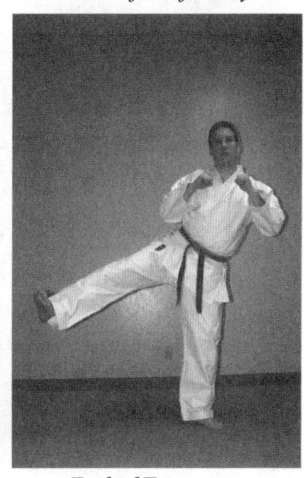

End of Trajectory

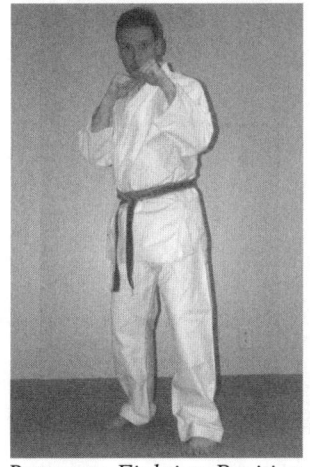

Return to Fighting Position

115

Switch Wheel Kick

The Switch Wheel Kick is identical in execution to the Turning Wheel Kick, with one notable exception. A switching motion of the feet, which is performed immediately prior to the execution of the kick. The switch is used to confuse the opponent and can also increase the power in this kick due to the added momentum of switching your feet. The starting position is the same as for Spinning Wheel Kick, with your kicking leg in the forward position rather than in the rear position. The actual switching of the feet prior to execution of the kick is performed by simultaneously switching the position of both feet utilizing a straight line or scissors type motion. With the end result being a fighting position with the kicking leg now in the rearward position. When executing the switch, be sure and move your feet first without moving your upper body in order to avoid telegraphing the switch to your opponent. Your hips and upper body will begin to move immediately after your feet, but not before.

Fighting Position:
1. Your fighting position for this kick is the exact same as for Spinning Wheel Kick. That is your kicking leg will be in the forward position to begin with rather than in the rear.
2. This stance is approximately shoulder width apart with the heel of your rear foot in a direct line with the heel of your front foot.
3. Your front or lead foot should be pointing directly at your opponent.
4. Your rear foot is angled towards the left at approximately a 45-degree angle. Your weight should be distributed evenly over the balls of both feet.

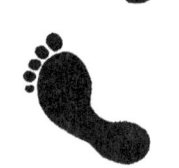

Fighting Position Foot Position

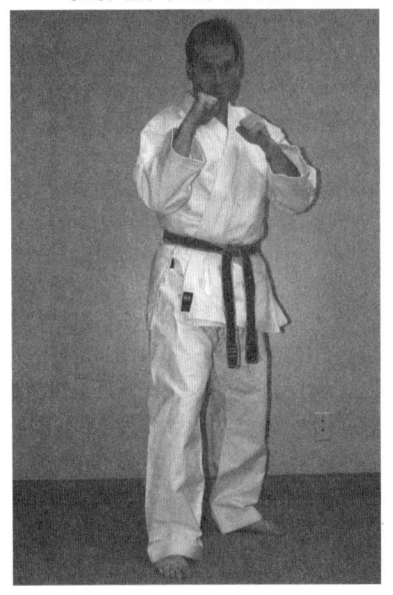

Fighting Position Front View

Fighting Position Side View

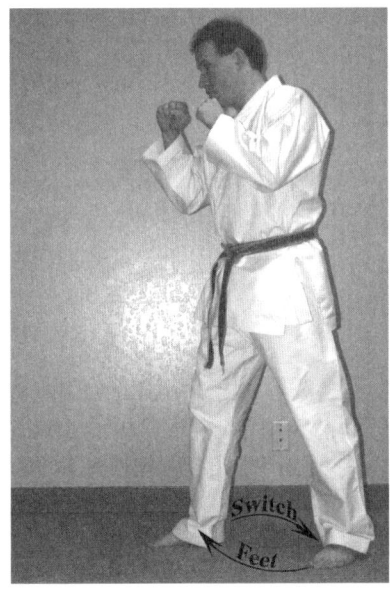

5. Your knees are slightly, but not noticeably bent. They should not be locked or rigid.
6. Your body should be facing at a 45-degree angle toward your opponent. This presents a smaller target area and also facilitates a faster switch-and-turn when utilizing this kick.
7. Your hands should be held up (like a boxer's), with the elbows tucked in to protect the ribs and your hands up to protect your head. Your hands should remain as close to this position as possible throughout the entire kick.
8. Your head should be facing your opponent with your chin tucked down and protected by your lead shoulder.
9. Your eyes should be centered on your opponents chest.

Switch Feet & Turn Back:

10. Utilizing a scissors type motion of your legs and feet, simultaneously switch your front foot with your rear foot. After you have begun the switching of the feet, turn your back towards your opponent. After switching, the heels of both of your feet should be pointed towards your opponent.
11. Prior to turning your back, your head should be turned over your kicking leg shoulder and your eyes should be looking at your opponent.
12. Your back should be facing directly toward your opponent.

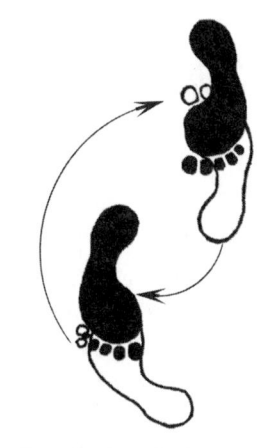

Switch Feet & Turn Back Foot Position

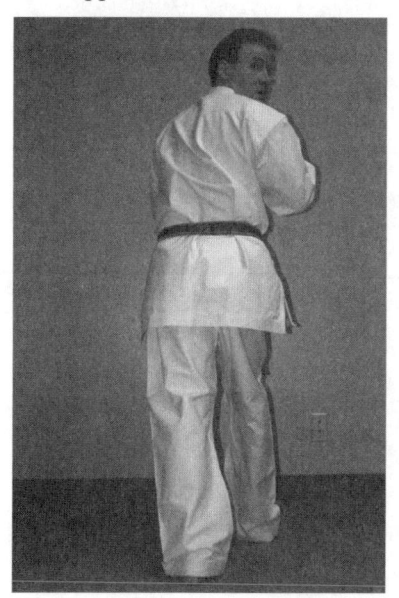

Switch Feet & Turn Front View

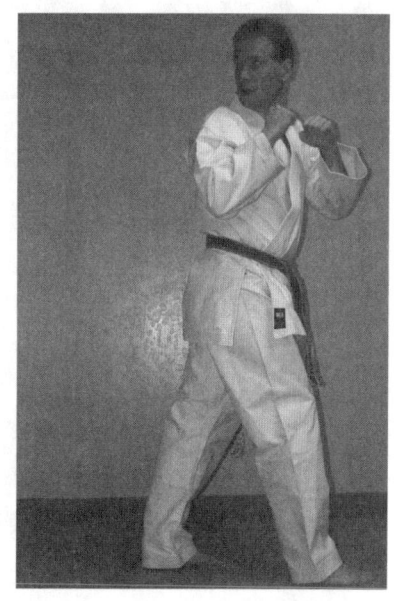

Switch Feet & Turn Side View

117

Begin Trajectory:

13. Using the toes of your kicking foot, push off the floor and bring your kicking leg up at a 45-degree angle between the direction your body is facing and your right hand side. Your leg should be straight, with a slight bend in the knee. In this position, your kicking foot should already be in the correct position to strike your opponent.
14. As you bring your kicking leg up, your upper body should start bending over slightly, from the waist, to the left. Your back will remain straight.
15. Your head is still up and turned over your kicking shoulder, your eyes should always remain in contact with your opponent throughout the entire kick.
16. Your back should no longer be facing directly towards your opponent, but should start turning, along with your shoulders, in the direction of the kick.

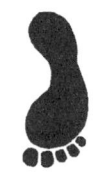

Begin Trajectory Foot Position

Note: When executing a "Switch" kick of any kind, compare it to the shooting action of a rifle. For example; the switching motion is the trigger on the rifle, while the ground is the firing pin, the ball of your kicking foot is the primer in the bullet casing, the combination of muscular speed, strength and proper technique is the gunpowder, and finally, the heel of your kicking foot is the bullet. As you squeeze the trigger (switch your feet), it releases the firing pin striking the primer in the casing...

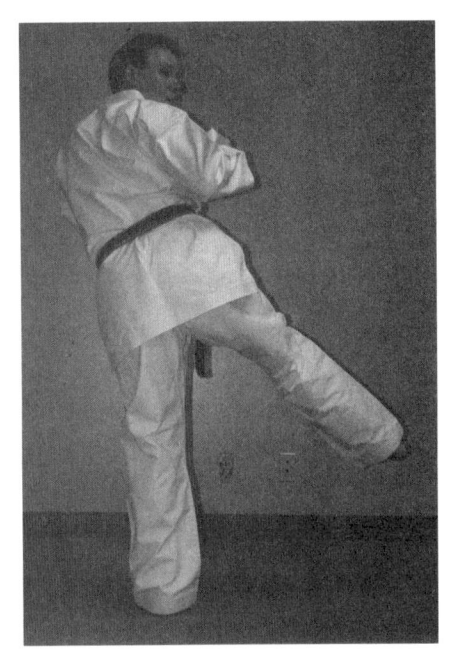

Begin Trajectory Front View   *Begin Trajectory Side View*

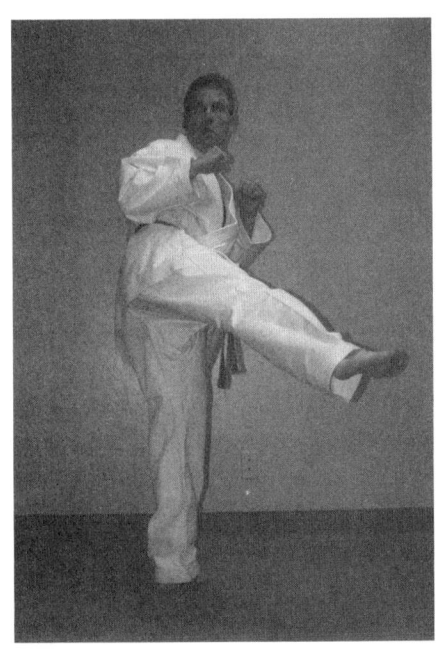

Peak of Trajectory:

17. Your base leg foot should now have moved approximately 45-degrees (clockwise) by pivoting on the ball of your foot. While your kicking leg, with the knee slightly bent, has now moved up to the correct height to strike your target.
18. The heel of the kicking foot should follow a straight line of trajectory from the "Peak of Trajectory" through the target (Impact), to the "Follow Through" position.
19. Your upper body should now be leaning to your left at almost a 75-degree angle in relation to your bodys upright position, and almost parallel with the ground.
20. Although your body is now in the above position, your head should still be looking over your kicking leg shoulder at your opponent.
21. Your back is no longer facing toward your opponent. It should now be facing at a 45-degree angle to your opponent's left in approximately the same direction that your kicking leg will be in, when it is in the "Follow Through" position.

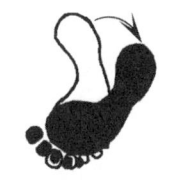

Peak of Trajectory Foot Position

Note: ...**(the ball of your kicking foot touching the ground), and ignites the gunpowder, which fires the bullet (execute your kick) along its path of trajectory, where it <u>STRIKES THROUGH</u> its target.**

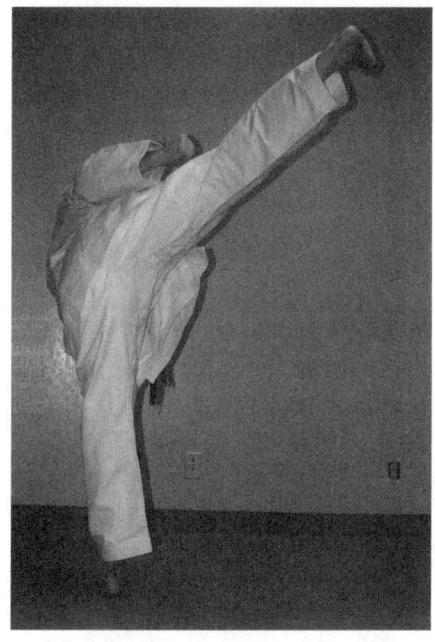

Peak of Trajectory Front View   *Peak of Trajectory Side View*

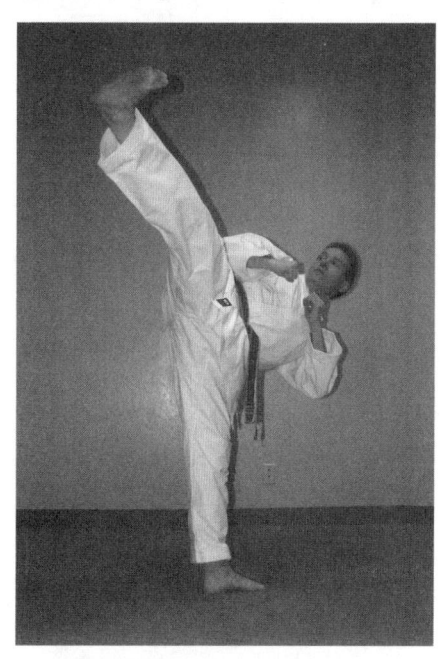

119

Impact:
22. Your base leg foot has now moved another 45-degrees (clockwise), by pivoting on the ball of the foot, with the arch of your foot now facing towards your opponent.
23. Your upper body should still be leaning to your left at almost a 75-degree angle in relation to your bodys upright position, and almost parallel with the ground. Although it has moved clockwise prior to the movement of your kicking leg and foot. At the moment of impact, your entire body should tighten to add power to the kick, as your foot continues to travel through the target.
24. Notice how your kicking foot, kicking leg (with knee slightly bent), hips, back, shoulders and head are all in a straight line at the initial moment of "Impact". Also, notice how the toes of the kicking foot are pulled back towards your body and pointed. This helps insure that contact with the target is made with the back of the heel.
25. Your head should still be up and looking over the kicking leg shoulder. Eye contact with your opponent is maintained at all times.

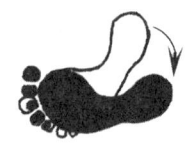

Impact Foot Position

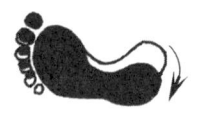

Impact (ADVANCED) Foot Position

Note: Utilize deception when fighting. Make sure your opponent believes that you are going to do one thing, when you really intend to do another.

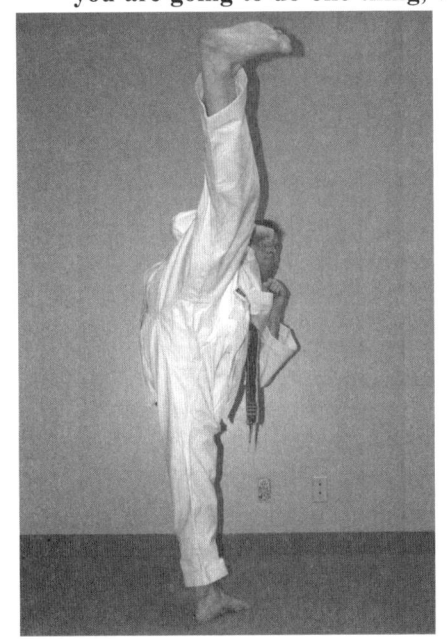

Impact Front View   *Impact Side View*

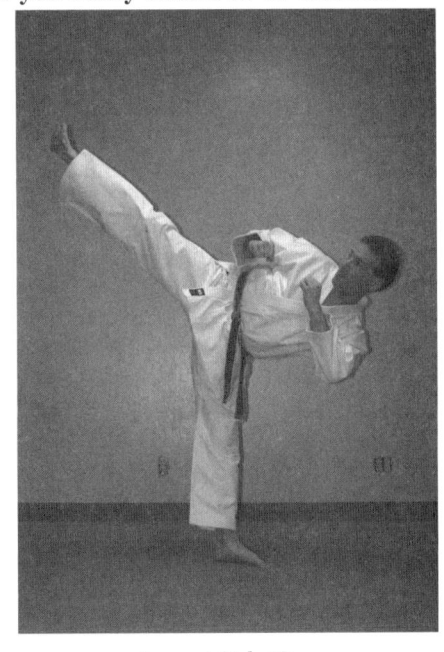

Follow Through:

26. Your base leg foot should have moved another 45-degrees (clockwise) by pivoting on the ball of the foot.
27. Your upper body should still be leaning to your left at almost a 75-degree angle in relation to your bodys upright position, and almost parallel with the ground. Although it has once again moved clockwise prior to the movement of your kicking leg and foot. Your back is straight and the front of your body is now at approximately a 45-degree angle to the front of your opponent.
28. Your kicking leg foot should continue along exactly the same path it followed from the "Peak of Trajectory" to "Impact." Your foot should be approximately 45-degrees past your target.
29. Your head should no longer be looking over your kicking leg shoulder. However, your eyes are still looking at your opponent.

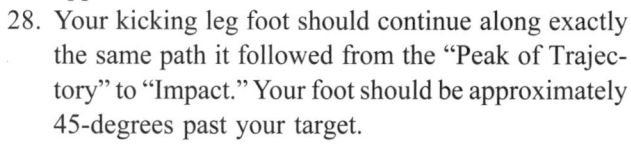

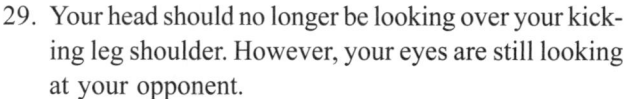

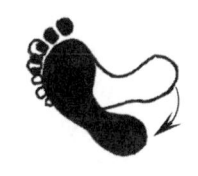

Follow Through Foot Position

Note: Not turning your upper body and lower body together in the same direction when executing a Wheel Kick, can also be likened to the act of "ringing out" a wet hand towel as previously described on page 114. However, the pressure is not on your knee in this case, but your lower back. Always adhere to proper form and technique when executing any kick, not just the Wheel Kick.

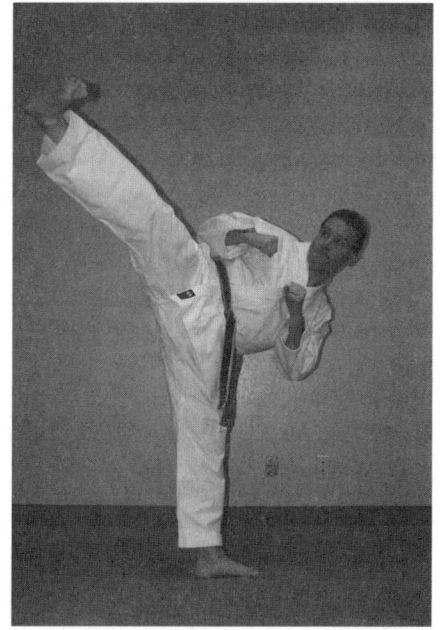

Follow Through Front View   *Follow Through Side View*

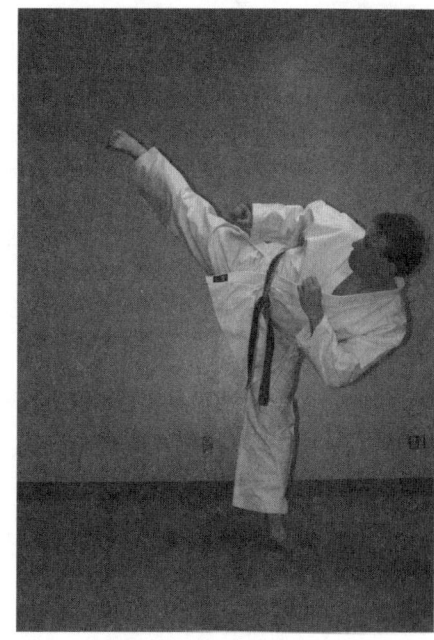

End of Trajectory:
30. Your base leg foot should have moved another 45-degrees (clockwise) by pivoting on the ball of the foot. The toes of your base leg foot should now be pointing directly at your opponent.
31. Your kicking leg remains straight with the knee slightly bent. Your kicking foot is now slightly in front of you and to your right at approximately the height of your base leg knee.
32. Your upper body will straighten up from the approximately 75-degree bent over position you were in when kicking. Your back remains straight and your upper body is now facing directly toward your opponent.
33. Your head should still be up and looking directly over the center of your chest. Your eyes are still in contact with your opponent, whether he is still standing, or lying on the ground..

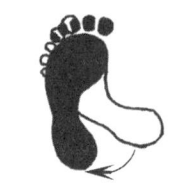

End of Trajectory Foot Position

Note: In the illustration on the right, the bullet, which represents your kicking foot, has begun its initial expansion as it penetrated through the target area and into the target.

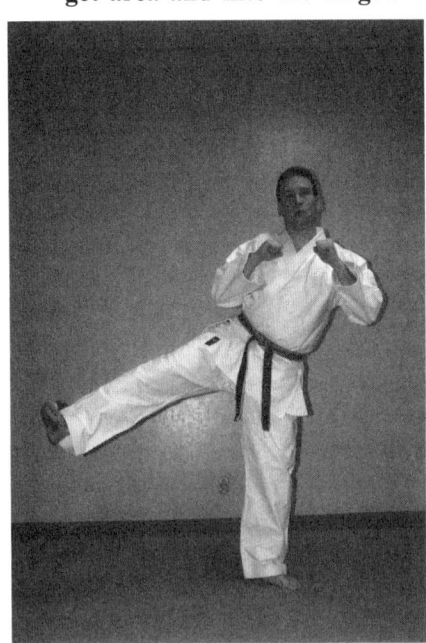

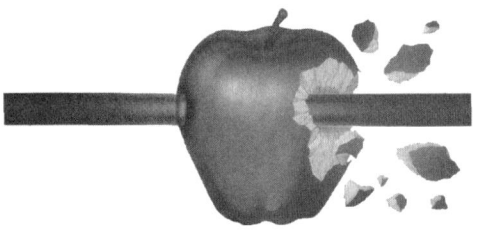

End of Trajectory Front View   *End of Trajectory Side View*

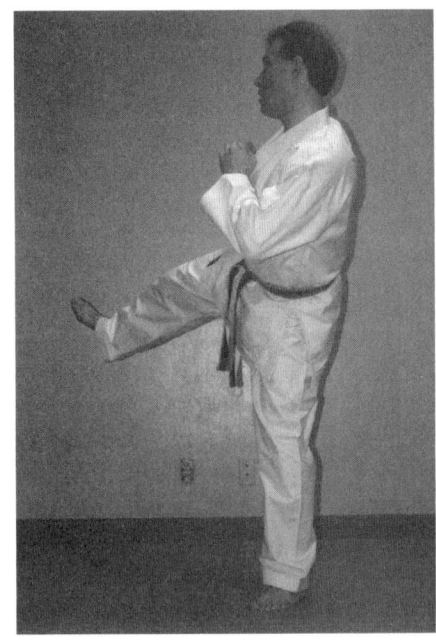

122

Return to Fighting Position:

34. Your entire body from your head to your toes, should be in exactly the same fighting position that you would be in if you were going to execute a Turning Wheel Kick with your right leg. Although, you won't be in exactly the same location.
35. Your kicking leg foot continues the 360-degree motion and returns to its original starting position. Although your kicking leg knee will remain slightly bent as it returns to the starting position.
36. Your hands, which should have remained as close to this position as possible throughout the entire kick, are held up (like a boxer's), with the elbows tucked in to protect the ribs and your hands up to protect your head.
37. Your head should now be looking over your lead leg shoulder with your eyes in contact with your opponent.

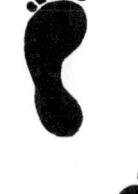

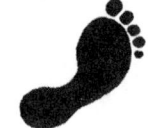

Return to Fighting Position Foot Position

Note: The bullet continues to expand as it travels through the target and out the opposite side, continuing along its initial "Path of Trajectory" with no visible signs of losing speed. This illustration represents the correct way of utilizing all of the proper principles involved in order to maximize the effectiveness of your kicks.

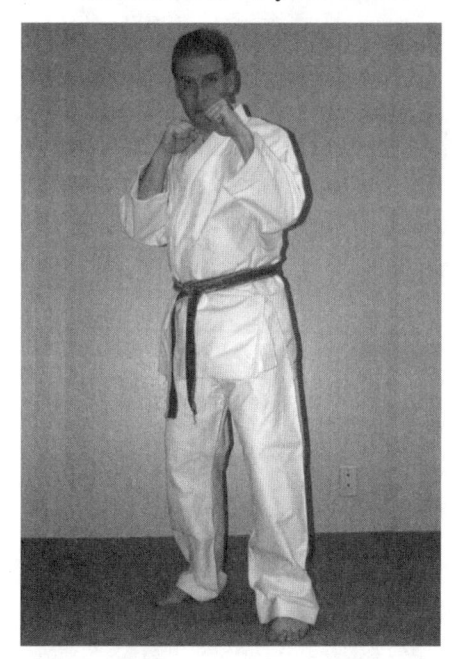

Return to Fighting Position Front View   *Return to Fighting Position Side View*

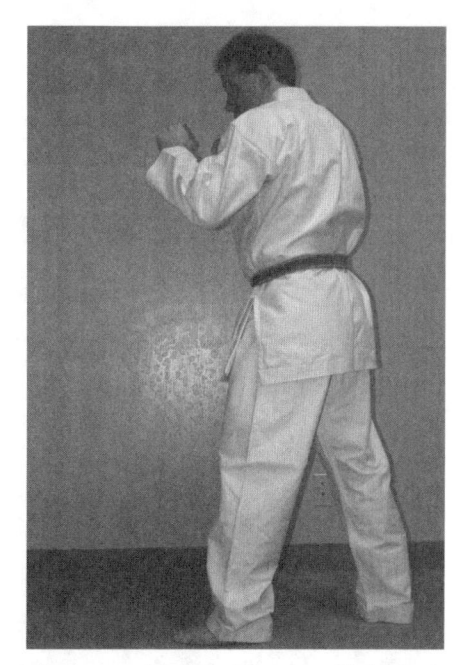

123

Pictorial Overview:

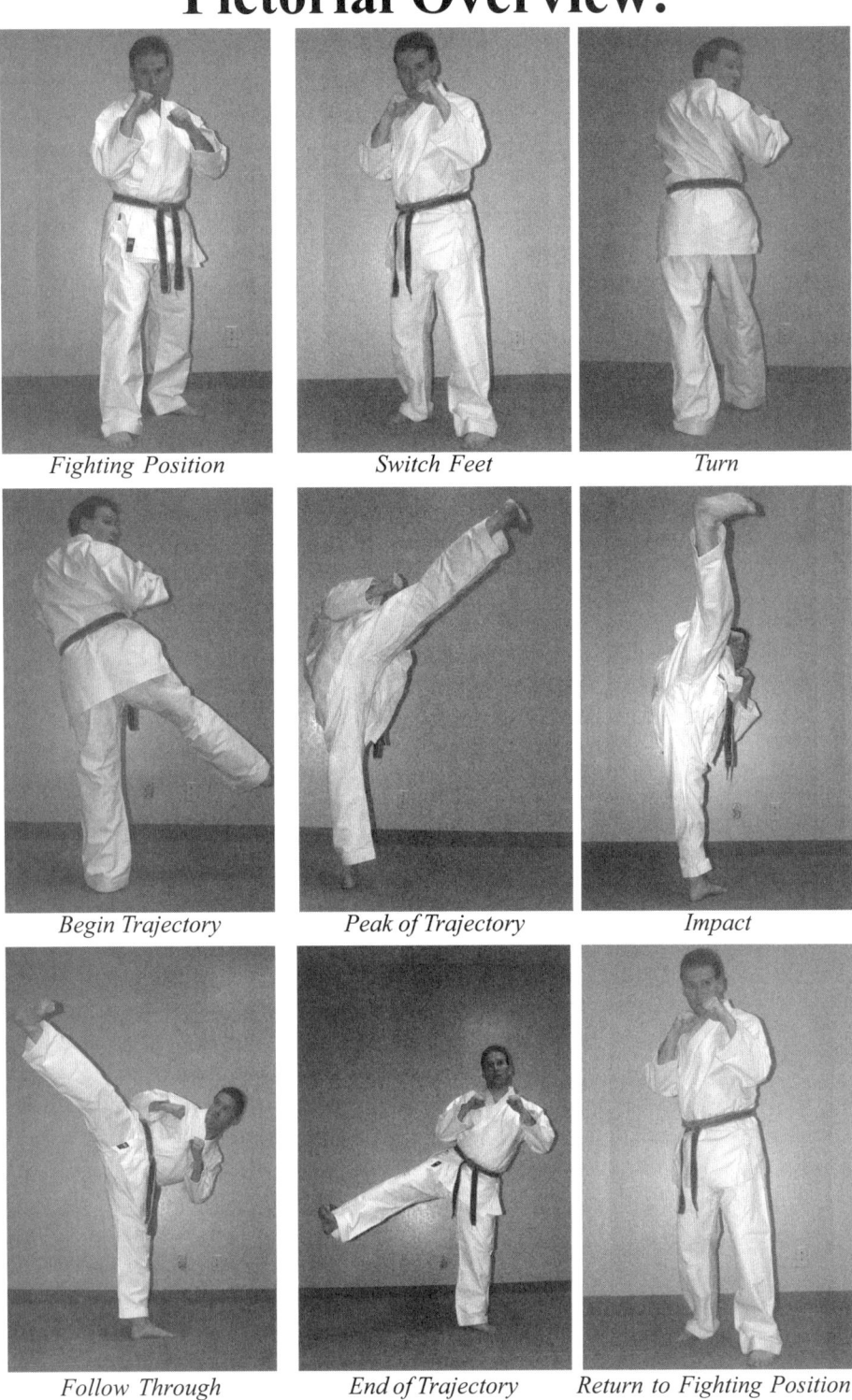

Fighting Position   *Switch Feet*   *Turn*

Begin Trajectory   *Peak of Trajectory*   *Impact*

Follow Through   *End of Trajectory*   *Return to Fighting Position*

Off-Setting Wheel Kick

The Off-Setting Wheel Kick is identical in execution to the Turning Wheel Kick, with one notable exception. A quick double step motion to the side (which puts you at a 45-degree angle from your original starting position), which is performed immediately prior to executing the kick. The starting position is the same as Turning Wheel Kick, in that your kicking foot is in the rear position. The actual double-step motion of the feet prior to the execution of the kick is performed by first moving the rearward foot and then the forward foot off at a 45-degree angle to the side of your opponent. When executing the double-step motion, be sure and move your rearward foot first, then your forward foot, without initially moving your hips and upper body in order to avoid telegraphing the move to your opponent. Your hips and upper body will begin to move when you begin to place the forward foot back onto the ground.

Fighting Position:
1. Your fighting position for this kick is the exact same as Turning Wheel Kick, in that your kicking leg will be in the rearward position.
2. This stance is approximately shoulder width apart with the heel of your rear foot directly in line with the heel of your front foot
3. Your front or lead foot should be pointed directly at your opponent.
4. Your rear foot is angled toward the right at approximately a 45-degree angle. Your weight should be distributed evenly over the balls of both feet.
5. Your knees are slightly, but not noticeably bent. They should not be locked straight or rigid.

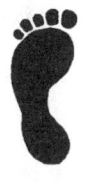

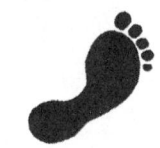

Fighting Position Foot Position

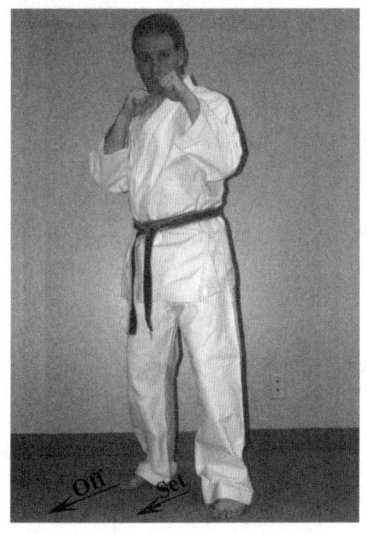

Fighting Position Front View

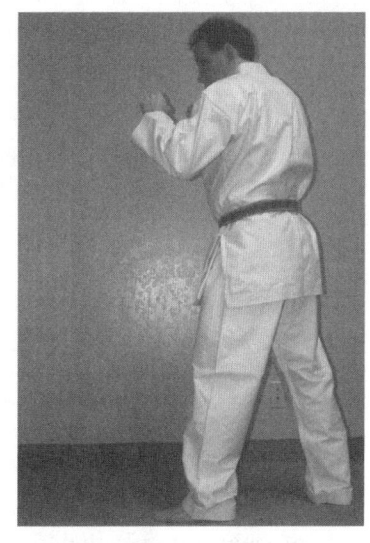

Fighting Position Side View

125

6. Your body should be facing at a 45-degree angle towards your opponent. This presents a smaller target area and also facilitates a faster turn when utilizing this kick.
7. Your hands should be held up (like a boxer's), with the elbows tucked in to protect the ribs and your hands up to protect your head. Your hands should remain as close to this position as possible throughout the entire kick.
8. Your head should be facing your opponent with your chin tucked down and protected by your lead shoulder.
9. Your eyes should be centered on your opponent's chest.

Off-Set (part one):

10. Move your rear foot to the right (approximately 2-3 feet), and slightly forward (approximately 8 to 10 inches).

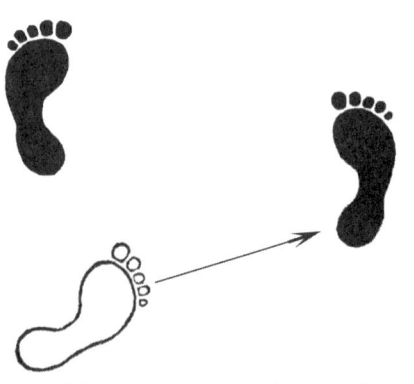

Off-Set Foot Position (part one)

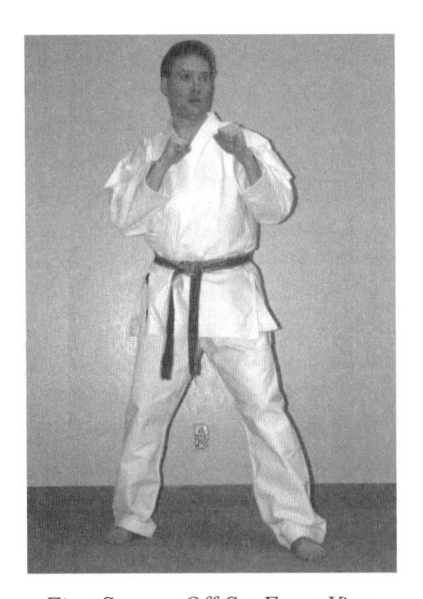

First Step on Off-Set Front View

First Step on Off-Set Side View

Off-Set (part two) & Turn:

11. Move your front foot to the right approximately 12 to 18 inches. While moving your front foot, pivot on the ball of your rear foot. This will turn your back towards your opponent. As you set your front foot down, the heel of your front foot should now be fac-

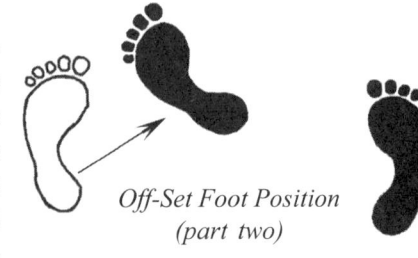

Off-Set Foot Position (part two)

ing towards your opponent. However, when first learning this kick, make the off-setting and the turn two separate moves.

12. Your body should now be at a 45-degree angle from its original starting position, and you should be ready to execute a Turning Wheel Kick.

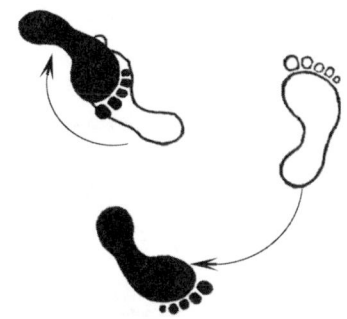

Turning Foot Position

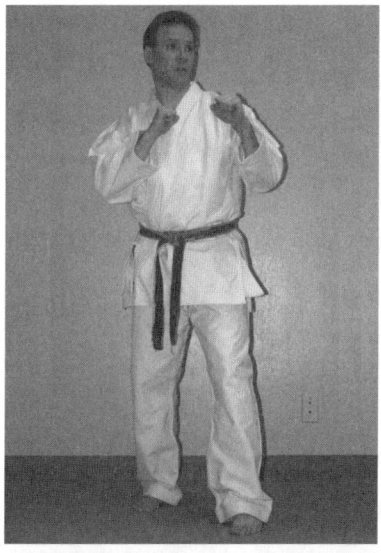

Second Step on Off-Set Front View

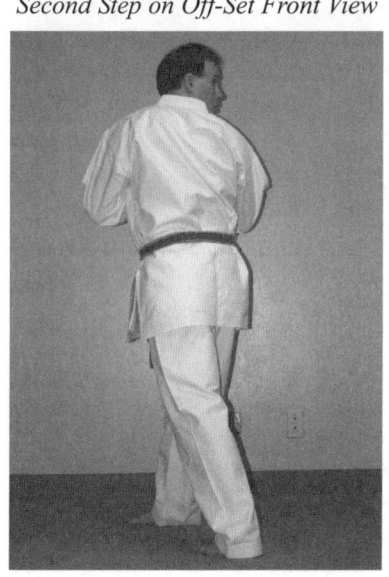

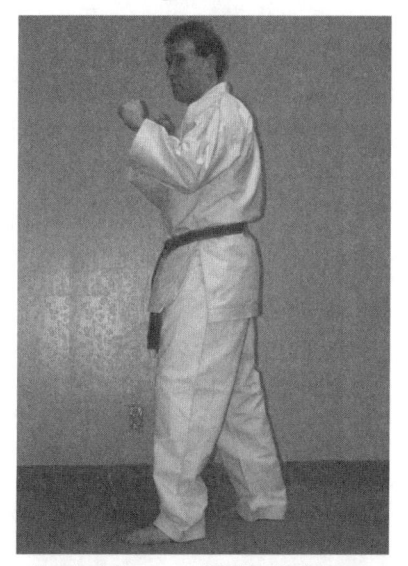

Second Step on Off-Set Side View

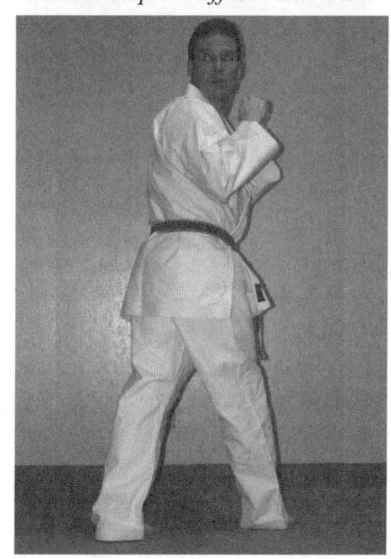

Turning Front View

Turning Side View

127

Begin Trajectory:

13. Using the toes of your kicking foot, push off the floor and bring your kicking leg at a 45-degree angle between the direction your body is facing and your right hand side. Your leg should be straight, with a slight bend in the knee. In this position, your kicking foot should already be in the correct position to strike your opponent.
14. As you bring your kicking leg up, your upper body should start bending over slightly, from the waist, to the left. Your back will remain straight.
15. Your head is still up and turned over your kicking shoulder, your eyes should always remain in contact with your opponent throughout the entire kick.
16. Your back should no longer be facing directly towards your opponent, but should start turning, along with your shoulders, in the direction of the kick.

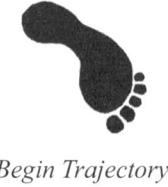

Begin Trajectory Foot Position

Note: In order to generate the maximum amount of power possible when executing the Wheel Kick, you must adhere to the correct execution of movement throughout the entire kicking sequence. Just as is boxing, power must first be generated by the movement of the feet, legs, hips, body, and shoulders prior to <u>STRIKING THROUGH</u> your target.

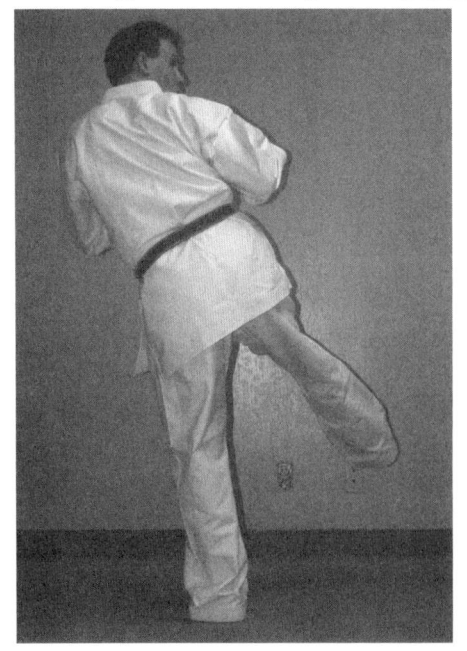

Begin Trajectory Position Front View   *Begin Trajectory Position Side View*

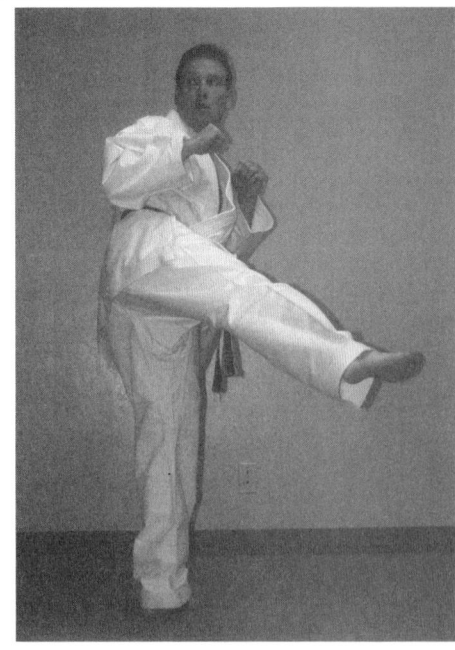

Peak of Trajectory:

17. Your base leg foot should now have moved approximately 45-degrees (clockwise) by pivoting on the ball of your foot. While your kicking leg, with the knee slightly bent, has now moved up to the correct height to strike your target.
18. The heel of the kicking foot should follow a straight line of trajectory from the "Peak of Trajectory" through the target (Impact), to the "Follow Through" position.
19. Your upper body should now be leaning to your left at almost a 75-degree angle in relation to your bodys upright position, and almost parallel with the ground.
20. Although your body is now in the above position, your head should still be looking over your kicking leg shoulder at your opponent.
21. Your back is no longer facing toward your opponent. It should now be facing at a 45-degree angle to your opponent's left in approximately the same direction that your kicking leg will be in, when it is in the "Follow Through" position.

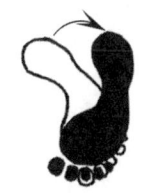

Peak of Trajectory Foot Position

Note: The "Off-Setting" movement is one of the primary techniques utilized in the "8 Direction of Attack" strategy. This is a very important strategic technique and one that can be utilized in any martial art.

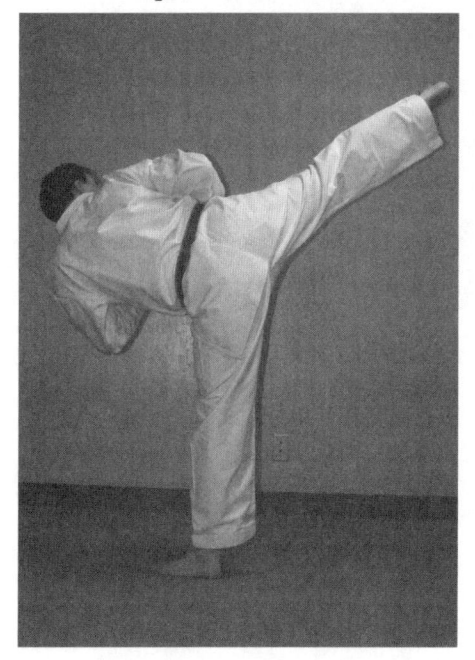

Peak of Trajectory Front View *Peak of Trajectory Side View*

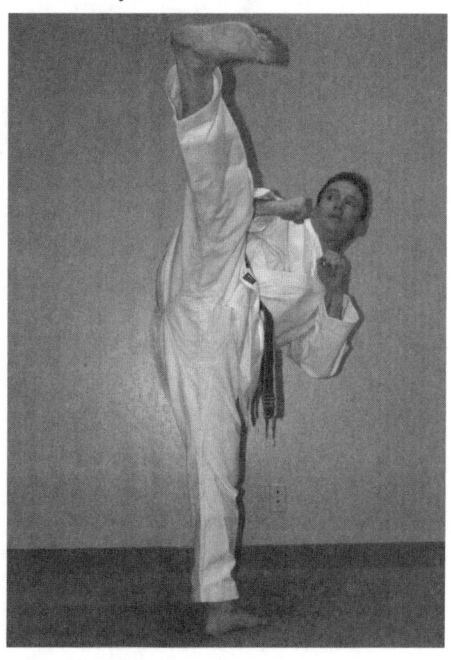

Impact:

22. Your base leg foot has now moved another 45-degrees (clockwise), by pivoting on the ball of the foot, with the arch of your foot now facing towards your opponent.
23. Your upper body should still be leaning to your left at almost a 75-degree angle in relation to your bodys upright position, and almost parallel with the ground. Although it has moved clockwise prior to the movement of your kicking leg and foot. At the moment of impact, your entire body should tighten to add power to the kick, as your foot continues to travel through the target.
24. Notice how your kicking foot, kicking leg (with knee slightly bent), hips, back, shoulders and head are all in a straight line at the initial moment of "Impact". Also, notice how the toes of the kicking foot are pulled back towards your body and pointed. This helps insure that contact with the target is made with the back of the heel.
25. Your head should still be up and looking over the kicking leg shoulder. Eye contact with your opponent is maintained at all times.

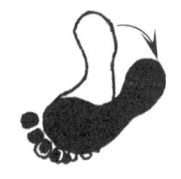

Impact Foot Position

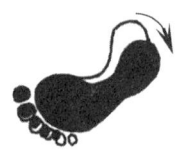

Impact (ADVANCED) Foot Position

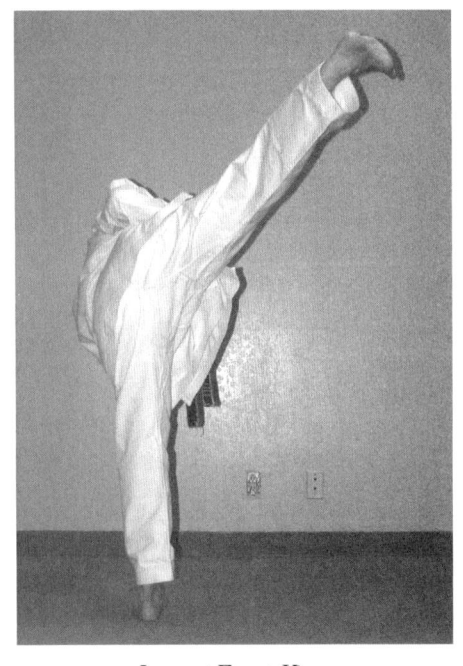

Impact Front View

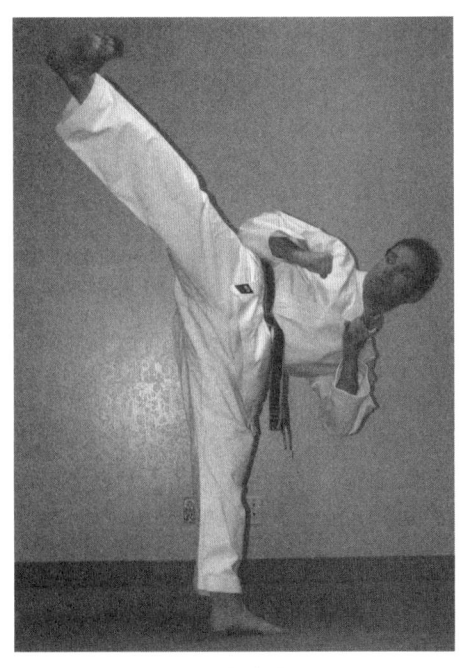

Impact Side View

Follow Through:

26. Your base leg foot should have moved another 45-degrees (clockwise) by pivoting on the ball of the foot.
27. Your upper body should still be leaning to your left at almost a 75-degree angle in relation to your bodys upright position, and almost parallel with the ground. Although it has once again moved clockwise prior to the movement of your kicking leg and foot. Your back is straight and the front of your body is now at approximately a 45-degree angle to the front of your opponent.
28. Your kicking leg foot should continue along exactly the same path it followed from the "Peak of Trajectory" to "Impact." Your foot should be approximately 45-degrees past your target.
29. Your head should no longer be looking over your kicking leg shoulder. However, your eyes are still looking at your opponent.

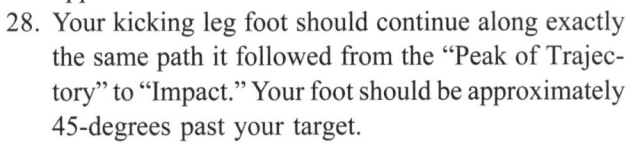

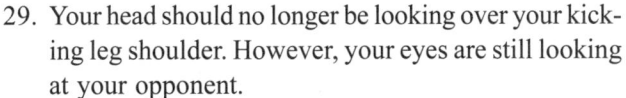

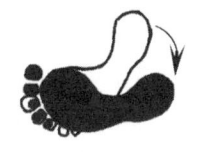

Follow Through Foot Position

Note: **The ability to effectively and efficiently utilize high section kicks depends primarily on the following four factors. A: Your expertise in kicking. B: Your overall flexibility and physical condition. C: Your environment at the time. D: Your opponent.**

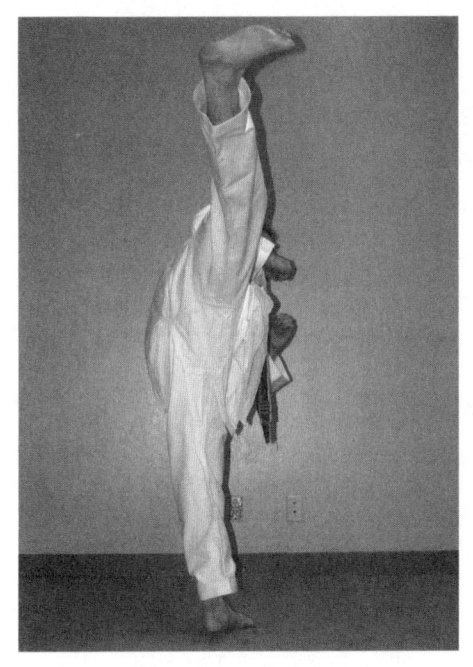

Follow Through Front View   *Follow Through Side View*

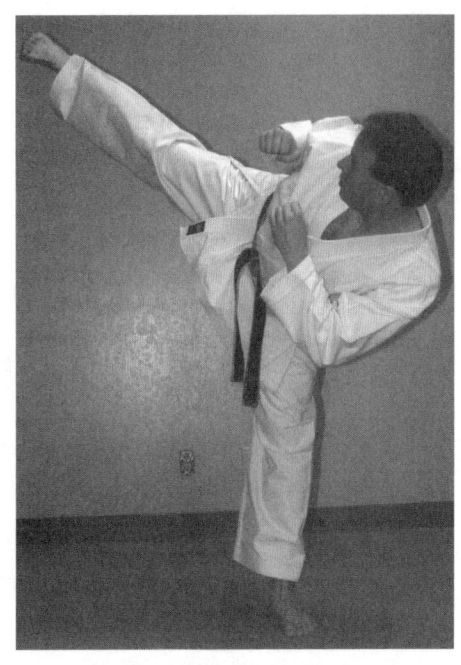

End of Trajectory:

30. Your base leg foot should have moved another 45-degrees (clockwise) by pivoting on the ball of the foot. The toes of your base leg foot should now be pointing directly at your opponent.
31. Your kicking leg remains straight with the knee slightly bent. Your kicking foot is now slightly in front of you and to your right at approximately the height of your base leg knee.
32. Your upper body will straighten up from the approximately 75-degree bent over position you were in when kicking. Your back remains straight and your upper body is now facing directly toward your opponent.
33. Your head should still be up and looking directly over the center of your chest. Your eyes are still in contact with your opponent, whether he is still standing, or lying on the ground.

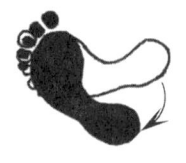

End of Trajectory Foot Position

Note: If you leave your kicking foot hanging in the air after "STRIKING THROUGH" your target, you have not only executed the kick improperly, but you have also left yourself in a very vulnerable position. One that your opponent may very easily exploit to his advantage. As I have stated before, in order to maximize the effectiveness of your kicks, you must, correctly, apply <u>all of the proper principles outlined in this book</u>.

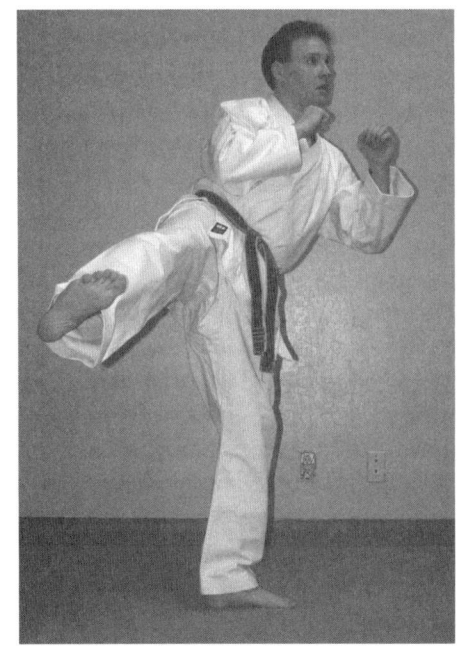

End of Trajectory Front View   *End of Trajectory Side View*

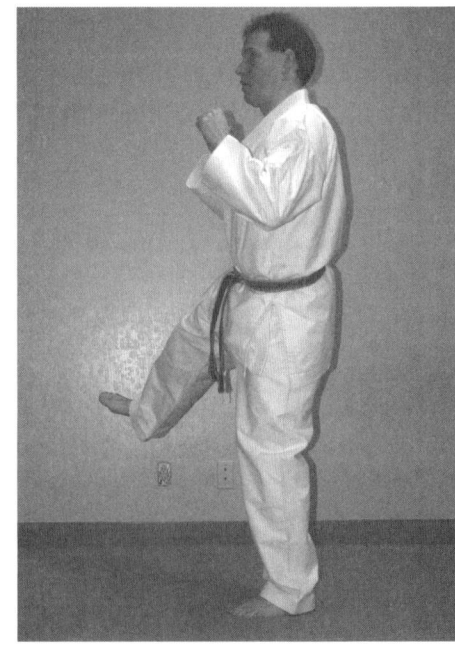

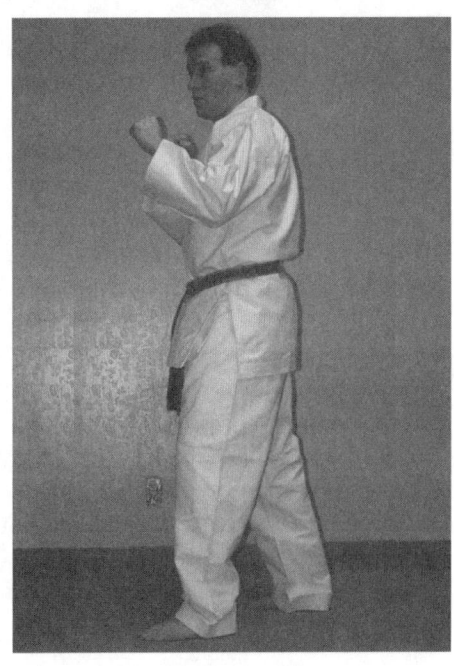

Return to Fighting Position:
34. Your entire body from your head to your toes, should be in exactly the same position that you initially started in (refer to the Fighting Position section of this kick), prior to executing this kick. Although, you won't be in exactly the same location.
35. Your kicking leg foot continues the 360-degree motion and returns to its original starting position. Although your kicking leg knee will remain slightly bent as it returns to the starting position.
36. Your hands, which should have remained as close to this position as possible throughout the entire kick, are once again in the same position they were in prior to executing the kick.
37. Your head should now be looking over your lead leg shoulder with your eyes in contact with your opponent.

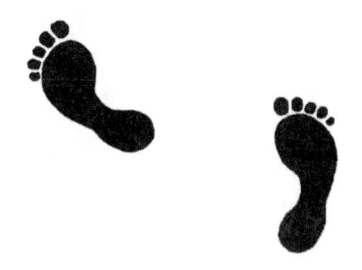

Return to Fighting Position Foot Position

Note: You should now be in the exact same position that you were in after executing the off-setting movement.
Note: When properly applied, the footwork motion of off-setting prior to kicking can greatly increase the power generated in a Wheel Kick.

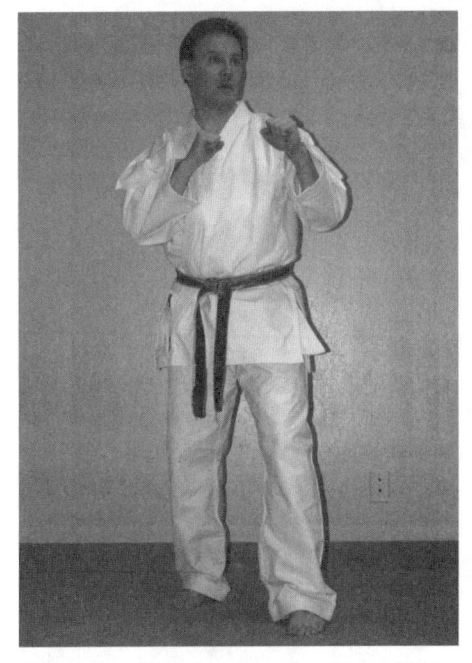

Return to Fighting Position Front View *Return to Fighting Position Side View*

133

Pictorial Overview:

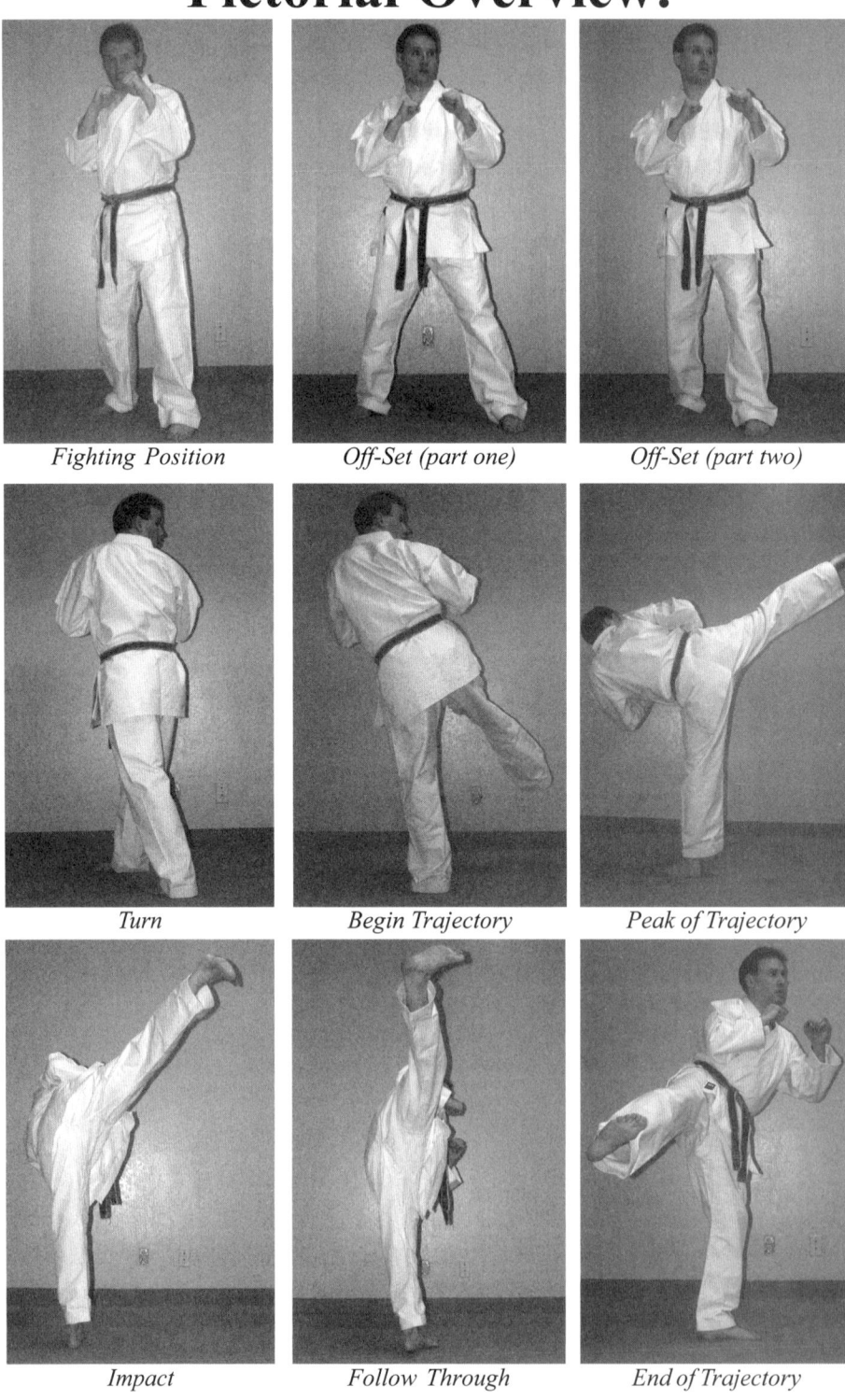

Fighting Position

Off-Set (part one)

Off-Set (part two)

Turn

Begin Trajectory

Peak of Trajectory

Impact

Follow Through

End of Trajectory

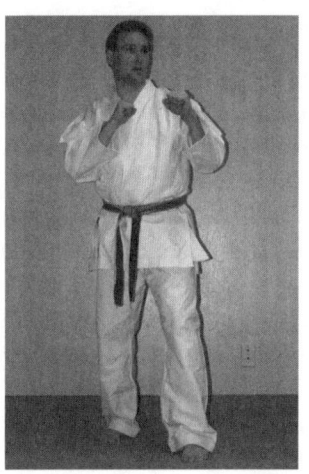

Return to Fighting Position

Note: If you look closely at the photograph of the pocketwatch below, you will see a cutout view of the face of the watch, which exposes a number of gears in various sizes and positions that you normally would not see. These gears are representative of all of the various aspects of a Wheel Kick, which like each individual component of a Wheel Kick, are of a very high quality and that, like a finely crafted pocketwatch, are skillfully combined with one another to create an exquisitely efficient product.

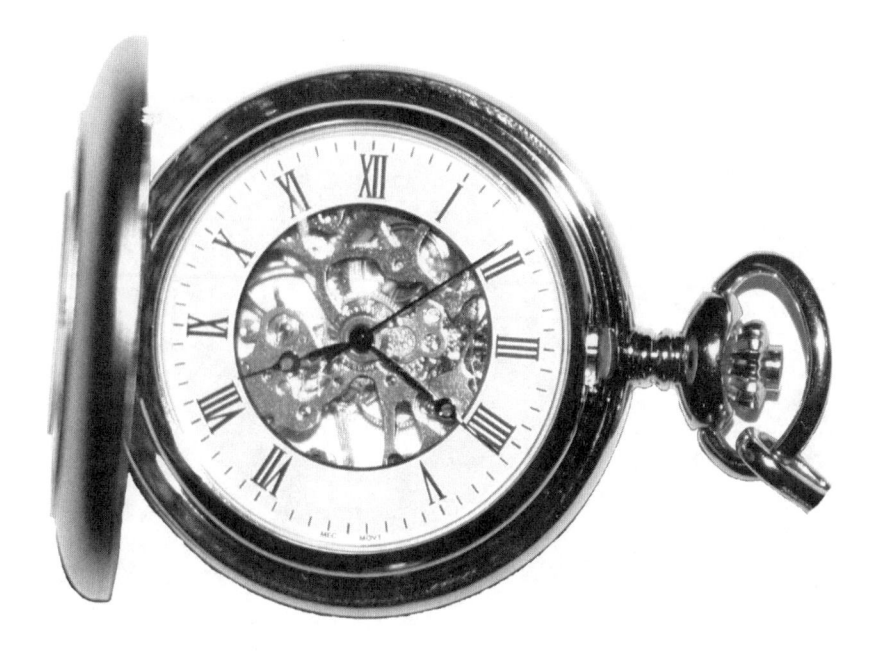

Jump Turning Wheel Kick

The Jump Turning Wheel Kick is identical in execution to the Turning Wheel Kick, with one notable exception. That being a jumping motion that is performed immediately prior to executing the kick. This motion can be used to gain height in your kick, and it can also be used to gain distance either towards or away from your opponent. It can also increase the power in the kick due to the added momentum of jumping and kicking. The actual jump turning motion is executed by bending your knees slightly and leaping either straight up, forward, or even backward, depending on the situation and your opponent, in order to execute the kick. The jump itself should be practiced independently of the kick until you can execute the jump without telegraphing the kick by utilizing any unnecessary movements, such as hunching of the back and shoulders, bending of the knees too deeply, or winding up of the upper body.

Fighting Position:
1. This stance is approximately shoulder width apart with the heel of your rear foot in a direct line with the heel of your front foot.
2. Your front or lead foot should be pointed directly at your opponent.
3. Your rear foot is angled towards the right at approximately a 45-degree angle. Your weight should be distributed evenly over the balls of both feet.
4. Your knees are slightly, but not noticeably bent. They should not be locked straight or rigid.

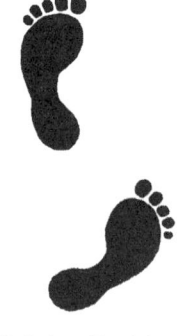

Fighting Position Foot Position

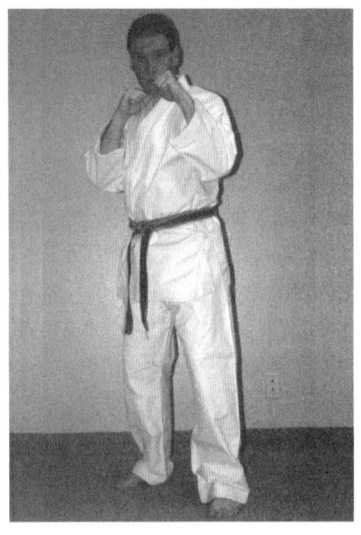

Fighting Position Front View

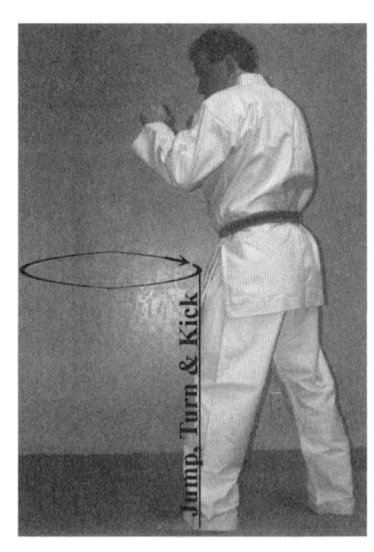

Fighting Position Side View

5. Your body should be facing at a 45-degree angle toward your opponent. This presents a smaller target area and also facilitates a faster jump-turn when utilizing this kick.
6. Your hands should be held up (like a boxer's), with the elbows tucked in to protect the ribs and your hands up to protect your head. Your hands should remain as close to this position as possible throughout the entire kick.
7. Your head should be facing your opponent with your chin tucked down and protected by your lead shoulder.
8. Your eyes should be centered on your opponent's chest

Jump, Turn & Begin Trajectory:

9. Moving both feet simultaneously, jump straight up and begin turning your body in a clockwise motion. While you are in the air, the following things should be done simultaneously. They are as follows:
9a. Turn your head and look over your kicking shoulder. Eye contact with your opponent is maintained at all times.
9b. Bring your kicking leg up to the begin trajectory position.
9c. Keep your hands up throughout the entire kick.
9d. Your body, which should lean slightly to the left, should make a complete 360-degree turn while in the air. Execute the kick.

Note: If you execute the entire kick correctly, from the initial jump, to the "Follow Through" position, your kicking foot should start returning to the ground before your non-kicking foot touches the ground.

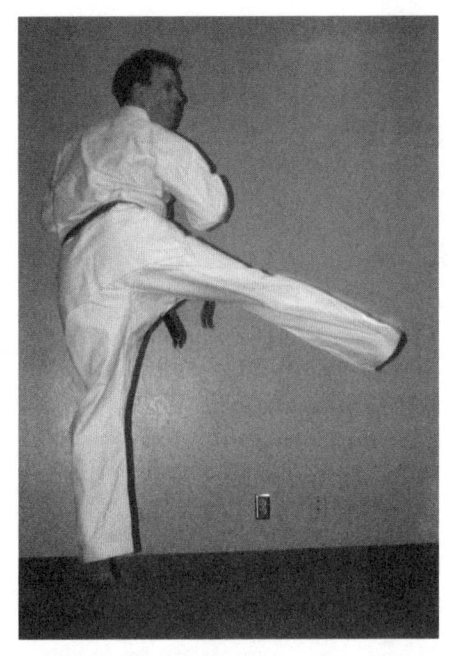

Jump, Turn & Begin Trajectory Front   *Jump, Turn & Begin Trajectory Side*

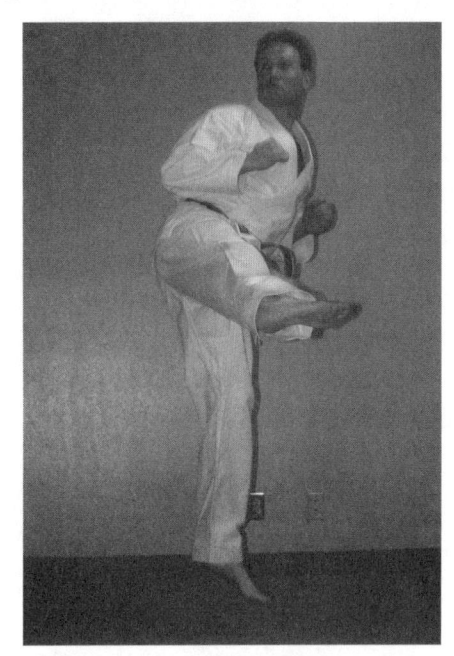

Peak of Trajectory:

10. Your kicking leg, with the knee slightly bent, has now moved up to the correct height to strike your target.
11. Even though you are in the air, the heel of your kicking foot should follow a straight line of trajectory from the "Peak of Trajectory" through the target (Impact), to the "Follow Through" position.
12. Your upper body should be leaning slightly to your left, although nowhere near the almost 75-degree angle you would be in if you were executing a ground based Wheel Kick.
13. Although your body is now in the above position. Your head should still be looking over your kicking leg shoulder. Eye contact with your target is maintained at all times.
14. Your back is currently facing in the same direction that your kicking leg will be in, when it is in the "Follow Through" position.

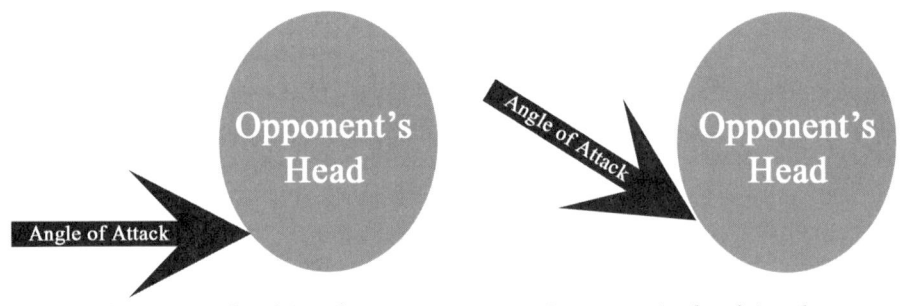

*Correct Angle of Attack
Top & Front View*

*Incorrect Angle of Attack
Top & Front View*

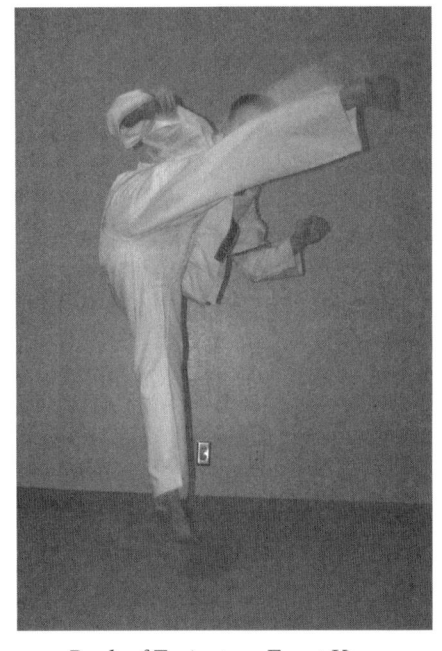

Peak of Trajectory Front View

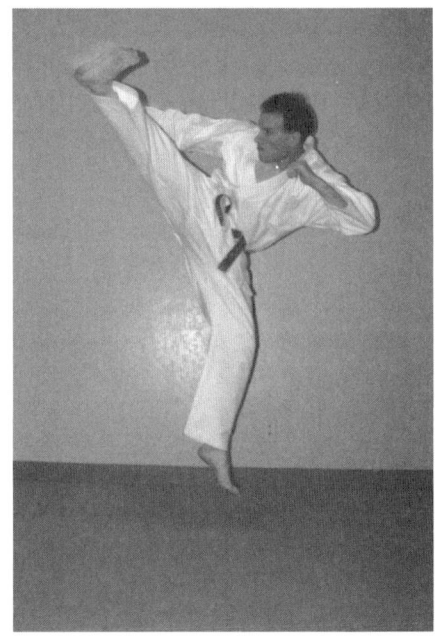

Peak of Trajectory Side View

Impact:
15. At the moment of impact, your entire body should tighten to add power to the kick. Notice how the toes of the kicking foot are pulled back towards your body and pointed. This helps insure that contact with the target is made with the back of the heel.
16. Your upper body should still be leaning slightly to your left.
17. Notice how your body is now sideways to your opponent. However, it is at a slight angle due to the actions of the kicking leg and the continuous 360-degree turning motion of the entire body.
18. Your head should still be up and looking over your kicking leg shoulder. Eye contact with your target is maintained at all times.

Note: As you can see in the illustrations presented on the previous page, the optimum angle for impact in relation to your opponent's head is a 90-degree angle. Therefore, the further away you are from a 90-degree angle, the less effective your kick is going to be. For example, as you look at the illustrations on the previous page, imagine that you have not only an overhead view, but also a front view of your opponent's head. The black arrows are Wheel Kicks delivered to your opponent's jaw. Which one is going to be more effective, the one on the left? Or the one on the right?

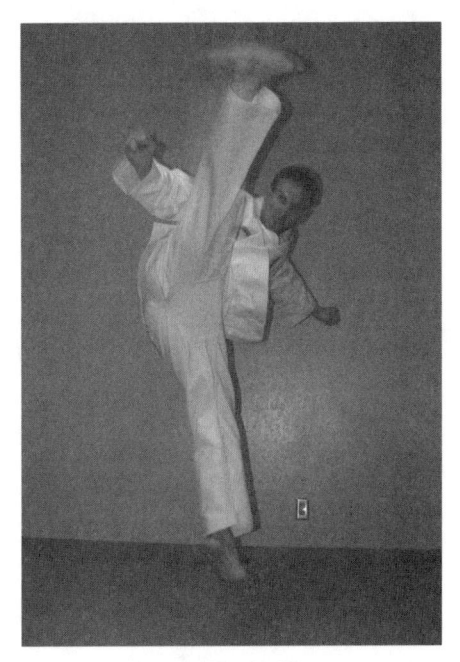

Impact Front View   *Impact Side View*

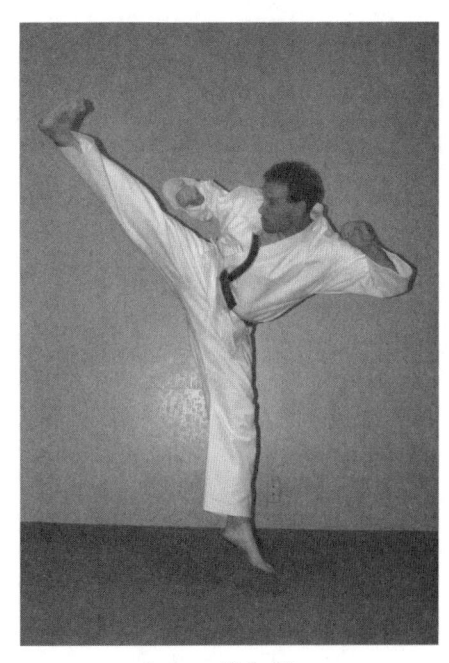

139

Follow Through:
19. Your kicking foot should continue along exactly the same path it followed from the "Peak of Trajectory" to "Impact". Your foot should be approximately 45-degrees past your target.
20. Your upper body should still be leaning slightly to the left, although you will start to straighten your body at this point. The front of your body is now at approximately a 45-degree angle to the front of your opponent.
21. Your hands, which should have remained as close to the original starting position as possible, should still be up to protect your head and body. Did you notice my hand position in the "Side View" photograph? This is very incorrect!
22. Your head should no longer be looking over your kicking leg shoulder. However, your eyes are still looking at your opponent.

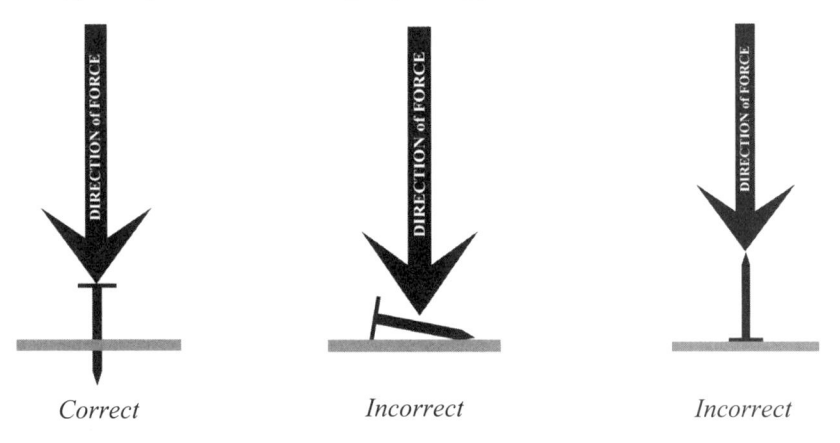

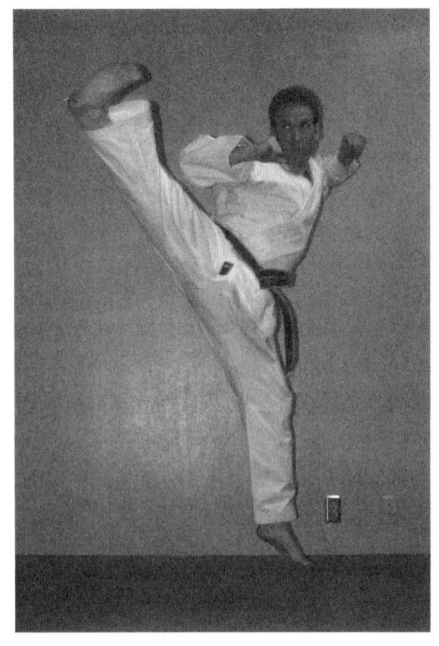

Correct *Incorrect* *Incorrect*

Follow Through Front View *Follow Through Side View*

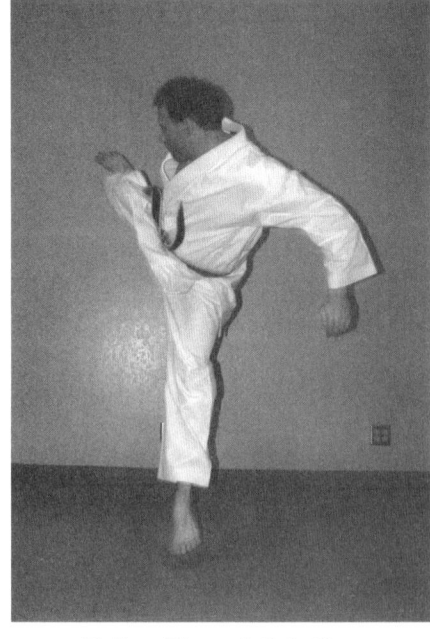

End of Trajectory:
23. Your base leg foot should have just touched down on the ground, and the toes of your base leg foot should now be pointing directly at your opponent.
24. Your kicking leg remains straight with the knee slightly bent. Your kicking foot is now slightly in front of you and to your right at approximately the height of your base leg knee.
25. Your upper body will straighten up from the slightly bent over position you were in when kicking. Your back remains straight and your upper body is now facing directly toward your opponent.
26. Your head should still be up and looking directly over the center of your chest. Your eyes are still in contact with your opponent, whether he is still standing, or lying on the ground..

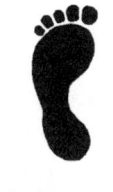

End of Trajectory Foot Position

Note: As I explained to you on page 26, and have illustrated for you on the previous page, if you apply the correct surface area to the correct target, it is like driving a nail into a board. If however, you strike the target incorrectly without applying all of the proper principles and correct techniques, your effectiveness will be greatly reduced and you may cause more damage to yourself rather than your opponent.

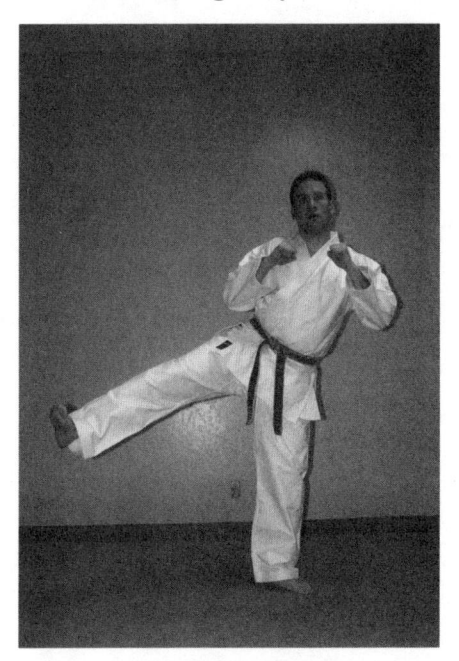

End of Trajectory Front View   *End of Trajectory Side View*

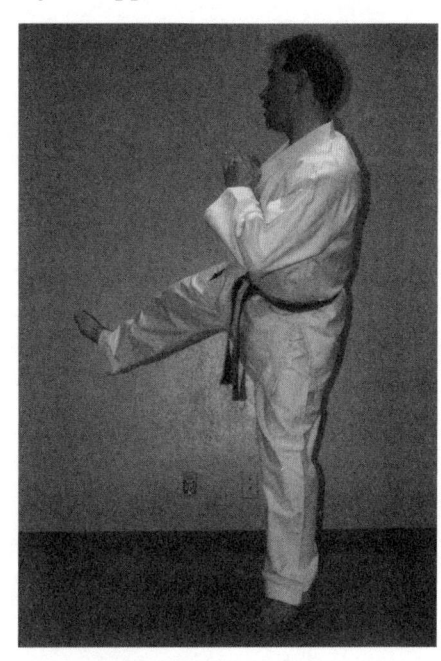

Return to Fighting Position:
27. Your entire body from your head to your toes, should be in exactly the same position that you initially started in (refer to the Fighting Position section of this kick), prior to executing this kick.
28. Your kicking leg foot continues the 360-degree motion and returns to its original starting position. Although your kicking leg knee will remain slightly bent as it returns to the starting position.
29. Your hands, which should have remained as close to this position as possible throughout the entire kick, are once again in the same position they were in prior to executing the kick.
30. Your head should now be looking over your lead leg shoulder with your eyes in contact with your opponent.

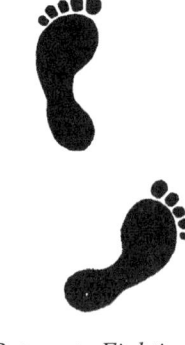

Return to Fighting Position Foot Position

Note: The overhead view of the path of trajectory of your kicking foot throughout the entire execution of this kick, is identical to the primary kick Turning Wheel Kick. Even though you are jumping up in the air, it will still look like the face of a clock or, as pictured on the right, a wagon wheel.

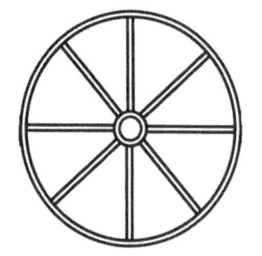

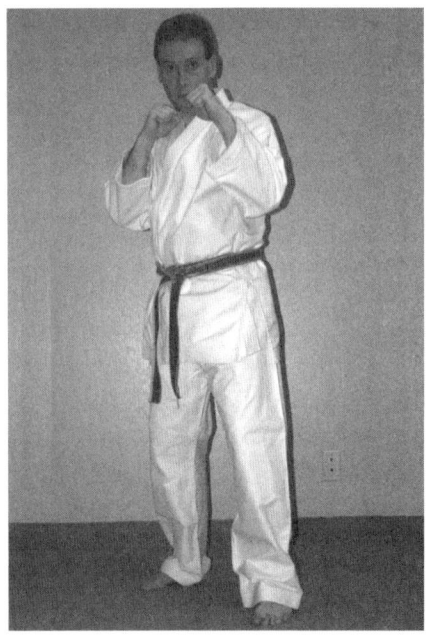

Return to Fighting Position Front View   *Return to Fighting Position Side View*

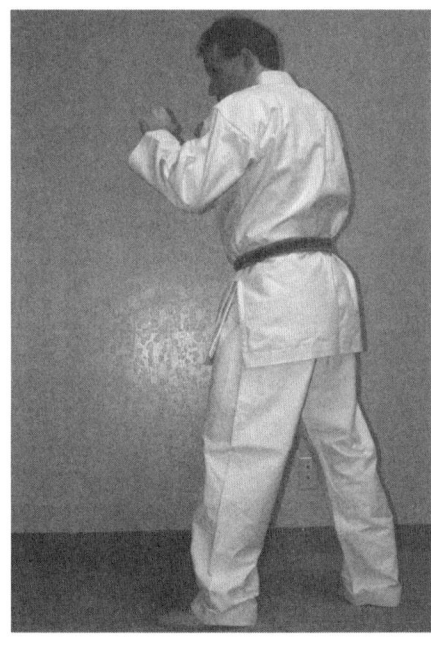

142

Pictorial Overview:

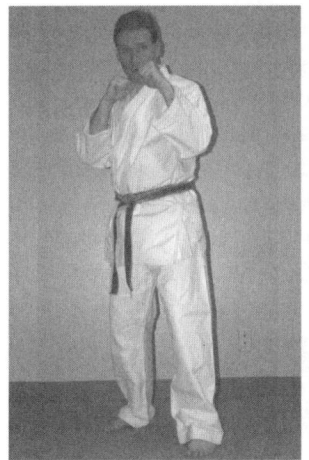

Fighting Position

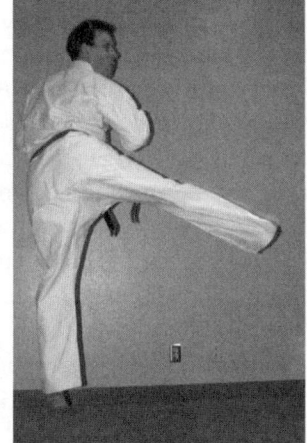

Jump, Turn & Begin...

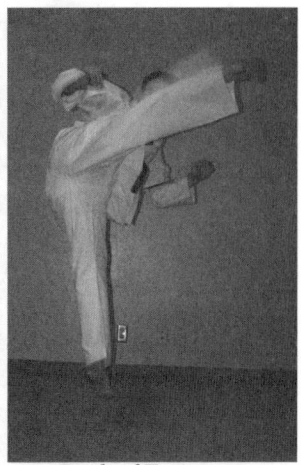

Peak of Trajectory

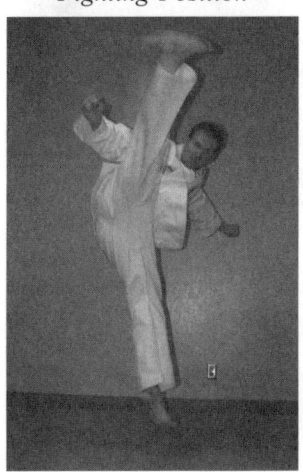

Impact

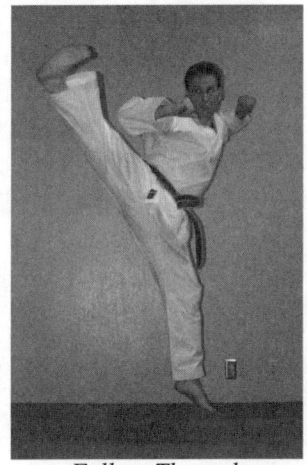

Follow Through

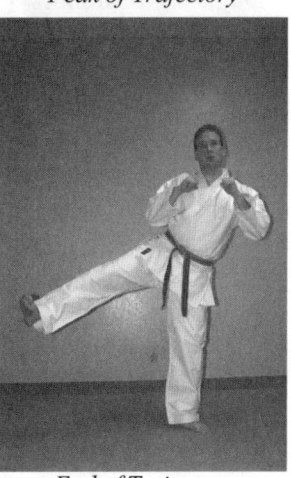

End of Trajectory

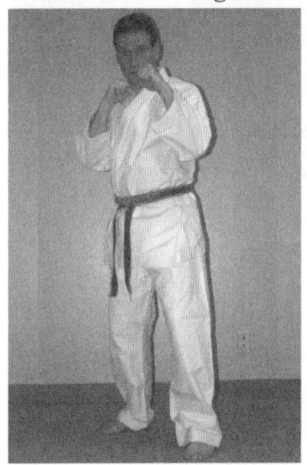

Return to Fighting Position

143

540-Degree Jump Turning Wheel Kick

The 540-Degree Jump Turning Wheel Kick is identical in execution to the Spinning Wheel Kick, with one notable exception. That being a stepping forward-jumping motion that is performed immediately prior to executing the kick. This motion is used to close the distance with an opponent; it can also increase the power in the kick due to the added momentum of the stepping forward and jumping. The actual step forward, jumping motion is executed by bringing your rearward leg knee up and around the front of your body and keeping it in the air, while pivoting to the side on the ball of your base foot. As you are doing this, jump up into the air off of your base leg and execute the kick. The initial bringing of your rearward leg knee up and around the front of your body should be practiced independently of both the jumping motion and the kick itself. They should only be brought together after you have learned the three separate movements, and when you can sufficiently execute each movement without telegraphing them to your opponent.

Fighting Position:
1. Your fighting position for this kick is exactly the same as for Spinning Wheel Kick. With your kicking leg in the forward position, rather than in the rearward position.
2. This stance is approximately shoulder width apart with the heel of your rear foot in a direct line with the heel of your front foot. Your front or lead foot should be pointed directly at your opponent.
3. Your rear foot is angled towards the left at approximately a 45-degree angle. Your weight should be distributed evenly over the balls of both feet.

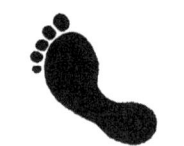

Fighting Position Foot Position

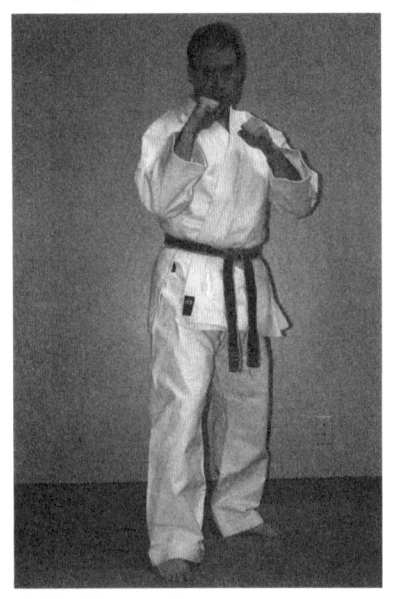

Fighting Position Front View

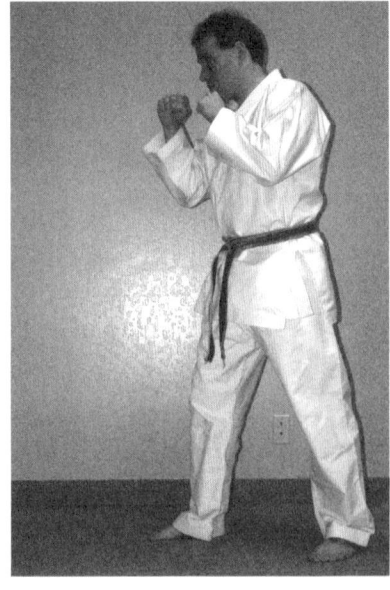

Fighting Position Side View

144

4. Your knees are slightly, but not noticeably bent. They should not be locked straight or rigid.
5. Your body should be facing at a 45-degree angle towards your opponent. This presents a smaller target area and also facilitates a faster step-forward-jump-turning motion when utilizing this kick.
6. Your hands should be held up (like a boxer's), with the elbows tucked in to protect the ribs and your hands up to protect your head. Your hands should remain as close to this position as possible throughout the entire kick.
7. Your head should be facing your opponent with your chin tucked down and protected by your lead shoulder.
8. Your eyes should be centered on your opponent's chest.

Step Forward & ...:

9. Bring your rear leg knee up and around in front of you, while simultaneously pivoting on the ball of your base leg foot, as if you were preparing to do a Side Kick off of your back leg. Your side that was previously facing away from your opponent should now be facing towards your opponent.
10. As you reach the above position, jump straight up off of your base leg. While you are in the air, the following things should be done simultaneously. They are as follows:

10a. Turn your head and look over your kicking shoulder at your target. Eye contact with your opponent is maintained at all times.

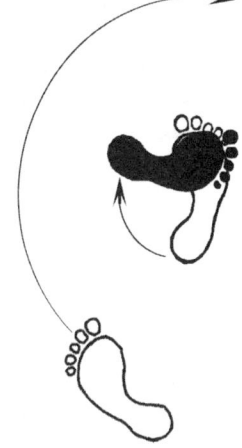

Step Forward &...
Foot Position

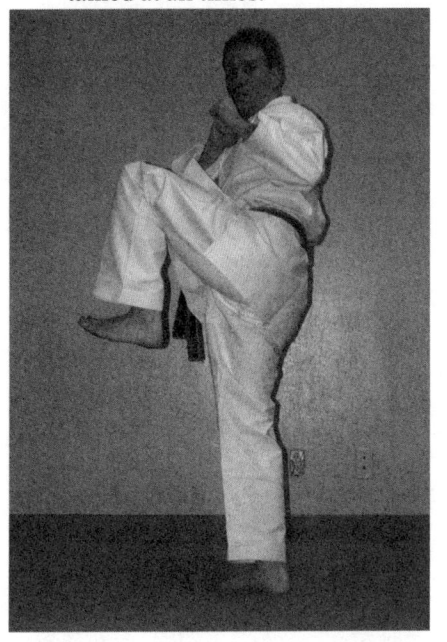

Step Forward &... Front View

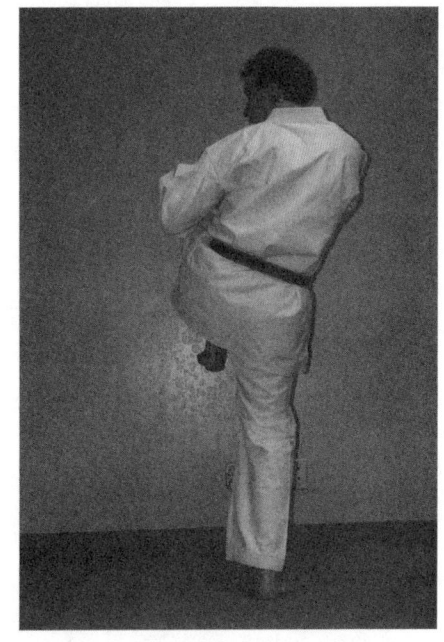

Step Forward &... Side View

145

...Jump, Turn & Begin Trajectory:
10b. Bring your kicking leg up to the begin trajectory position.
10c. Keep your hands up throughout the entire kick.
10d. Your body, which should lean slightly to the left, should make a complete 360-degree turn while in the air. Execute the kick.

Note: When executing any Wheel Kick, whether it is a ground based kick or an aerial kick, you want to have your body weight centered over the axis point of your 360-degree turn. Your axis point, will run in a straight "up and down" line from the ball of your base foot, through your base leg and up through your hips. If your weight is centered over your axis point, your body should "spin" just like the top which is pictured on the upper right, when you execute a 360-degree turn.

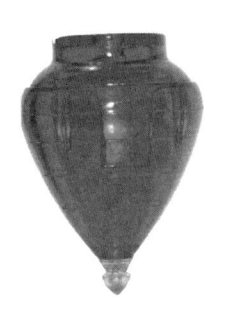

Note: However, if your weight is not centered over the axis point, say for example you have leaned to far over, then your "spin" will look more like a wobble, like the top which is pictured on the bottom right, when you execute a 360-degree turn.

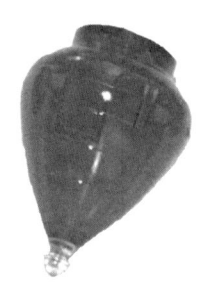

Note: When executing this or any jumping kick, keep your arms held up and as close to your body as possible. Don't let them flap around like a bird.

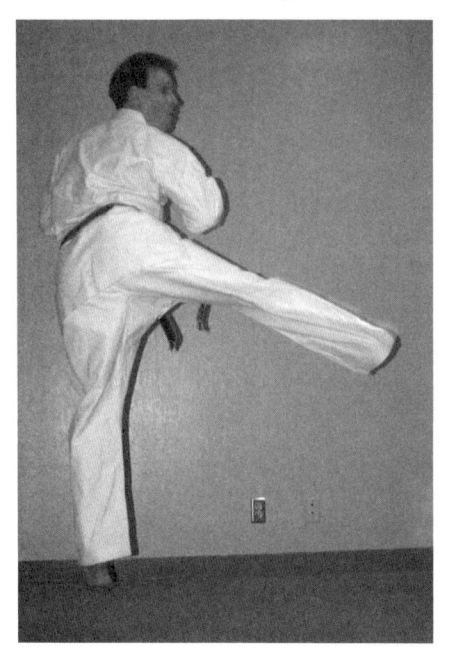

Jump, Turn & Begin Trajectory Front   *Jump, Turn & Begin Trajectory Side*

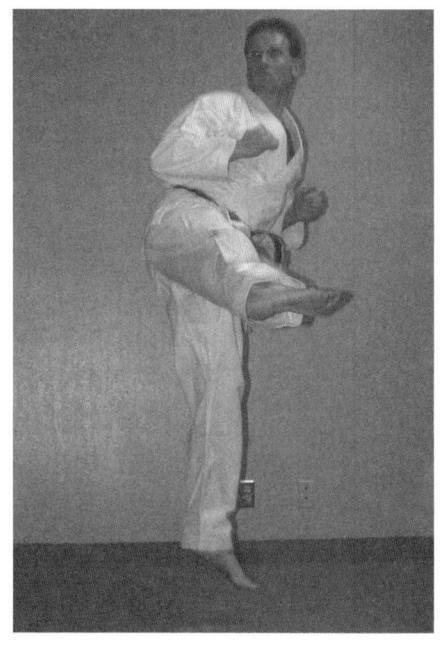

Peak of Trajectory:

11. Your kicking leg, with the knee slightly bent, has now moved up to the correct height to strike your target.
12. Even though you are in the air, the heel of your kicking foot should follow a straight line of trajectory from the "Peak of Trajectory" through the target (Impact), to the "Follow Through" position.
13. Your upper body should be leaning slightly to your left, although nowhere near the almost 75-degree angle you would be in if you were executing a ground based Wheel Kick.
14. Although your body is now in the above position. Your head should still be looking over your kicking leg shoulder. Eye contact with your target is maintained at all times.
15. Your back is currently facing in the same direction that your kicking leg will be in, when it is in the "Follow Through" position.

Note: As I described earlier on page 7, "A properly executed Wheel Kick performed by a man (or woman), is likened to the swing of a professional golfers golf club as he hits a golfball off a tee." Now keeping this in mind, you can envision your opponents head as the golfball, his neck as the tee, and his body as the ground when executing a Wheel Kick. Hit the ball (opponent's head) in the correct spot (vital point) with the correct technique, and the...

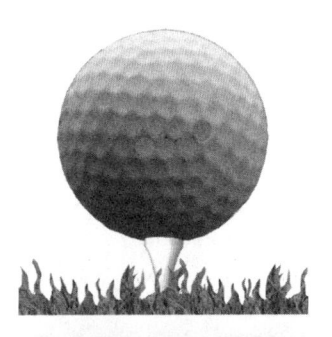

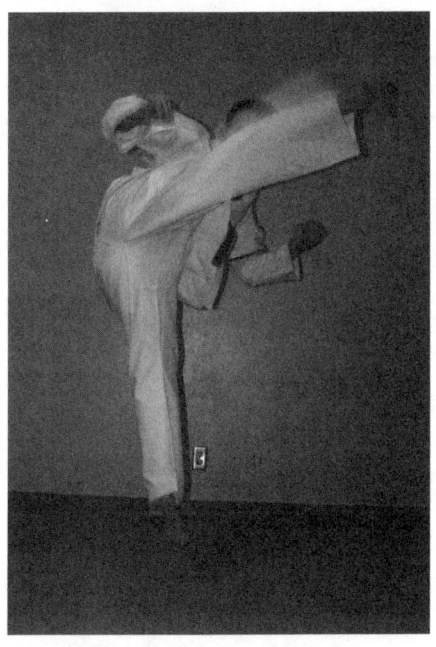

Peak of Trajectory Front View *Peak of Trajectory Side View*

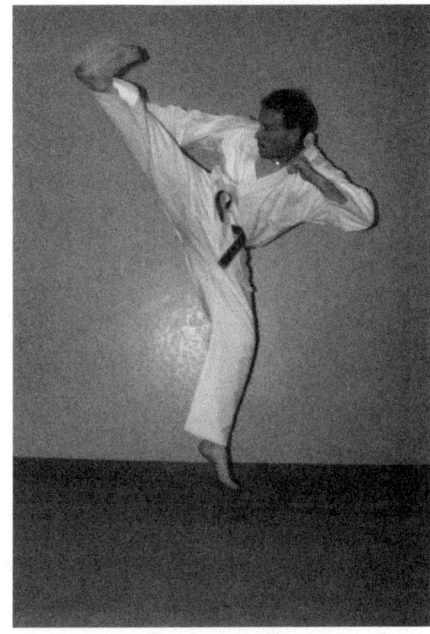

Impact:

16. At the moment of impact, your entire body should tighten to add power to the kick. Notice how the toes of the kicking foot are pulled back towards your body and pointed. This helps insure that contact with the target is made with the back of the heel.
17. Your upper body should still be leaning slightly to your left.
18. Notice how your body is now sideways to your opponent. However, it is at a slight angle due to the actions of the kicking leg and the continuous 360-degree turning motion of the entire body.
19. Your head should still be up and looking over your kicking leg shoulder. Eye contact with your target is maintained at all times.

Note: ...results are obvious, the ball flies down the fairway (your opponent is no longer a threat). If however, you strike incorrectly and say, hit the ground (opponent's body) instead of the ball (opponent's head), you not only risk bending or damaging your golf club (kicking leg, knee, or hip), but your ball will not move at all (have little or no effect on your opponent), as demonstrated in the photograph on the right.

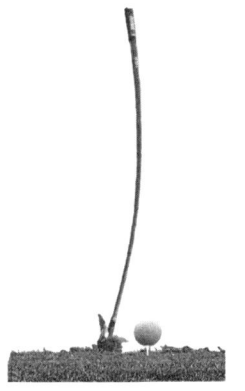

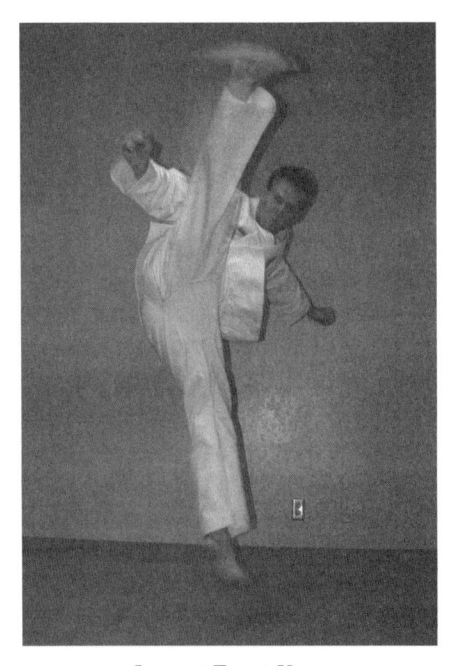

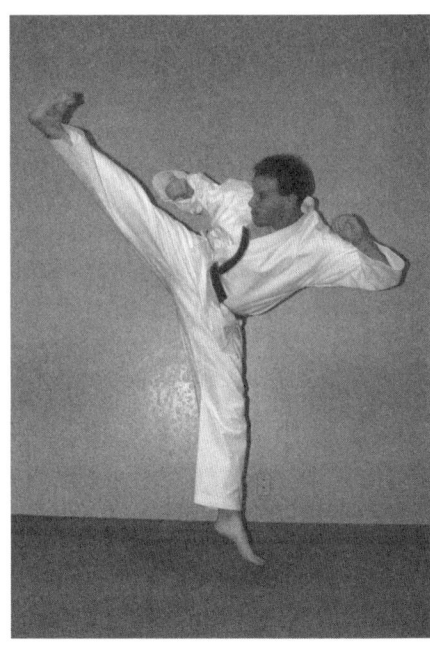

Impact Front View　　　　　　　　*Impact Side View*

148

Follow Through:
20. Your kicking foot should continue along exactly the same path it followed from the "Peak of Trajectory" to "Impact". Your foot should be approximately 45-degrees past your target.
21. Your upper body should still be leaning slightly to the left, although you will start to straighten your body at this point. The front of your body is now at approximately a 45-degree angle to the front of your opponent.
22. Your hands, which should have remained as close to the original starting position as possible, should still be up to protect your head and body. Did you notice my hand position in the "Side View" photograph? This is very incorrect!
23. Your head should no longer be looking over your kicking leg shoulder. However, your eyes are still looking at your opponent.

Note: If you were to look at the basic outline of your body during the "Peak of Trajectory" through "Follow Through" phase of any Wheel Kick, it would have the basic appearance of a capital "Y". Which you can see in the much larger illustration on the right.

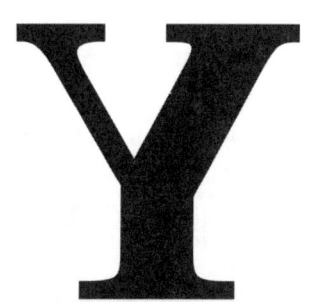

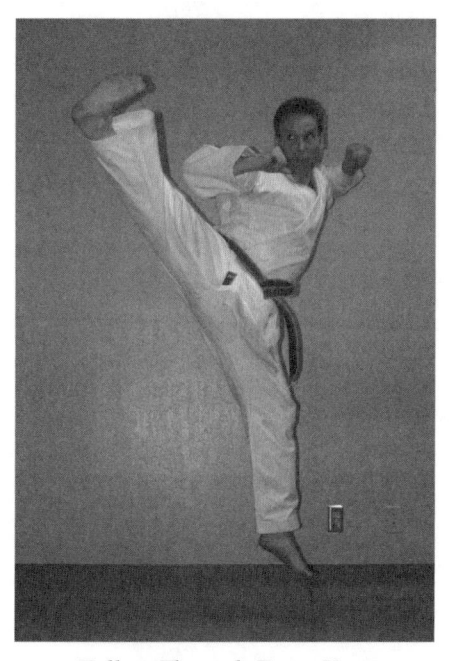

Follow Through Front View   *Follow Through Side View*

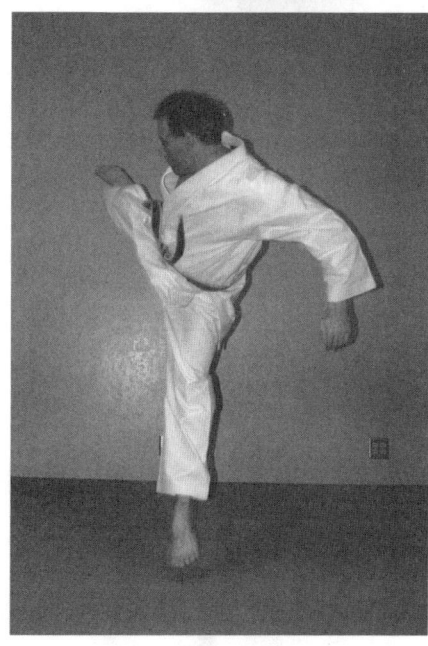

149

End of Trajectory:

24. Your base leg foot should have just touched down on the ground, and the toes of your base leg foot should now be pointing directly at your opponent.
25. Your kicking leg remains straight with the knee slightly bent. Your kicking foot is now slightly in front of you and to your right at approximately the height of your base leg knee.
26. Your upper body will straighten up from the slightly bent over position you were in when kicking. Your back remains straight and your upper body is now facing directly toward your opponent.
27. Your head should still be up and looking directly over the center of your chest. Your eyes are still in contact with your opponent, whether he is still standing, or lying on the ground.

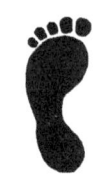

End of Trajectory Foot Position

Note: **Although I have broken down all of the kicks in this book into various steps, you must remember that eventually you will be executing these kicks without thought in one fluid movement while adhering to every principle and technique described in this book in order to maximize the effectiveness of your kick.**

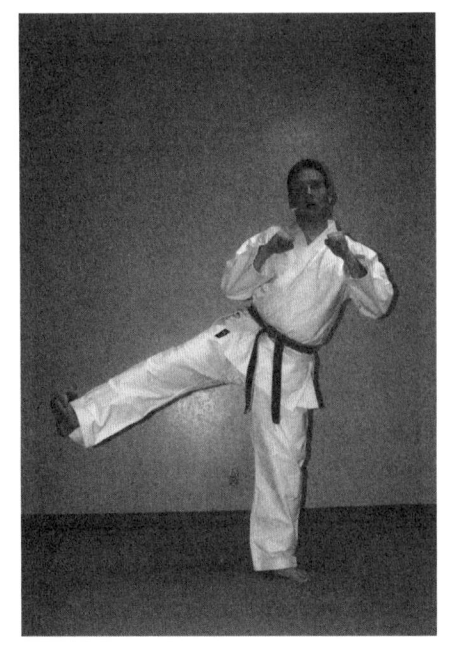

End of Trajectory Front View   *End of Trajectory Side View*

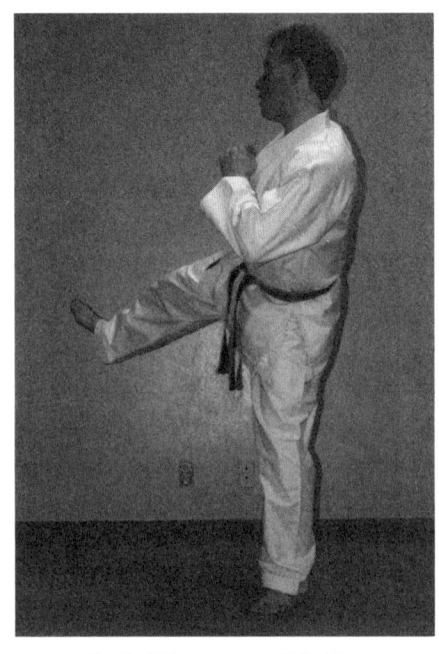

Return to Fighting Position:

28. Your entire body from your head to your toes, should be in exactly the same fighting position that you would be in if you were going to execute a Turning Wheel Kick with your right leg. Although, you won't be in exactly the same location.
29. Your kicking leg foot continues the 360-degree motion and returns to its original starting position. Although your kicking leg knee will remain slightly bent as it returns to the starting position.
30. Your hands, which should have remained as close to this position as possible throughout the entire kick, are held up (like a boxer's), with the elbows tucked in to protect the ribs and your hands up to protect your head.
31. Your head should now be looking over your lead leg shoulder with your eyes in contact with your opponent.

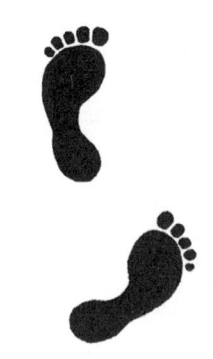

Return to Fighting Position Foot Position

Note: Although this book details only one of the ten primary kicks and ten of its main variations. You must remember that there are nine more primary kicks, and many more variations of each of those kicks. Kicking is only one aspect of becoming a complete and effective fighter. One should also study and practice hand and elbow techniques, throwing, grappling, and joint techniques.

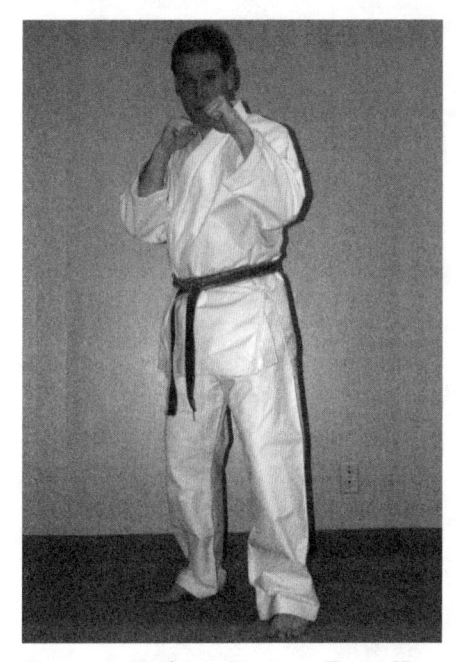

Return to Fighting Position Front View   *Return to Fighting Position Side View*

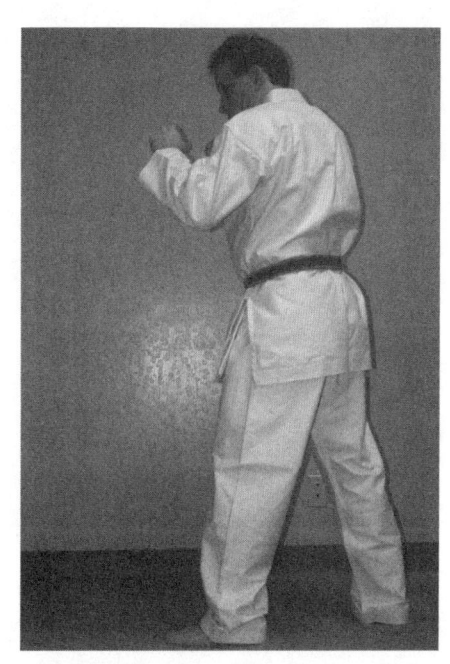

151

Pictorial Overview:

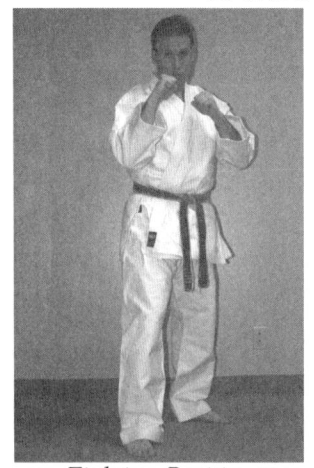

Fighting Position

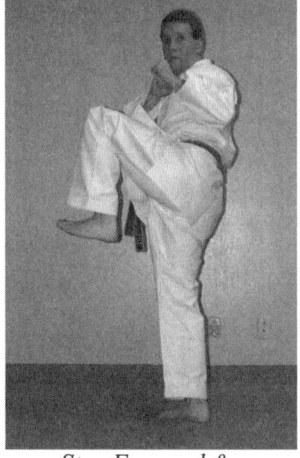

Step Forward &...

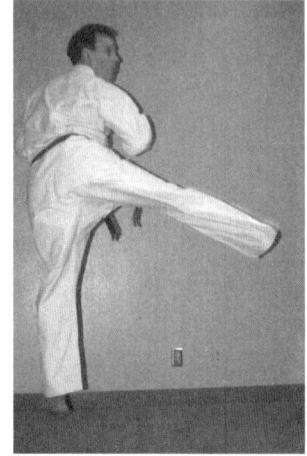

Jump, Turn & Begin...

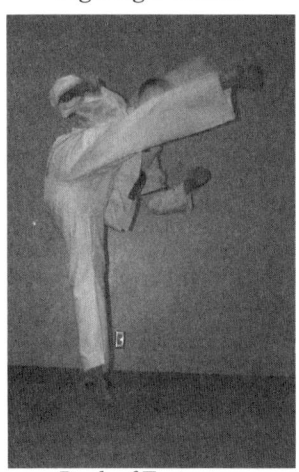

Peak of Trajectory

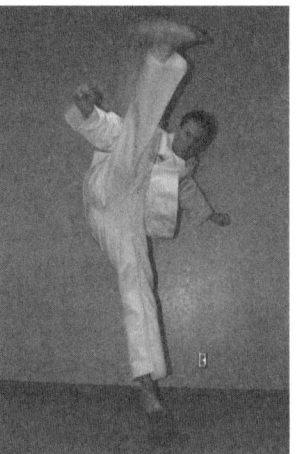

Impact

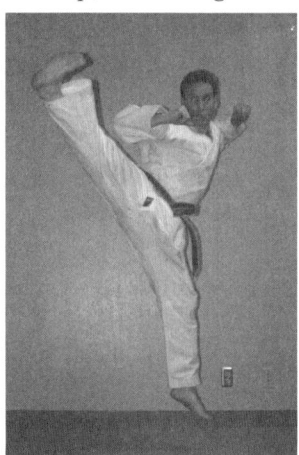

Follow Through

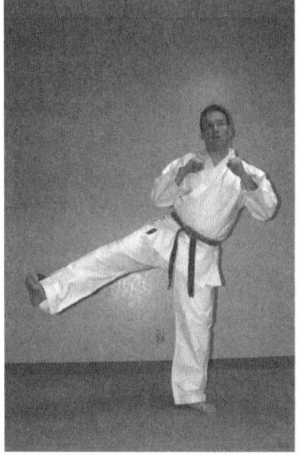

End of Trajectory

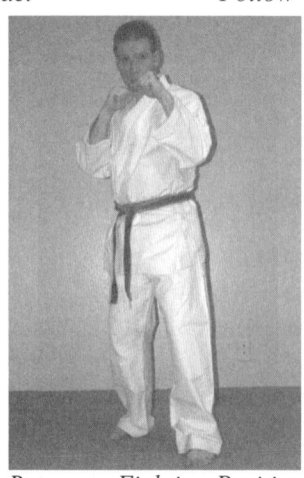

Return to Fighting Position

Spinning Wheel Kick
(With the left leg)

Here is an example on how to change the instructions presented in this book in order to execute the exact same kicks with the left leg. First of all you're going to be kicking with the left leg rather than the right, so your rear foot and body position will be exactly opposite of those that you would use if you were kicking with the right leg. And finally, your direction of movement will change from clockwise when kicking with the right leg, to counterclockwise when kicking with the left leg. To put it simply, kicking with the left leg should mirror exactly those kicks performed with the right leg and vice versa.

Fighting Position:
1. Your fighting position for this kick is the exact same as for Turning Wheel Kick. That is your kicking leg will be in the forward position to begin with rather than in the rear.
2. This stance is approximately shoulder width apart with the heel of your rear foot in a direct line with the heel of your front foot.
3. Your front or lead foot should be pointing directly at your opponent.
4. Your rear foot is angled towards the right at approximately a 45-degree angle. Your weight should be distributed evenly over the balls of both feet.
5. Your knees are slightly, but not noticeably bent. They should not be locked or rigid.

Fighting Position Foot Position

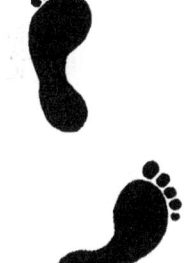

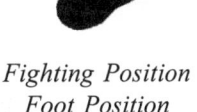

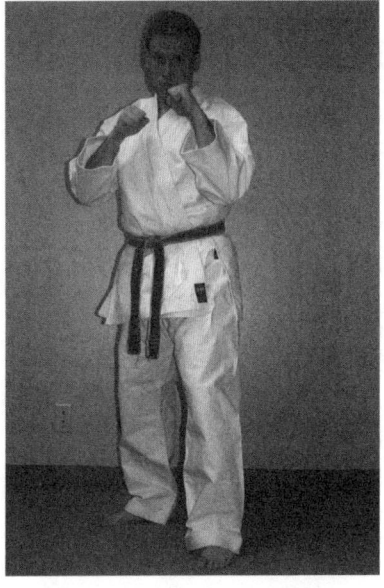

Fighting Position Front View

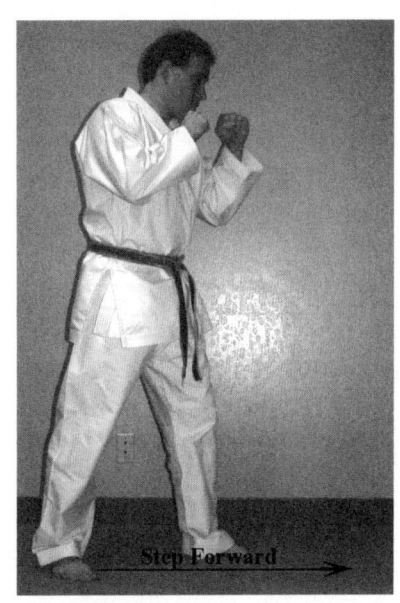

Fighting Position Side View

6. Your body should be facing at a 45-degree angle towards your opponent. This presents a smaller target area and also facilitates a faster step-and-turn when utilizing this kick.
7. Your hands should be held up (like a boxer's), with the elbows tucked in to protect the ribs and your hands up to protect your head. Your hands should remain as close to this position as possible throughout the entire kick.
8. Your head should be facing your opponent with your chin tucked down and protected by your lead shoulder.
9. Your eyes should be centered on your opponent's chest.

Step Forward & Turn Back:
10. Take a step forward with your rear foot. And...
11. As you step forward with your rear leg, pivot on the ball of your base leg foot. This will have the effect of turning your back toward your opponent.
12. Your eyes should still be centered on your opponent's chest
13. When you set your rear foot down, it should be not only in front of you, but also approximately 8 inches to the side. This allows for better balance and a more accurate kick. Your back should now be toward your opponent, and the heel of your now-base leg foot should also be pointed toward your opponent.

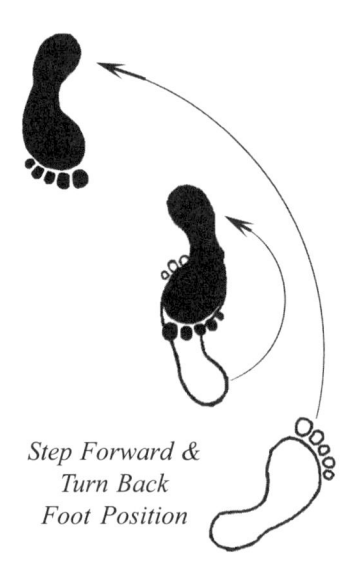

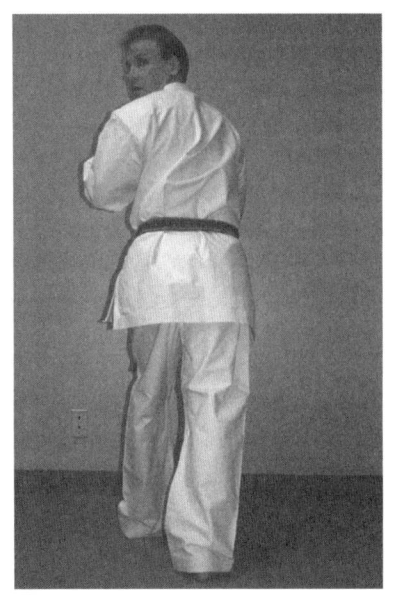

Step Forward & Turn Back Foot Position

Step Forward & Turn Front View

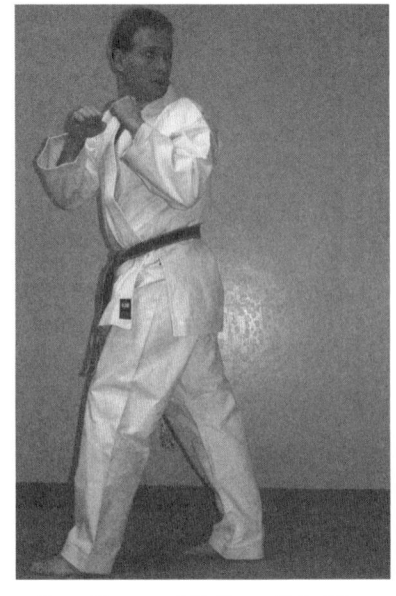

Step Forward & Turn Side View

Begin Trajectory:

14. Using the toes of your kicking foot, push off the floor and bring your kicking leg up at a 45-degree angle between the direction your body is facing and your left hand side. Your leg should be straight, with a slight bend in the knee. In this position, your kicking foot should already be in the correct position to strike your opponent.
15. As you bring your kicking leg up, your upper body should start bending over slightly, from the waist, to the right. Your back will remain straight.
16. Your head is still up and turned over your kicking shoulder, your eyes should always remain in contact with your opponent throughout the entire kick.
17. Your back should no longer be facing directly towards your opponent, but should start turning, along with your shoulders, in the direction of the kick.

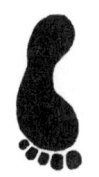

Begin Trajectory Foot Position

Note: The available vital points that are open to attack is going to be determined by your opponent. However, you can create your own openings on your opponent if you correctly utilize deception prior to, and during your attack.

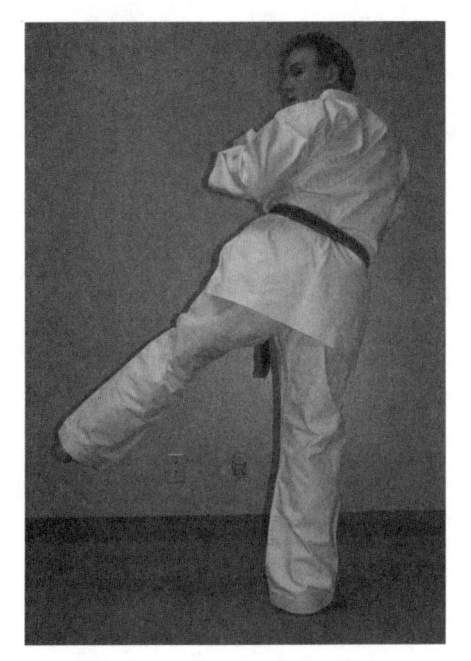

Begin Trajectory Front View   *Begin Trajectory Side View*

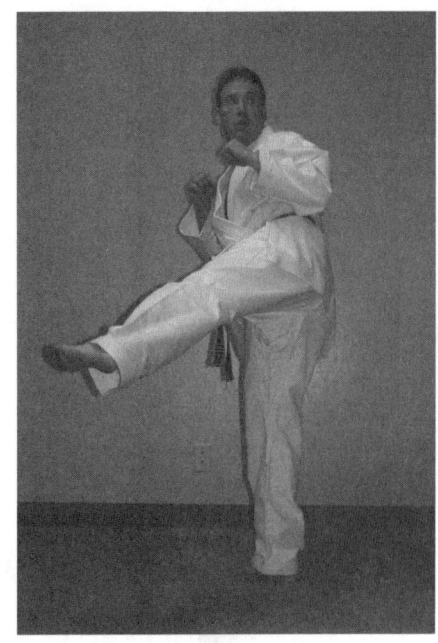

Peak of Trajectory:

18. Your base leg foot should now have moved approximately 45-degrees (counterclockwise) by pivoting on the ball of your foot. While your kicking leg, with the knee slightly bent, has now moved up to the correct height to strike your target.
19. The heel of the kicking foot should follow a straight line of trajectory from the "Peak of Trajectory" through the target (Impact), to the "Follow Through" position.
20. Your upper body should now be leaning to your right at almost a 75-degree angle in relation to your bodys upright position, and almost parallel with the ground.
21. Although your body is now in the above position, your head should still be looking over your kicking leg shoulder at your opponent.
22. Your back is no longer facing toward your opponent. It should now be facing at a 45-degree angle to your opponent's right in approximately the same direction that your kicking leg will be in, when it is in the "Follow Through" position.

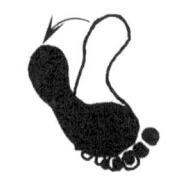

Peak of Trajectory Foot Position

Note: At the end of your workout, execute a Wheel Kick as slow as you can, while maintaining strict form and control. Pay close attention to how each body part feels while executing each individual phase of the kick.

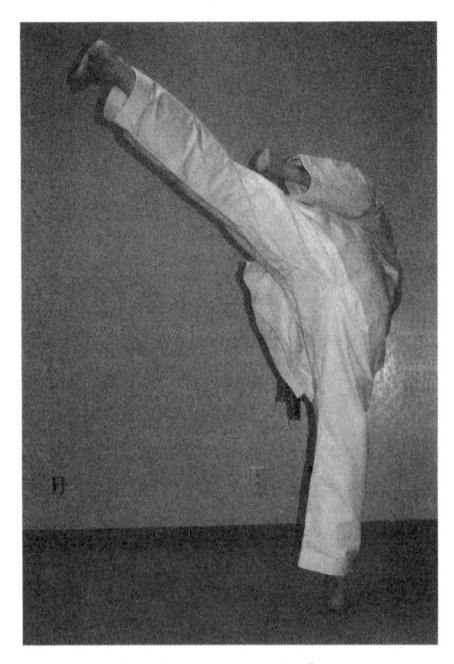

Peak of Trajectory Side View   *Peak of Trajectory Front View*

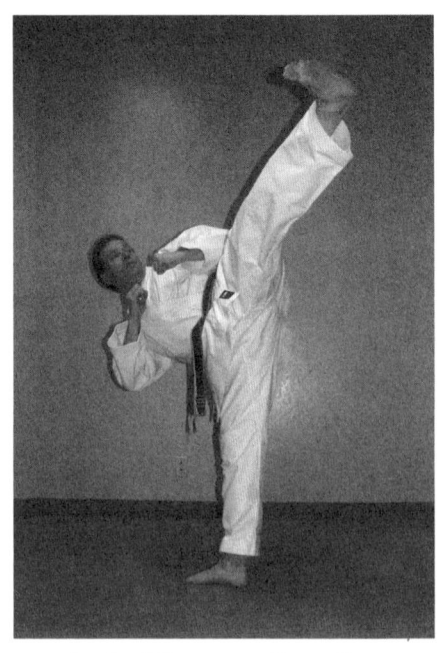

Impact:

23. Your base leg foot has now moved another 45-degrees (counterclockwise), by pivoting on the ball of the foot, with the arch of your foot now facing towards your opponent.
24. Your upper body should still be leaning to your right at almost a 75-degree angle in relation to your bodys upright position, and almost parallel with the ground. Although it has continued to move counterclockwise prior to the movement of your kicking leg and foot. At the moment of impact, your entire body should tighten to add power to the kick, as your foot continues to travel through the target.
25. Notice how your kicking foot, kicking leg (with knee slightly bent), hips, back, shoulders and head are all in a straight line at the initial moment of "Impact". Also, notice how the toes of the kicking foot are pulled back towards your body and pointed. This helps insure that contact with the target is made with the back of the heel.
26. Your head should still be up and looking over the kicking leg shoulder. Eye contact with your opponent is maintained at all times.

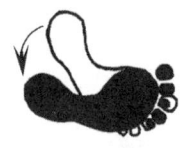

Impact Foot Position

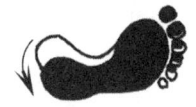

Impact (ADVANCED) Foot Position

Note: Don't kick over your opponent's head, kick through it!

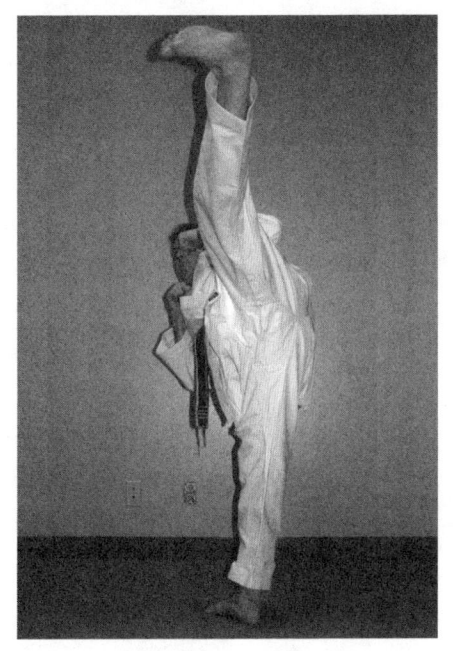

Impact Front View

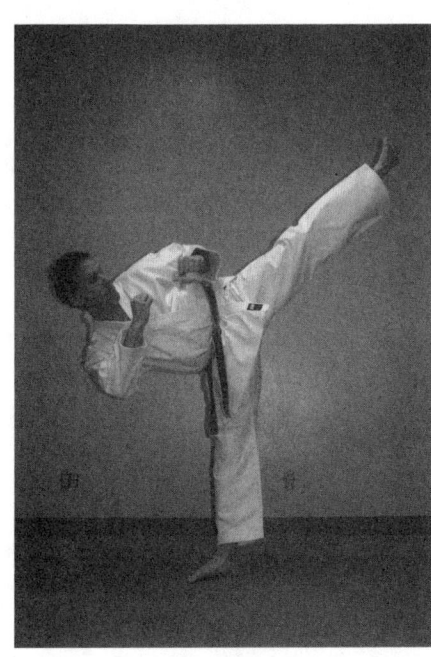

Impact Side View

157

Follow Through:

27. Your base leg foot should have moved another 45-degrees (counterclockwise) by pivoting on the ball of the foot.
28. Your upper body should still be leaning to your right at almost a 75-degree angle in relation to your bodys upright position, and almost parallel with the ground. Although it has once again moved counterclockwise prior to the movement of your kicking leg and foot. Your back is straight and the front of your body is now at approximately a 45-degree angle to the front of your opponent.
29. Your kicking leg foot should continue along exactly the same path it followed from the "Peak of Trajectory" to "Impact." Your foot should be approximately 45-degrees past your target.
30. Your head should no longer be looking over your kicking leg shoulder. However, your eyes are still looking at your opponent.

Note: If you look closely at the illustration on the right, you will see that from your initial "Fighting Position", you will pivot on the ball of your base leg foot approximately 270-degrees counterclockwise, before setting your entire foot...

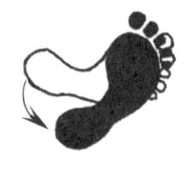

Follow Through Foot Position

Counterclockwise with the Left Leg

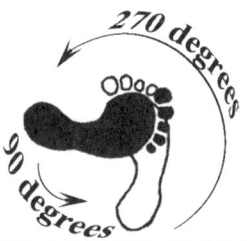

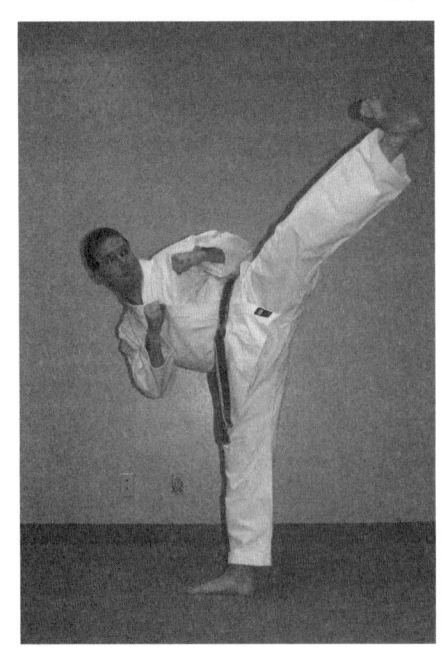

Follow Through Front View   *Follow Through Side View*

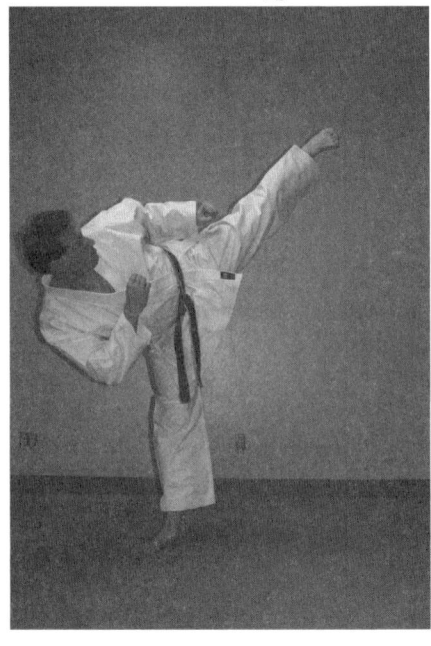

End of Trajectory:

31. Your base leg foot should have moved another 45-degrees (counterclockwise) by pivoting on the ball of the foot. The toes of your base leg foot should now be pointing directly at your opponent.
32. Your kicking leg remains straight with the knee slightly bent. Your kicking foot is now slightly in front of you and to your left at approximately the height of your base leg knee.
33. Your upper body will straighten up from the approximately 75-degree bent over position you were in when kicking. Your back remains straight and your upper body is now facing directly toward your opponent.
34. Your head should still be up and looking directly over the center of your chest. Your eyes are still in contact with your opponent, whether he is still standing, or lying on the ground.

Note: ...back down on the ground at the initial moment of impact. Immediately after the initial moment of impact, you will complete the 360-degree turn and return to your original starting position by pivoting the remaining 90-degrees on the ball of your base leg foot. When kicking with the right foot, you will move clockwise.

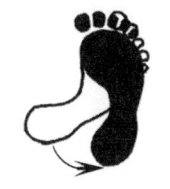

End of Trajectory Foot Position

Clockwise with the Right Leg

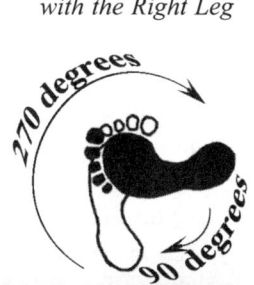

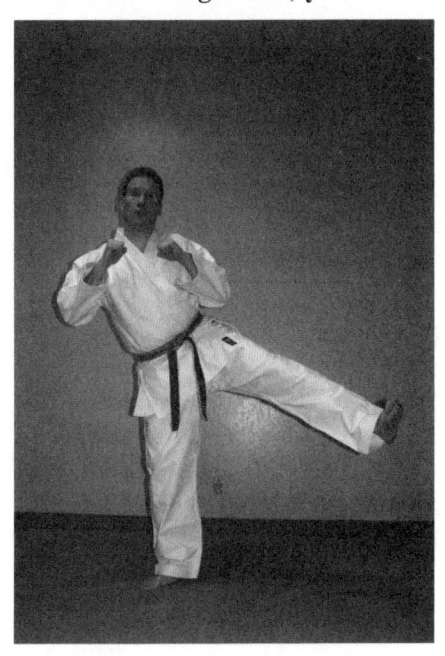

End of Trajectory Front View

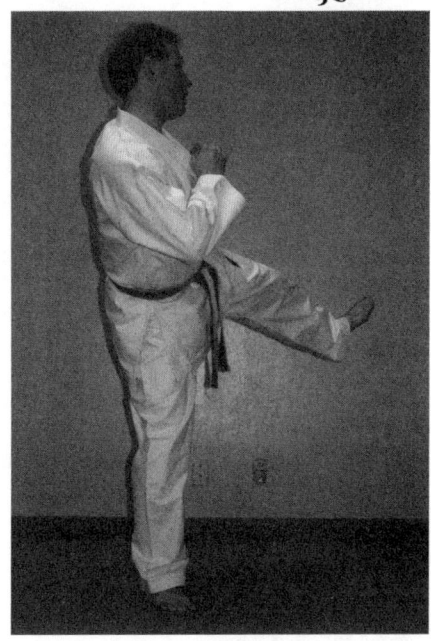

End of Trajectory Side View

Return to Fighting Position:

35. Your entire body from your head to your toes, should be in exactly the same fighting position that you would be in if you were going to execute a Turning Wheel Kick with your left leg. Although, you won't be in exactly the same location.
36. Your kicking leg foot continues the 360-degree counterclockwise motion and returns to its original starting position. Although your kicking leg knee will remain slightly bent as it returns to the starting position.
37. Your hands, which should have remained as close to this position as possible throughout the entire kick, are held up (like a boxer's), with the elbows tucked in to protect the ribs and your hands up to protect your head.
38. Your head should now be looking over your lead leg shoulder with your eyes in contact with your opponent.

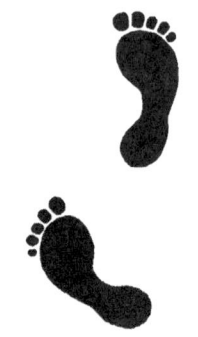

Return to Fighting Position Foot Position

Note: If you are like the vast majority of martial artists, you will have one leg that is very good at kicking and the other that seems to lag behind. One thing that I do to correct this, is to perform 15 repetitions on my weak leg for every 10 repetitions that I perform with my strong leg. This works well for me and is a training technique you may want to try yourself.

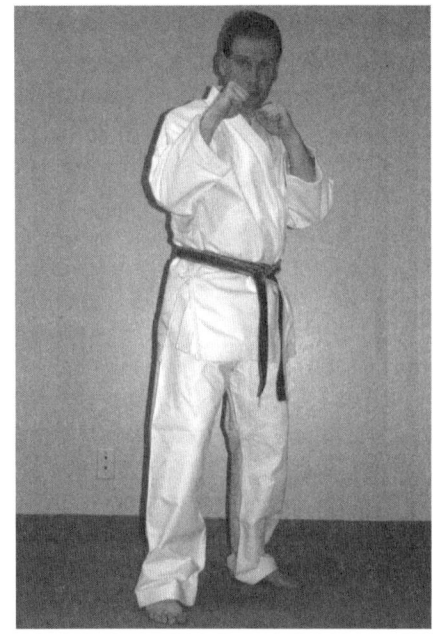

Return to Fighting Position Front View   *Return to Fighting Position Side View*

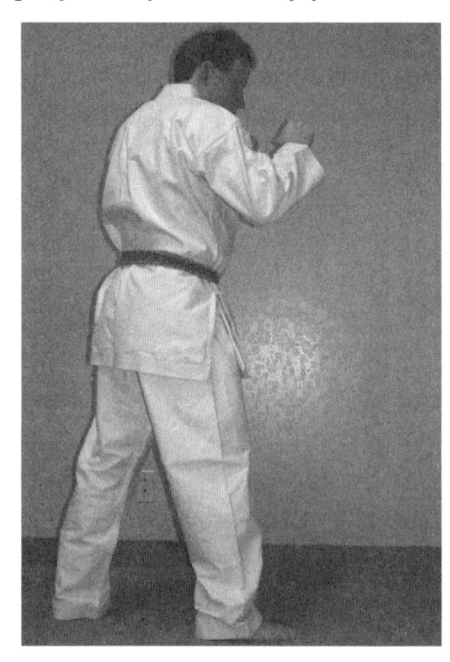

Pictorial Overview:

Fighting Position

Step Forward

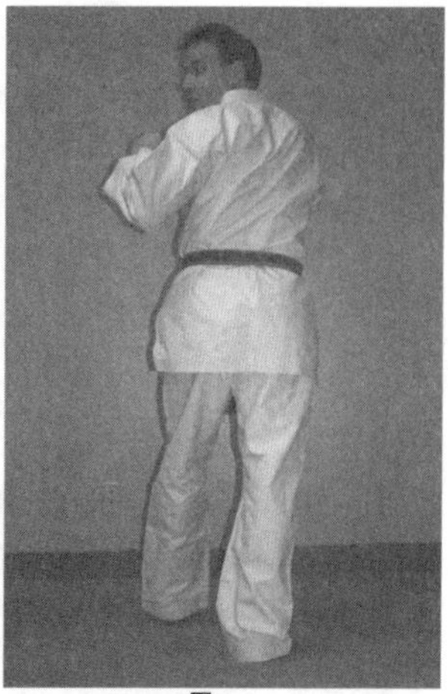

Turn

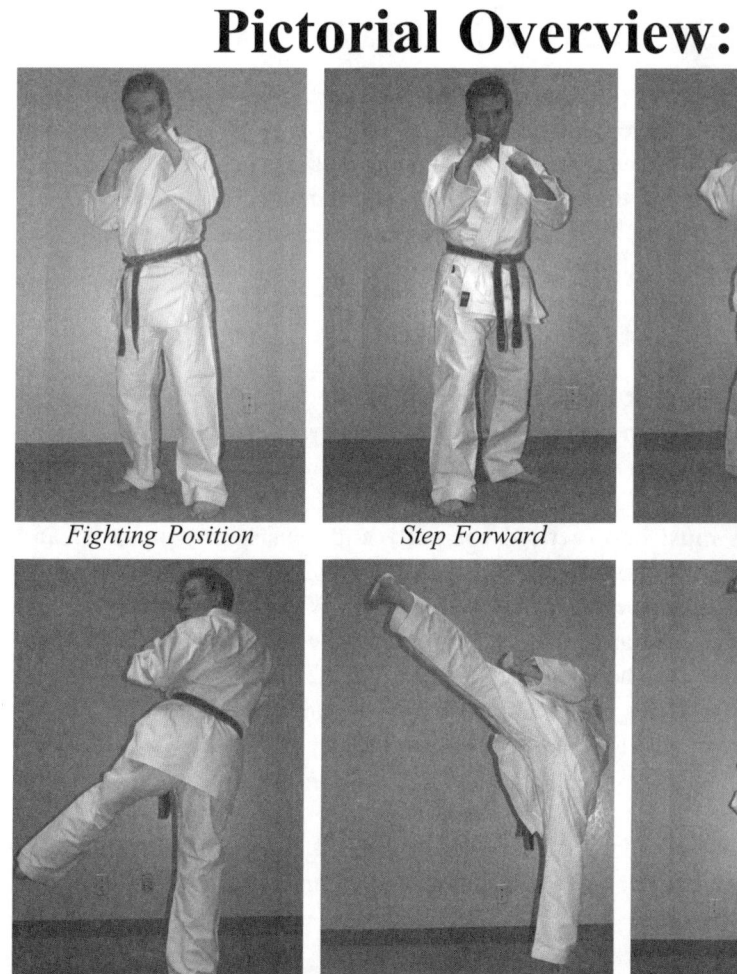

Begin Trajectory

Peak of Trajectory

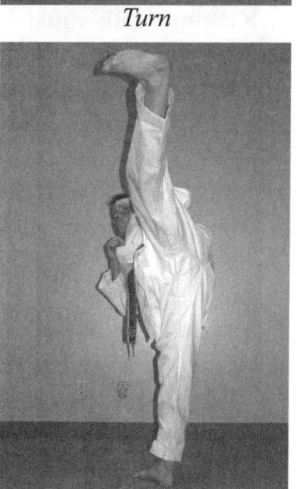

Impact

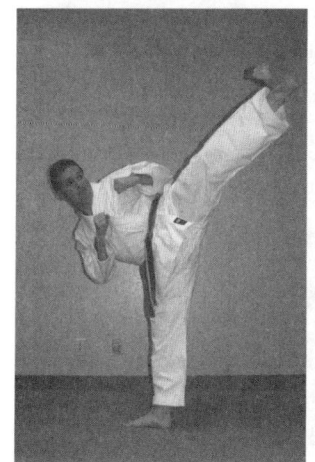

Follow Through

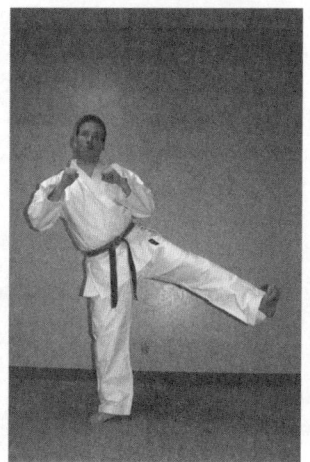

End of Trajectory

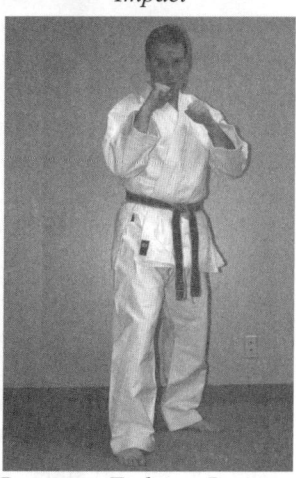

Return to Fighting Position

Training and Practice Methods

The following practice methods in this section, when performed correctly and consistently, are designed to improve your skill, speed, and power when executing the Wheel Kick. However, whether or not you improve is dependent solely upon you and your commitment to your training. When performing the exercises and drills that follow, concentrate on form and technique rather than speed or power.

Skill

The precise movement and skill you wish to obtain in the ring and on the street should be practiced correctly and consistently during training.

In other words, how you practice and train in the dojo is how you will react in the ring or on the street.

Kicking skills must be practiced correctly and consistently or speed and technique will begin to deteriorate.

Your kicking skills can be likened to an automobile. With proper maintenance and care, your automobile will last a lifetime. However, if you neglect your automobile, it will break down on you when you need it most. You never can tell when you will suddenly need those skills. Now let's take a look at some of my favorite training exercise that I use in order to improve my Wheel Kick.

Mirror:

The mirror is without a doubt my favorite training aid. It enables me to see myself clearly and analyze my technique in minute detail. I can then correct any flaws as they become evident.

Training Partner:

Training with a partner is an invaluable way to practice as a partner can tell you if you are making a mistake when executing your kick. Partners can also hold bags and pads for kicking as well as making the entire work out more enjoyable. A word of caution though, if your training partner spends a good deal of time talking and less time working out, then perhaps it is time to search for a new partner. Idle chatter should have no place in your training regimen. A focused workout session on your own is infinitely preferable to one spent with a poor partner.

Three Dimes:

Begin by taking three dimes and placing them on the floor, one under the pivot point on the ball of your base leg foot, the second under the center of your base leg heel. The third dime is placed in the exact position where your base leg heel will make contact with the ground during the moment of impact. Execute a Turning Wheel Kick. At the moment of impact, your base leg heel should have come to rest exactly on the third dime. As you continue with your kick, your base leg heel should return to its original starting position by once again coming to rest exactly on the second dime. This exercise, when practiced correctly and consistently, will greatly improve the pivoting skills needed to properly execute a Wheel Kick.

Wall Practice:

This exercise to improve my Wheel Kick was first demonstrated to me over twenty years ago. It is still valid today and should be an important part of your training program. This exercise is very simple to perform and focuses primarily on the "Peak of Trajectory," "Impact," and the "Follow Through" of the kicking leg.

Start by placing your base leg hand on the wall at approximately shoulder height, while looking over your kicking leg shoulder. Bring your kicking leg up at a 45-degree angle to the "Peak of Trajectory" position, and continue along the "Path of Trajectory" by bringing your kicking leg back to the "Impact" position and continuing through to the "Follow Through" position. And finally, returning your foot back down on the ground to its original starting position.

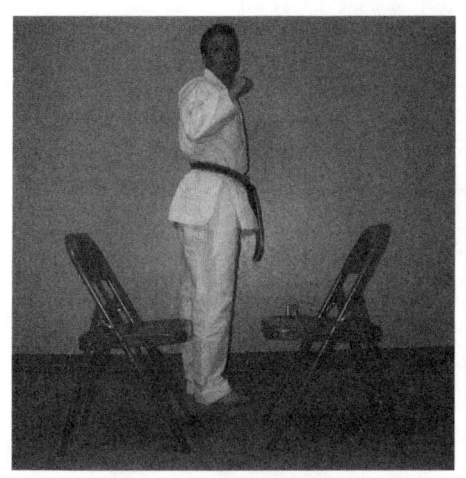

Starting & Finishing Position

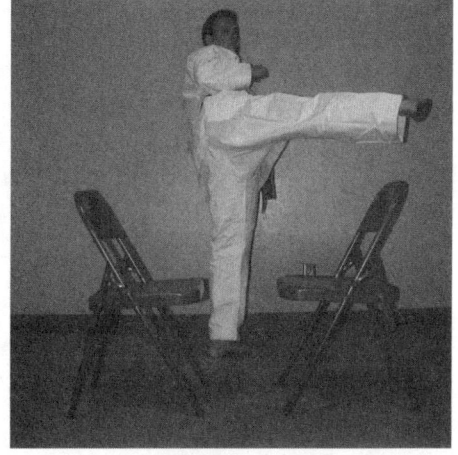

Peak of Trajectory

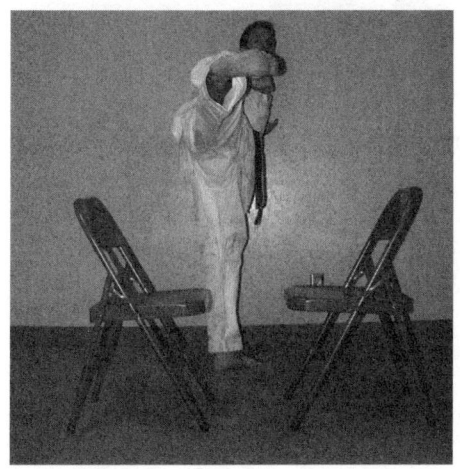

Impact

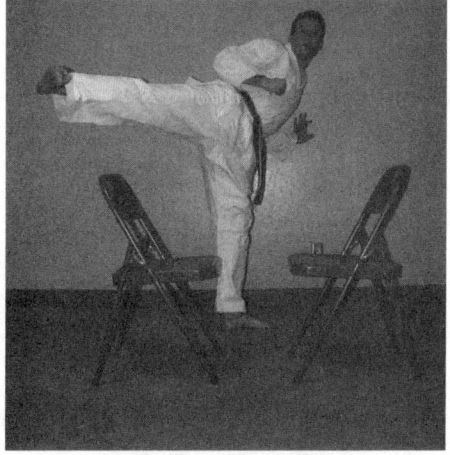

Follow Through

Chair Practice:

This is a terrific practice method to perform in order to perfect your turning skills when utilizing the Wheel Kick. Perform a Turning Wheel Kick like you normally would, and then utilize the chair to maintain your balance while working to perfect your technique. As with the wall practice method, you should concentrate on improving your form and technique rather than speed or power. You can increase the level of difficulty when performing the wall or

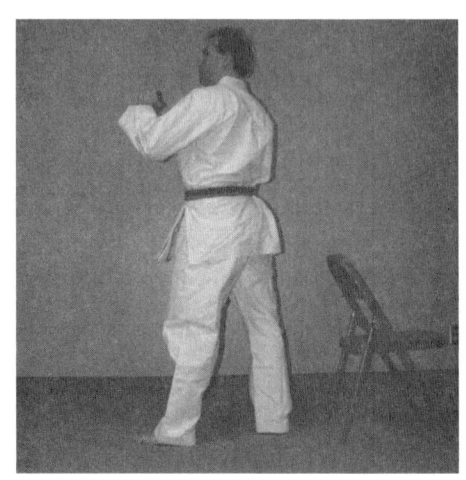

Fighting Position

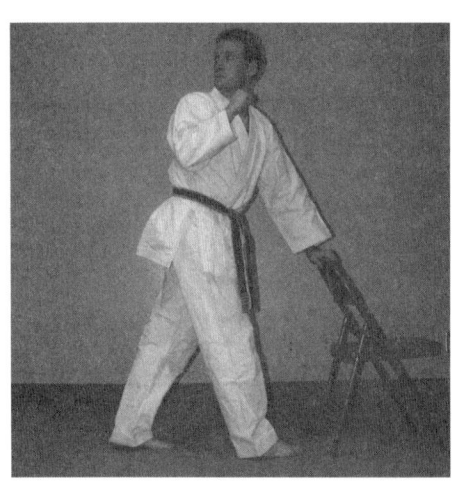

Turn & Grab Chair

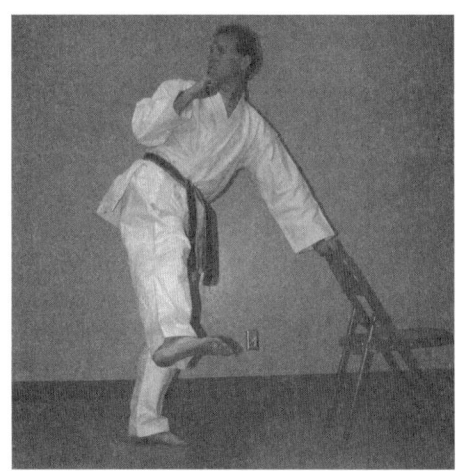

Begin Trajectory

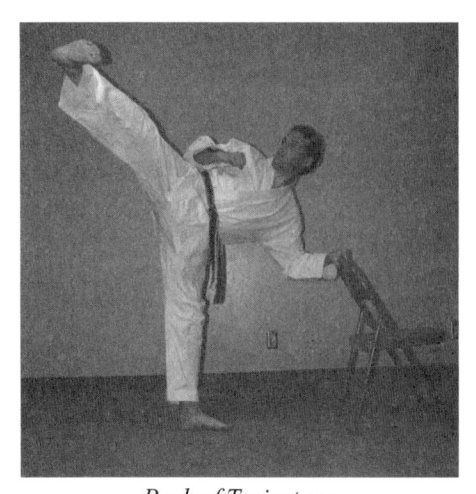

Peak of Trajectory

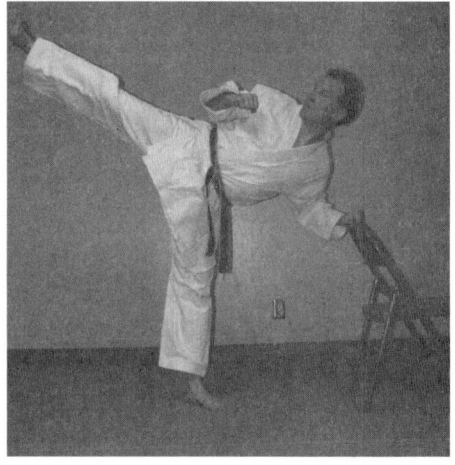

Impact

Follow Through *End of Trajectory*

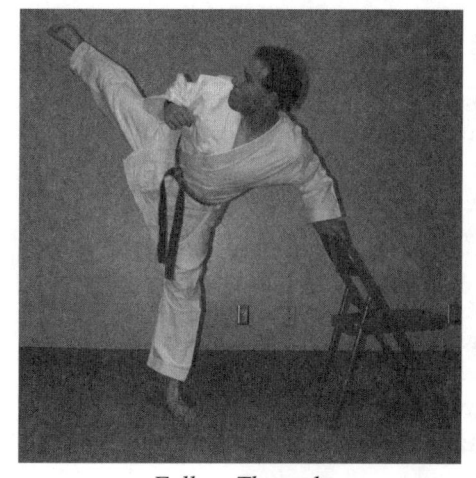

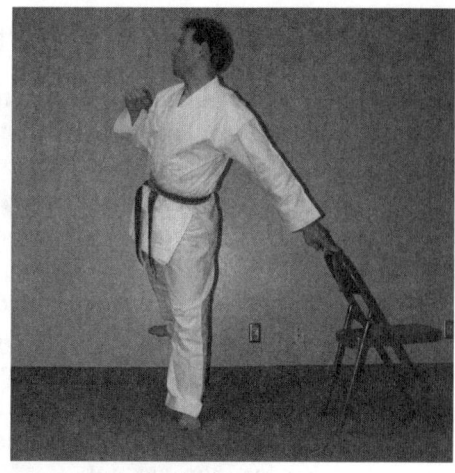

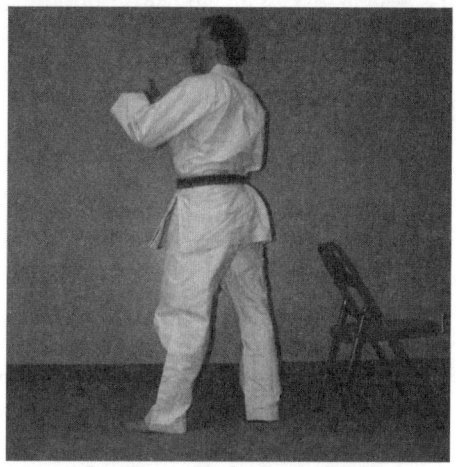

Return to Fighting Position

chair practice method by attaching ankle weights to your legs before performing the exercises. **However, a word of caution.**

You must practice your kicks more slowly and pay very close attention to form. **Do Not** perform the Wheel Kick at full speed with ankle weights on. If you do, you are asking for trouble and a possible knee or hip injury. Practice hard, but practice smart. Another variation is to practice total relaxation of the body throughout the entire kicking sequence, except at the moment of impact. Upon impact tighten every muscle in your body from your toes to your fingertips. As soon as you have impacted with your target, relax your body again. Start slow, and gradually increase speed. This will help prepare your body to deliver the maximum amount of force to the target. This takes a lot of practice, be patient and the results will come.

Remember that you must practice each kick that you learn 5,000 to 10,000 times correctly, before you can be proficient at it. And then you must practice on a regular basis to maintain that skill level. Practice does not make you perfect, but it sure does help.

Strength

Nearly every movement in the martial arts is carried out in opposition to a resistance. Therefore, an increase in strength means an improvement in performance.

"Stronger muscles give the athlete greater movement potential. If everything is equal, the stronger athlete will be bigger, faster, more flexible, more enduring, and less prone to injury." —Dr. Ellington Darden

"One of the benefits of strength is that it acts as a shock absorber for a muscle. Most injuries, such as tennis elbow, are caused by a force or succession of forces that cause the muscle to exceed its tensile strength. When that happens, the muscle tears. The stronger you are, the less likely that is to happen." —Michael Quinn

In order to increase muscular strength and endurance, the muscles must be worked harder than normal.

Your legs carry you everywhere you go, and are approximately 10 times stronger than your arms. Therefore the stronger your legs are, the stronger you are.

Although I have included only a few specific leg exercises in this volume, I consider the following exercises to be some of the best available for adding strength to not only your Wheel Kicks, but all of your other kicks as well. In subsequent volumes in the Achieving Kicking Excellence series, I will include several additional leg exercises which, depending on how you perform them, can develop either strength or endurance depending on the amount of weight used and repetitions performed. As with all exercises, train hard, but train smart.

Hack Squat Machine:

Squats are perhaps the single best overall strength building exercise there is for the entire body, and most assuredly the best exercise there is for the lower body. The muscles emphasized during the squat are the quadriceps, gluteus maximus, lower back and the hamstrings. The Hack Squat is a variation of the basic squat, and is an excellent means of isolating the leg muscles. This exercise is used by many weightlifters when they have no spotter available, or when they can no longer safely perform free weight squats because their back or legs are too tired or sore. Remember, you should always wear shoes, weight lifting gloves and a weight lifting belt for support when you are weight lifting.

Before you begin, make sure that the weighted plates are securely fastened to the machine. Step into the machine and place your back against the padded surface, while wedging your shoulders beneath the padded yokes attached to the front of the machine. Your legs should be straight and your feet should be approximately 6 to 10 inches apart and parallel with each other. Firmly grasp the handles located on the sides of the machine. Keeping your back straight, reach down and release the safety bar.

From this position, slowly bend your legs, allowing your knees to move outward in the same direction as your toes. At the same time contract your back muscles in order keep your body rigid as your perform this exercise. Slowly squat down until you are in a full squat position with your thighs parallel to the ground. Once you have reached the full squat position, slowly stand up to the starting position. Repeat this movement as often and as safely as you can. This exercise primarily emphasizes the quadriceps. However, if you place your feet closer together, you will place more emphasis on the gluteal muscles. If you spread your feet further apart, you will place more emphasis on the adductors.

Remember:
1. Keep your back straight throughout the entire movement.
2. Focus your eyes on a spot at head level in order to help keep your head up.
3. Do not bounce at the bottom of the squat.
4. Do not squat lower than your thighs parallel to the foot, or base plate.
5. Inhale as you are performing the squat, and exhale as you are straightening your legs.

Training Routine:
1. For strength use a heavier weight and perform three sets of 8 to 12 repetitions.
2. For endurance use a lighter weight and perform three to five sets of 15 to 20 repetitions per set.
3. Perform this exercise no more than 3 times per week.

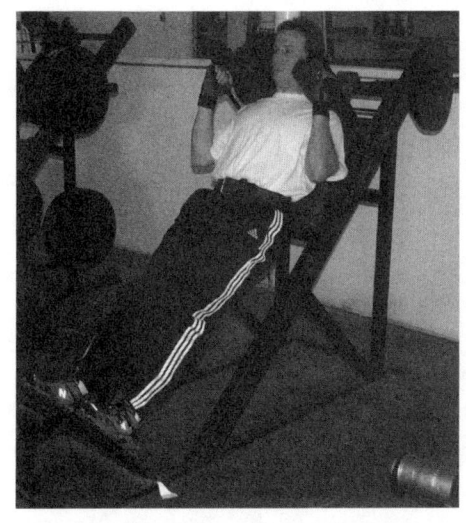

Starting & Finishing Position　　　　　　　　*Squat Position*

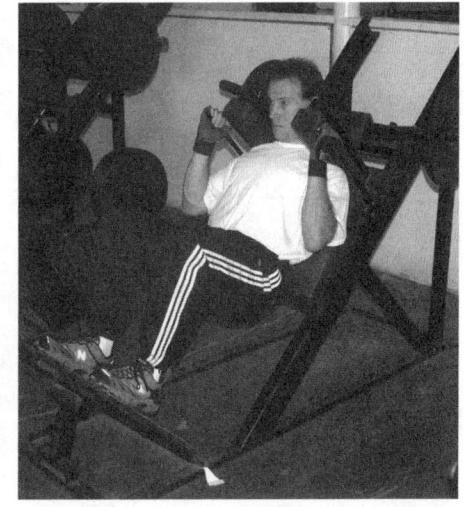

Seated Calf Machine:

This exercise places primary emphasis on the soleus muscle, which is located below the gastrocnemius, and is attached under the knee joint and connects with the calcaneus by the Achilles tendon. This exercise can be performed on a specially designed seated calf machine, or on a regular bench by placing your toes and the balls of your feet on a block of wood, and then placing a padded barbell across your lower thighs just above the knees. Before starting this exercise, make sure that the proper amount of weight is securely attached to the machine, or to the barbell.

Begin by sitting on the machine's seat and place the padded bar firmly across the lower portion of your thighs. Place your toes and the balls of your feet on the foot bar. Keeping your back straight, let your hands rest upon the top of the padded bar. Slowly raise your heels up and carefully release the safety bar located on the side of the machine. Slowly lower your heels as far below the level of your toes as possible. Hold this position for a moment. Then slowly raise them up as high as you can. Repeat this movement as often and as safely as you can.

Remember:
1. Perform this exercise slowly in order to obtain the maximum benefit.
2. Do not do partial movements. Utilize the entire range of motion on this exercise.

Training Routine:
1. For strength use a heavier weight and perform three sets of 8 to 12 repetitions.
2. For endurance use a lighter weight and perform three to five sets of 15 to 20 repetitions per set.
3. Perform this exercise no more than 3 times per week.

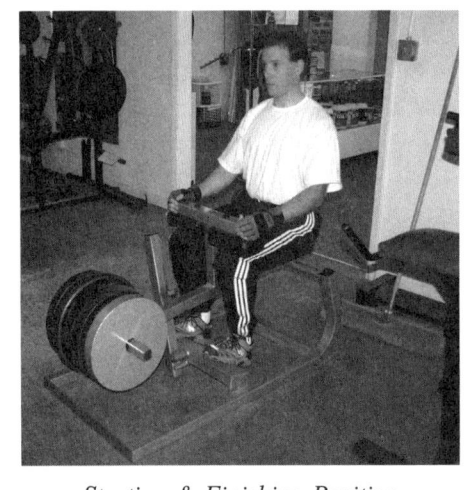

Starting & Finishing Position   *Toe Raise Position*

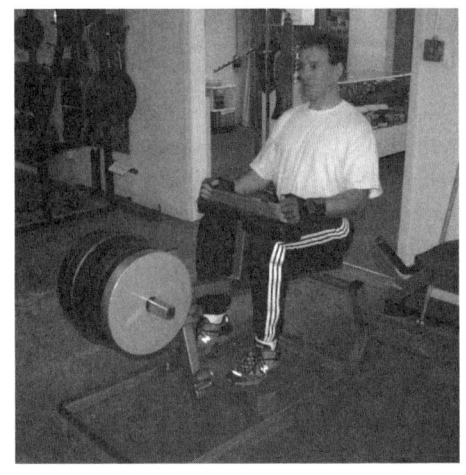

Side-to-Side Squats with weights:

Begin by standing with your feet approximately shoulder width apart, toes pointed out at a slight angle. Lift the barbell safely and place it behind your head and across your shoulders. Your hands should maintain a wide grip on the bar for better balance. Keep your back straight and your head up throughout the entire exercise. From this position, slowly spread your feet out to approximately two to three shoulder widths apart. Slowly squat down with one leg, until you are in a side squat position. Once you have reached the side squat position, your squatting leg thigh should be parallel with the floor, while your non-squatting leg is straight out to the side. Slowly return to the starting position, and repeat this movement on the opposite side. Repeat this movement as often and as safely as you can.

Remember:
1. Keep your back straight and rigid throughout the entire movement.
2. Focus your eyes on a spot at head level in order to help keep your head up.
3. **Use light weights only,** and do not bounce at the bottom of the squat.

Training Routine:
1. This is primarily an endurance building exercise and should be performed with a high number of repetitions (30 to 100) for several sets (3 to 10).
2. Perform this exercise no more than 3 times per week.

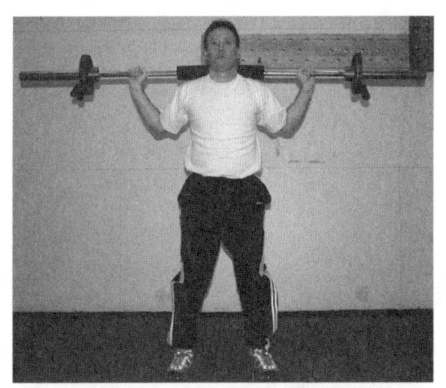

Starting & Finishing Position

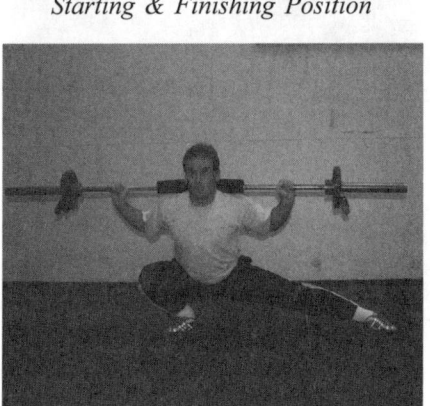

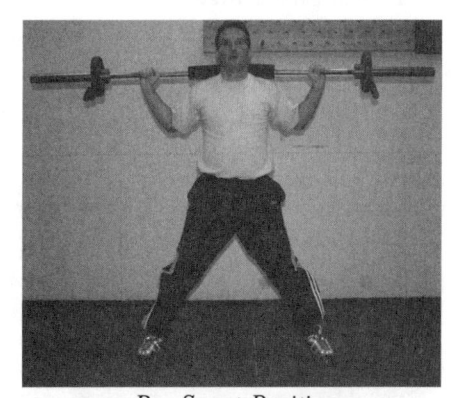

Pre-Squat Position

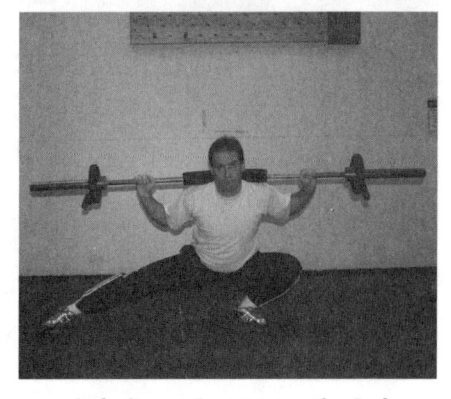

Side Squat Position to the Right

Side Squat Position to the Left

Cable Machine Leg Raises to the Side:

This exercise places primary emphasis on the gluteus maximus, the gluteus minimus, and the tensor fascia latae, all of which are located around the hip area. This exercise can be performed on a specially designed leg abduction machine, or on any cable weight machine with a floor level attachment. Before you begin, make sure that the ankle strap is securely attached to your ankle, and that the cable is securely attached to the ankle strap. It is also a good idea to have a thick sock on so that the ankle strap doesn't rub against your leg during the execution of this exercise. Start the exercise by first standing sideways to the machine with your back straight. Grasp the handle or the side of the machine for balance. **Do not grab the bars that the weights travel up and down on!** Lean your body to the side over your base leg and towards the weight machine, while slowly raising your opposite leg straight out to the side and as high as you can. Hold this position for a moment. Then slowly lower your leg back to the starting position. Repeat this movement as often and as safely as you can.

Remember:
1. Perform this exercise slowly in order to obtain the maximum benefit.
2. Do not do partial movements. Utilize the entire range of motion on this exercise.

Training Routine:
1. Use light weights to start with and perform three to five sets of 25 to 30 repetitions per set.
2. Perform this exercise no more than 3 times per week.

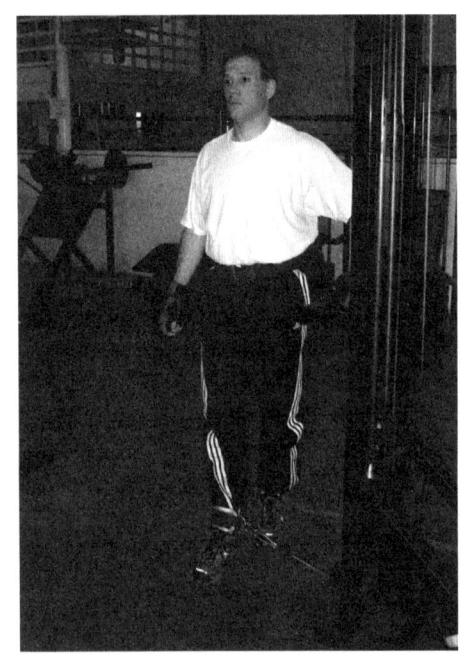

Starting & Finishing Position　　　　　*Leg Raise to the Side*

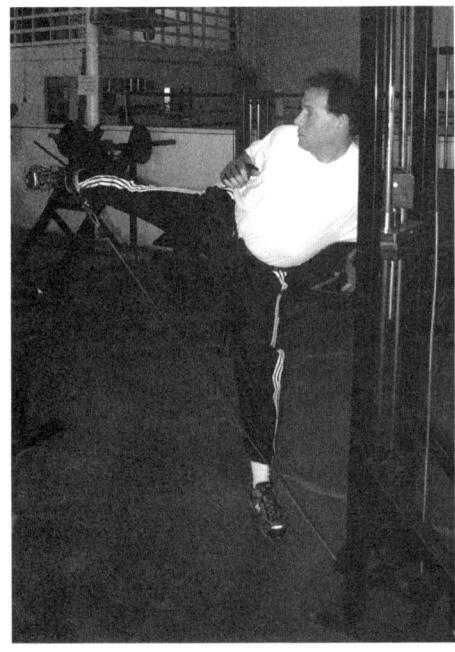

Seated Leg Curls:

This is another excellent exercise to perform in order to isolate your hamstring muscles, which are located at the back of your thighs. This exercise, for the most part, can only be performed effectively on a seated leg curl machine. Before starting, make sure the proper amount of weight is securely attached to the machine. Begin by sitting down on the padded seat with your back firmly against the padded back of the machine, be sure and keep your back straight at all times. **Do not hunch over or sit on the edge of the padded seat.** Place the back of your heels (Achilles Tendon area) over the lowermost padded rollers, while placing your shin (just below the front of your knees) under the uppermost set of padded rollers. Your legs should be straight at this point. Grab the sides of the bench with your hands in order to keep your upper body from moving during the course of this exercise. Utilizing your biceps femoris muscles, move your feet down and back in an arcing motion toward your hands, until your legs are back as far as possible. Hold this position for a moment, and then slowly raise your legs to the starting position. Repeat this movement as often and as safely as you can.

Remember:
1. As with all exercises, exhale during the execution of the movement, and inhale as you return to your original starting position.
2. Do not do partial movements. Utilize the entire range of motion on this exercise.

Training Routine:
1. For strength use a heavier weight and perform three sets of 8 to 12 repetitions.
2. For endurance use a lighter weight and perform three to five sets of 15 to 20 repetitions per set.
3. Perform this exercise no more than 3 times per week.

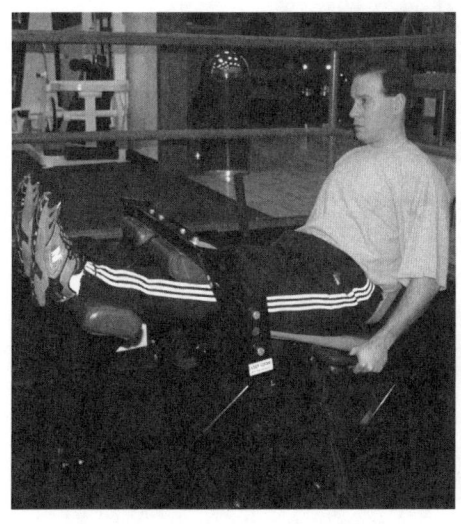

Starting & Finishing Position 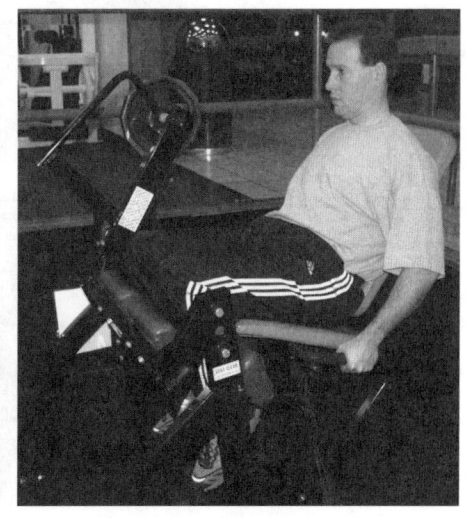   *Leg Curl Position*

Side-to-Side Squats:

This exercise, along with the variation using weights described on page 169, is perhaps the best overall leg exercise that you can do in order to improve the strength in your legs for kicking. Begin by standing with your feet approximately two to three shoulder widths apart, toes pointed out at a slight angle. Your hands can be either behind your head, or resting on your hips. Keep your back straight and your head up throughout the entire exercise. From this position, slowly squat down with one leg, allowing your knee to move outward in the same direction as your toes. At the same time contract your back muscles in order keep your body rigid as your perform this exercise. Slowly squat down until you are in a full side squat position with your squatting leg thigh parallel to the ground, and your non-squatting leg straight out to the side. Once you have reached the side squat position, slowly return to the starting position, and repeat this movement on the opposite side. Repeat this movement as often and as you safely can.

Remember:
1. Keep your back straight throughout the entire movement.
2. Focus your eyes on a spot at head level in order to help keep your head up.
3. Do not bounce at the bottom of the squat.
4. Do not squat lower than your thigh parallel with the floor.

Training Routine:
1. This is primarily an endurance building exercise and should be performed with a high number of repetitions (30 to 100) for several sets (3 to 10).
2. Perform this exercise no more than 3 times per week.

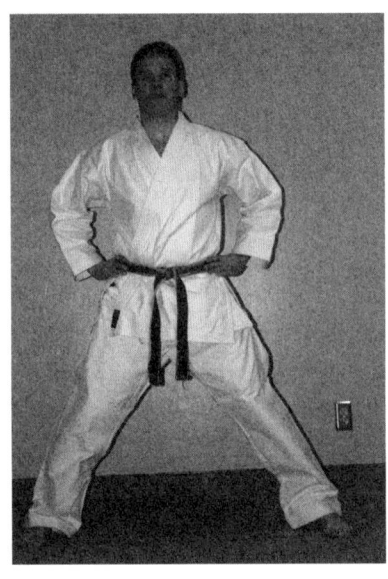

Starting & Finishing Position

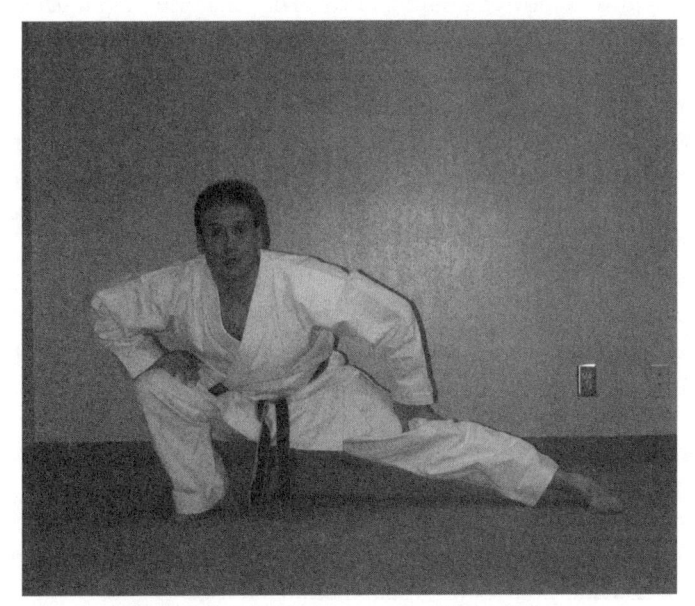

Side Squat Position to the Right Side

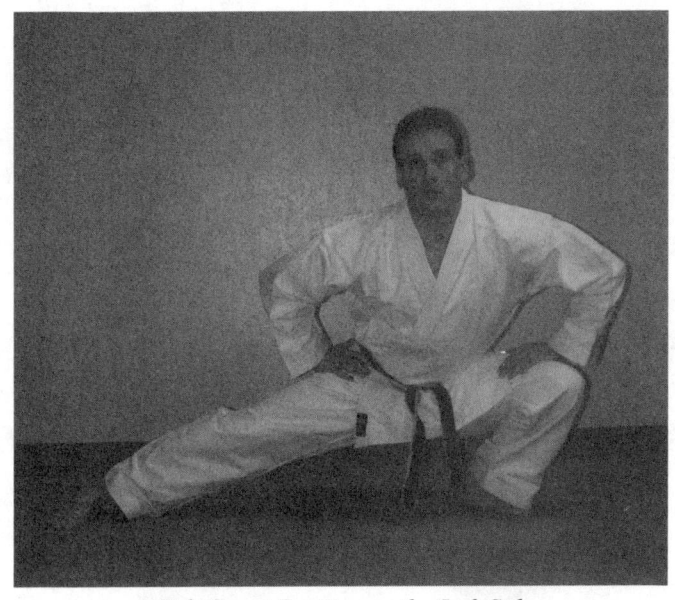

Side Squat Position to the Left Side

173

Plyometric Ski Jumps:

Plyometric ski jumps are without a doubt one of the best exercises to perform in order to add explosive power to your kicks. This exercise emphasizes all of the muscles of the leg to a certain degree, from the muscles of the foot all the way up to the gluteus maximus and lower back. When performing this or any other plyometric type exercise, you should exercise extreme caution due to the amount of stress that is placed on your body from these exercises. I would advise you to perform these exercises no more than two times per week, and to give yourself at least two days rest in between each plyometric training routine. Before you begin, make sure that the area around you is clear of any obstacles.

This exercise can be performed with or without shoes. Make sure that you are wearing gi bottoms or other loose fitting pants. Begin by standing with your feet approximately shoulders width apart and toes pointing slightly outward. Keeping your back straight, raise your hands up in front of you so that they are at shoulder level. From this position, jump up and to the side with both feet simultaneously bringing your knees up as high as possible, and your feet up underneath your buttocks, while jumping over the chosen obstacle, in this case, a weight bench. As soon as your knees reach their greatest height, straighten your legs back out as if you were reaching for the ground. When your feet hit the ground, only the balls of your feet should be touching the floor. Your knees should be slightly bent in order to absorb the impact. As soon as the balls of your feet hit the ground, jump up again and repeat the exercise. Repeat this movement as often and as safely as you can.

Remember:
1. Make sure that the area around you is free of any obstacles.
2. Focus your eyes on a spot at head level in order to help keep your head up.
3. Do not land with your legs locked or straight. Knees should be slightly bent.

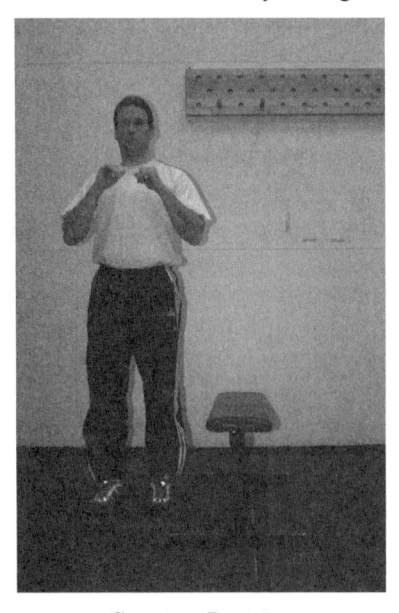

Starting Position　　　　　　　　　　*Coiling Position*

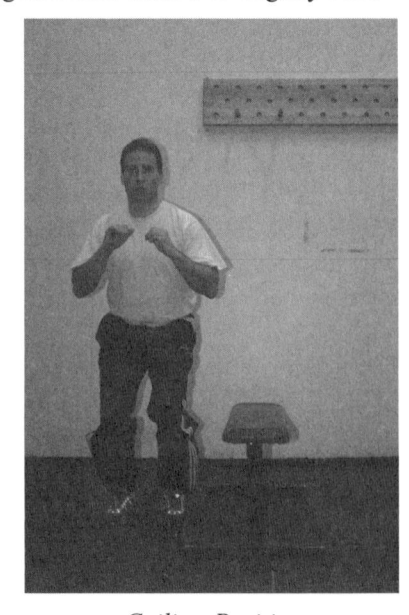

4. Your back should be kept as straight as possible at all times.
5. Do not pause between jumps.
6. Do not perform plyometric type exercises more than twice per week.

Training Routine:
1. Perform one set of 10 to 20 repetitions, no more than 2 times per week.
2. Work up to two sets of 20 to 50 repetitions, no more than 2 times per week.

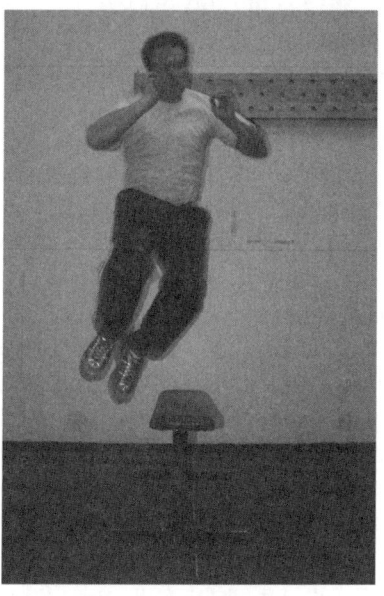

Mid-Jump Position

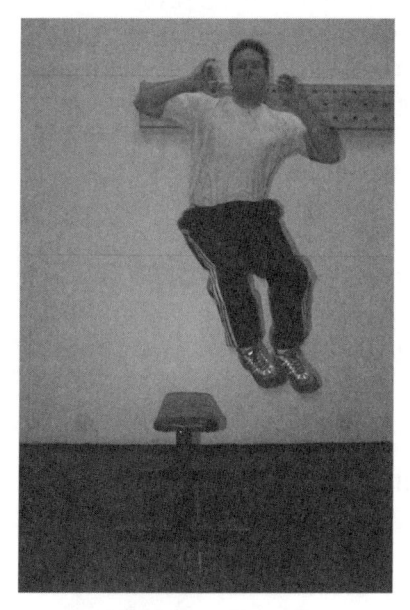

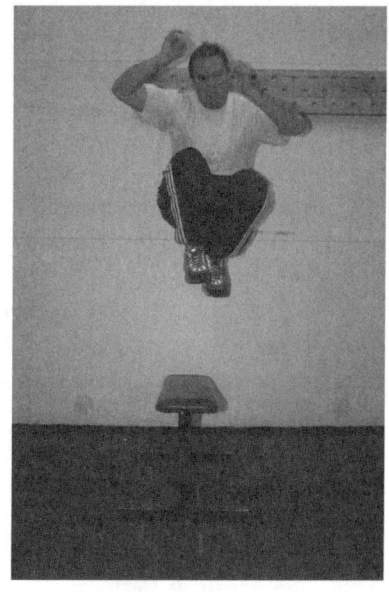

High Jump Position

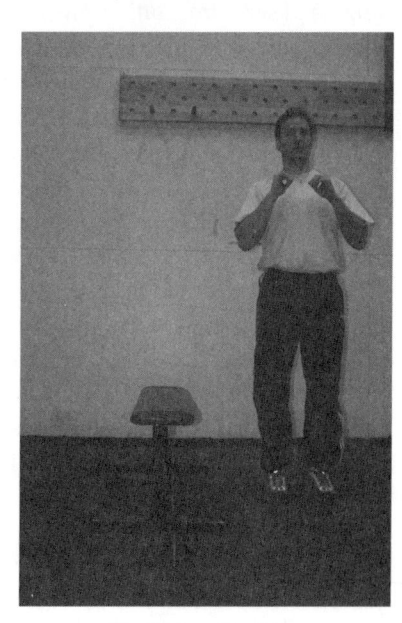

Midway to Ground

Finishing Position

Speed

The speed of your kicks during training should be at the same speed you plan to use during self-defense or during competition.

As I stated earlier in this section, how you practice and train in the dojo is how you will react in the ring or on the street.

The primary component of speed under pressure is not physical, but mental. Therefore, you must stay focused and concentrate.

Your mind controls your body; you must therefore keep control of your mind in order to perform at your optimum level.

If you think that you're slow, you will be slow. If however you believe that you can be faster, you will be faster.

Now let's take a look at some of my favorite speed training exercises that I use to increase the speed in my Wheel Kicks.

Ankle Weights:

This is my favorite piece of exercise equipment that I use in order to improve the speed of not only my Wheel Kicks, but all other kicks as well. Properly used ankle weights can improve your speed and hitting power in your legs as well as increasing muscular stamina. Improperly used however, they can cause a variety of injuries to the joints and connective tissues. This is not only detrimental to your body, but it also causes you to lose valuable training time. When practicing your kicks with ankle weights, you should make sure that they are securely fastened around your ankles and not loose. Start with 2 lbs. on each ankle and gradually build up the weight over time. Don't rush it. Perform your kicks no faster than 3/4 speed. Concentrate on technique and form. Remember that your legs will weaken faster utilizing the ankle weights. Therefore caution must be exercised so that you do not injure your knees or hips. Any kicking drill or exercise can be utilized with the ankle weights, with the notable exceptions of plyometric exercises and reactionary drills. I do not recommend using any kind of weight when performing plyometric exercises. These exercises are of such high intensity that no additional weight is needed. Reactionary drills require you to kick as fast as you can in response to an outside stimulus. Therefore ankle weights would be a hindrance rather than a benefit.

Quick Draw:

This is an excellent reactionary drill and requires the use of a training partner. I got the idea of this training method from watching western movies when I was a kid. Picture the following scene from any western movie.

The sheriff looks out the window of the saloon onto the dust-covered Main Street of town where the outlaw who killed his father stands waiting. A tied down six-gun slung low on his right thigh. The sheriff steps through the saloon doors and out onto the porch, his eyes never leaving the outlaw. He walks off the porch and out onto the street where he turns toward the outlaw. They stand facing each other from no more than 50 feet. Neither one moves. Suddenly the outlaw makes a move for his gun. BANG! The outlaw falls backward, dead, a .45 caliber bullet lodged in his brain. The sheriff holsters his Colt and walks back into the saloon.

Now you may be asking yourself how is this going to help your kicking skills. The answer is really quite simple. I have modified the classic western shoot out, or quick draw, by utilizing a training partner and your kicks instead of a Colt Peacemaker. Begin by having your training partner stand in front of you out of kicking range. You will be facing him in a fighting position. At your partner's discretion, he will make a prearranged movement, which will be the indicator for you to execute a kick as quickly as you can toward your partner. That indicator can be anything from a snapping of the fingers to the blinking of an eye. Use your imagination. Kicks can be performed one at a time, two or three at a time, using the same leg or alternating legs. Be creative and design your own unique routine. This exercise can also be utilized with a kicking paddle or force pad. However, extreme care must be utilized so that you do not accidentally miss your target and end up hitting your training partner. That doesn't seem to go over to well with training partners.

Water Training:

This particular training method requires a rather large piece of training equipment, a full-sized swimming pool. The deep end of the pool needs to be at least 6 feet deep in order for you to practice your kicks in mid-chest to shoulder deep water. This method of practicing your kicking technique is identical to the Wall Practice method, with the exception that there will be no chairs in which to kick over, as well as executing the primary kick and all of its variations in the air.

Start off by practicing your kicking technique at 1/4 speed until your kicking skills become easier and more natural. As you become progressively more efficient in your kicking skills, you will gradually increase your speed until you are performing your kicks at full speed. Even though you are practicing in the water, never sacrifice proper technique for speed or power.

It is imperative that you take all necessary precautions when practicing this technique. If at all possible, utilize this training method only with a training partner in case of any unforeseen accidents.

Proper Repetitive Practice:

Regardless of the activity, the more you practice the faster you will become, provided proper technique is maintained throughout the exercise. Notice the difference in the speed of your kick from the very first time you practice it, to the 1,000th time, the 5,000th time, the 10,000th time... Which one was faster?

Power

Force = Mass x Acceleration

In other words, the faster you are, multiplied by the greatest amount of muscular mass that you can generate behind your kick, equals striking power. Now let's take a look at my two favorite pieces of training equipment that I utilize in order to improve my kicking power when executing the Wheel Kick. They are the force bag (hand held kicking shield) and the kicking paddle.

Force Bag:

The force bag or kicking shield is a hand held pad or bag, that is usually made out of vinyl or leather with a foam filled core. There are usually two sets of handles located on the bag, two on the back portion of the bag, and one on each side of the bag. If utilized correctly, these bags are invaluable as training aids in order to increase the speed and power in your Wheel Kicks.

Begin by having your bag holder grasp the handles located on the sides of the bag. He should hold the bag straight out in front of him (one arm above the other), and perpendicular to the ground, with the bottom of the force bag at shoulder height. He should position himself in a parallel stance with his legs about one and a half to two shoulder widths apart. As the kicker, you want to aim your kicks about 4 inches in from the closest edge of the bag, and at the level of the vulnerable points you are striking at. At all times you must be extremely careful when kicking so that you do not accidentally kick your training partner. They tend to get a little grouchy when kicked.

As the bag holder, you do not want to get in the habit of being just a bag holder. Utilize this time to improve your defensive skills by relaxing your body the entire time until just before the moment of impact. Make sure that the bottom edge of the bag is perpendicular to the ground and facing directly at the kicker. It should not be at an angle. You can utilize any kicking routine you can think of with the force bag. You can practice single kicks, multiple kicks (one leg at a time or alternating legs), the Quick Draw method, etc. You are only limited by your own imagination.

Kicking Paddle:

The kicking paddle is a very versatile piece of training equipment that, when utilized correctly, can help improve not only the power in your Wheel Kick, but also your accuracy, speed, timing, and footwork. Another benefit of training with the kicking paddle is to help you to improve your ability to obtain and maintain the correct kicking distance between you and your opponent. Because it offers so much versatility in your training routine, the kicking paddle can also be used to simulate the offensive and defensive movements of an actual opponent.

You can utilize full force Wheel Kicks on the kicking paddles without worrying about damaging them. However, when using the kicking paddle or any other piece of training equipment, you must exercise caution so that you don't inadvertently hurt yourself by hyper-extending your knee, twisting an ankle, etc., or hurting your training partner by inadvertently hitting him or her. This is why the kicking paddle consists of the handle and the separate target area. Strike the target area when kicking, not the hands of your training partner. There are numerous routines, which you can utilize when working with the kicking paddle. Some of the routines I utilize in order to improve my Wheel Kicks are exactly the same as those utilized when kicking the force bag. While other routines are designed to simulate actual sparring conditions.

Running:

Running is a must for anyone who is serious about self-defense or competition. I will not go into any details about running itself other than to say that it should be an essential part of any martial artists training program. There are several good books on running available, and any one of them would be an invaluable addition to your library.

Running Stairs:

In addition to regular running, running stairs is an excellent method of building the muscles in the legs while at the same time building up your aerobic capacity and endurance. However, extreme caution must be exercised at all times to avoid injuring yourself while performing this or any exercise described in this book.

Relaxation and Tension:

Muscle contractions used during training should duplicate those used in self-defense or competition.

If you do not utilize the proper tension and relaxation principles in the dojo when kicking, you will not use them correctly on the street or in the ring. This principle is very simple yet seems to be very difficult for individuals to follow. Physiologically speaking a relaxed muscle is able to react faster than a tense muscle. Therefore you want to remain as relaxed as possible from the time you initiate your kick until just before the moment of impact. At this point your entire body should tighten up to add power to your kick. Immediately after the moment of impact, your muscles should once again relax in order to recoil as quickly as possible from your target. I have found that the best method for practicing this technique is to perform the wall method, which I described earlier in this section. Perform this technique slowly and concentrate on proper technique while remaining totally relaxed throughout the kicking process until just before the moment of impact. At this point tighten all of the muscles in your body and hold them that way for just an instant. Remember once impact has been made, relax immediately and recoil your kicking leg.

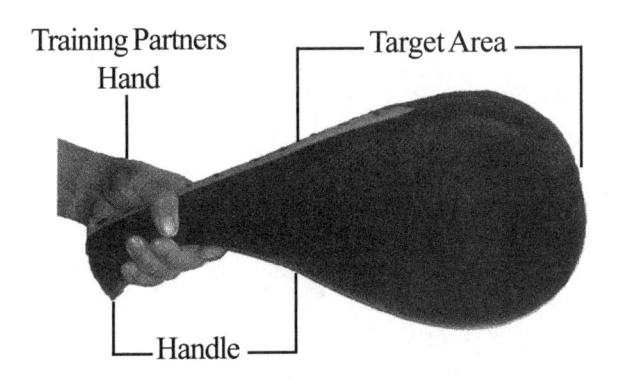

Kicking Paddle

Trouble Shooting Guide

In this chapter I will present some of the most common questions concerning mistakes that I have encountered from students when attempting to perform the Turning Wheel Kick or any one of its many variations. I will then attempt to provide a generalized answer to each of those questions. Although one must keep in mind that there is no way to provide the appropriate answer to each person without actually seeing him or her perform the kick in person. When you have a problem, always refer back to the instruction section that covers that particular movement in which you are having a problem. One of my instructors once imparted upon me a small piece of wisdom that I would now like to share with you concerning mistakes. "If you suddenly find yourself making mistakes, go back to the beginning". In other words, you can never practice or study the basic techniques enough, for they are the foundation in which all other techniques are based.

Why do I always seem to be hitting with the wrong part of my foot?
This is usually caused by one of three things. (1) You are not bringing your toes back and towards your shin exposing the back of your heel as the striking surface. This happens quite often when one tries to "reach" for the target, rather than having already created the proper striking distance prior to executing the kick. (2) Or, as I briefly mentioned in number one, you may even be too far away from your opponent and trying to "reach" for the target by extending your kicking foot towards your opponent, which would result in a strike with the toes or ball of your foot instead of the back of the heel. (3) You are too close to your opponent prior to executing the Wheel Kick and you end up striking your opponent with the back of your calf or Achille's heel, rather than the back of the heel. Remember to always create the proper striking distance before you execute your kick, not during the execution of the kick.

Why do I always seem to be hitting low every time I kick?
This particular problem is almost exclusively caused by one of three things, or a combination thereof. (1) You are attempting to kick from the ground in a "swooping" motion rather than having your kicking leg and foot follow the correct "Path of Trajectory." (2) You may not be leaning your body slightly backwards over your non-kicking leg during the execution of your Wheel Kick. (3) You may need to spend more time working on your flexibility.

Every time I try and use a Wheel Kick with a training partner, they always seem to see it coming and move out of the way!
This particular problem can be related not only to improper technique, but also to the inappropriate use of the Wheel Kick. Let's look at technique first. (1) You may not be turning fast enough prior to the execution of the technique, or you may be making some unconscious body movement prior to executing the kick, and therefore are telegraphing your intentions to you opponent. (2) Another possible problem

is that you may not yet have the entire sequence of movements flowing together to where they all are one continuous motion. You may be pausing during the execution of the kick and not be aware of it. The best way to correct both of these problems is to practice in front of a mirror. (3) The other possibility is that your technique is fine, but your application of the kick is incorrect. Are you attempting to use the Wheel Kick as your initial technique? Or as a finishing technique? Remember, that for the most part, the Wheel Kick is a finishing technique rather than an initial technique, although it can effectively be used in both instances. Try limiting your use of the kick when sparring and always try and set up the Wheel Kick by utilizing another technique before executing it. Whether it is another kick, punch or even simply footwork.

My Wheel Kick always seems to glance off the target whether it's in a tournament or in the dojo!
This problem is generally caused by one of two things. (1) You may not be pivoting enough, or perhaps too much, prior to executing your kick. Remember that the Wheel Kick (with the exception of Front Leg and Back Leg Wheel Kick), utilizes a "360-degree" circular "Path of Trajectory" during its execution rather than a straight line of trajectory. Therefore, you may not be striking your target at the appropriate point in your "360-degree" circular delivery of the kick. (2) Your primary target area is the head of your opponent which, (a) offers a lot smaller target area than the body and is circular in nature, (b) is located at the furthest and highest point from your kicking foot, and (c) is capable of a wide range of movement making it a difficult target to hit. Always, remember this old boxing adage, "Kill the body, and the head will follow."

Why do my Wheel Kicks miss the target more times than they hit it?
The most common solution to this problem is that you have to make sure that you are creating the correct distance between you and your opponent prior to executing the kick. Another possibility may be that you need to slow your kicks down and emphasize accuaracy over speed and power.

Why does my Wheel Kick slow down or sometimes stop all together after striking my target?
This can most often be attributed to a person hitting with a "surface" strike on his opponent, rather than "striking through" his opponent. In order to correct this you need to work on three primary areas. (1) A faster "Follow Through" with the kicking leg after impact. (2) A faster pivoting on the ball of the base leg foot after impact, and (3) Practicing the tension and relaxation movements before, during and after impact.

Why do I lose my balance every time I kick?
There are several possible reasons for this. (1) You may not be keeping your head up and looking over your kicking leg shoulder while executing the kick. (2) You may be attempting to imitate a bird by waving your arms all over the place instead of

having them in control and next to your body. (3) Your center of gravity may not be over your base leg. (4) Over-extending or "reaching" with the kicking leg. (5) Leaning to far backward with your upper body during the execution of the kick. (6) Not keeping your eyes focused on your opponent throughout the entire 360-degree circular motion.

How come I just can't seem to get any power into my Wheel Kick?

Power in a Wheel Kick is generated by the correct execution of all phases of the kick. The most important being proper technique. For arguments sake, let us assume (and you know what happens when you make an assumption) that you are performing all of the "movement" phases of the kick correctly. I would then have to say that you are probably not performing the tension and relaxation portion of the kick correctly, as this is the most difficult aspect of the kick to perform correctly. Remember that the entire body should be in a relaxed state throughout the entire execution of the kick, except immediately before impact. When the entire body should turn into a solid, rigid mass to support and add power to the kick, and then immediately relax again to add speed to the "Follow Through." Remember, that this is a 360-degree circular kick, your foot does not stop once it hits the target, it explodes through the target and continues along its "Path of Trajectory" until it returns to its original starting position.

Why is my Wheel Kick so slow?

Anything is slow the first few hundred or even a thousand times you do them. Speed is not important to learning, be patient and practice until the kick becomes instinctive in nature. After you become comfortable with the execution of the kick, then you can gradually add more speed when executing it. If you are still experiencing a slow kick, you may be too tense when executing the kick and this will greatly decrease your speed. Another potential problem could be that you "see" yourself as being slow. If you want to be fast, think fast!

I can do a Turning Wheel Kick fairly well, but when it comes to some of the other Wheel Kicks, I always seem to have problems!

The important thing to remember here is that all of the Wheel Kick variations are based on the primary kick, Turning Wheel Kick. If you are executing the Turning Wheel Kick correctly, then you need to focus more of your attention on not only the additional moves associated with each particular variation, but also in the ability to flow in one continuous motion from the additional portion of each particular Wheel Kick variation, to the Turning Wheel Kick itself.

Remember that often times we are unable to see clearly are own mistakes. That is why a qualified and competent instructor, and a good training partner is so vitally important to your martial arts training.

Wheel Kick Applications

In this chapter, I will discuss some of the basic applications for the Turning Wheel Kick and the ten variations discussed in this book. Please keep in mind that the numerous applications of each kick could fill an entire book. Therefore I will limit this section to one application per kick. A second series of books detailing the combat and tournament applications of each kick is in the works and will be published following the release of this ten volume series. Keep in mind that the photographs in this section are staged in order to give you the best possible view of each technique in order to help you learn from them. The actual execution of any of these kicks should be one continuous motion and should be executed instantaneously without thought. My assistant and I have intentionally made some errors that can be seen in some of these photographs in order to help you correct some common mistakes. See if you can spot them before I tell you them at the end of each kicking application.

For reference purposes, Ron Dunlap will be the attacker, while I will be the defender in this series of photographs. Ron is wearing a black uniform, while I am wearing a white uniform.

Turning Wheel Kick:

1. You and your opponent are facing each other in what is commonly referred to as a Closed Position, meaning that each of you has your left leg forward and the front of your bodies facing in different directions. In this case, the front of Ron's body is basically facing toward the camera, while the front of my body is facing away from the camera.

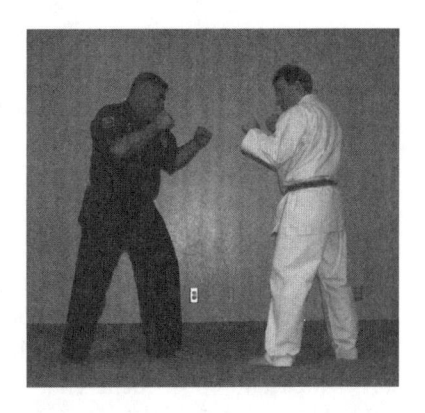

2. Your opponent starts to move forward in an attempt to deliver a punch to your head with his left hand. Notice how his weight shifts over his left leg as he moves forward. As soon as you sense a committed movement from your opponent, begin to execute your kick. Remember to protect yourself at all times and not to telegraph your intentions to your attacker.

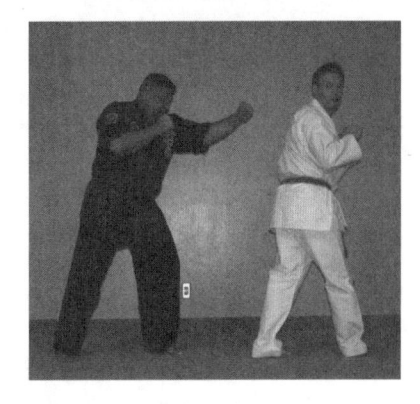

3. As you start to bring your leg up after you have first initiated your turn, you will start to bend over slightly at the waist. This has the added benefit of moving your upper body away from your opponents attack. Remember that all of these movements should be done instantaneously without thought and in one fluid motion.

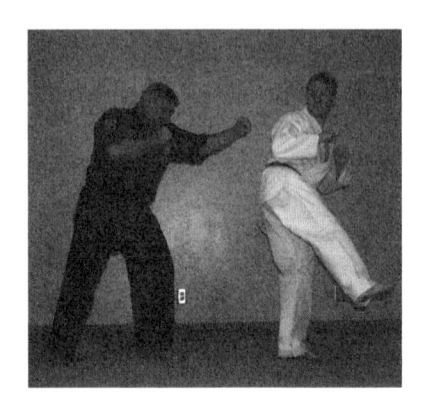

4. Execute the kick. Ideally you want to strike your opponent when he is midway through his committed technique. As seen in this picture. Notice how his weight is still shifted over his left leg while moving forward. This not only weakens his stance, but it also increases the impact effectiveness of your kick. Always keep in mind that your kick does not end upon striking the target, but when your foot has returned back to the ground, after going through your target..

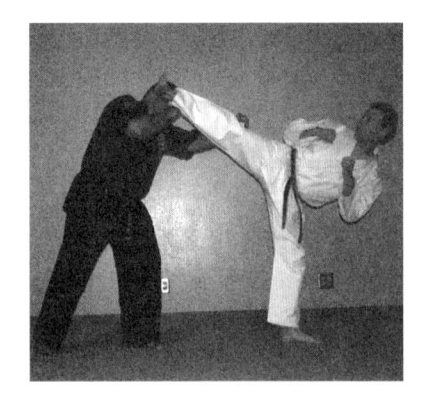

Did you notice anything wrong or improper in this series of photographs? Take another look. See them now?

Look at photograph number four; although the picture is small, pay particular attention to where I struck Ron with my foot. Rather then striking Ron in a particular target area and subsequent vital point, I struck Ron on the side of his head and behind his ear. Admittedly, striking this area will hurt, but my kick is no where near as effective as it would have been had I struck a vital point. Also, did you notice the position of my base leg foot in photograph number four? See how my heel is pointed at Ron, instead of the inside edge of my foot. This improper foot position not only causes a dramatic decrease in the effectiveness of my kick, but it is also prevents me from having an effective and speedy "Follow Through" after striking through my target. The results of this can be very disastrous to you. If you notice Ron's hand position, he can easily grab my kicking leg and put me in a world of hurt. That is why it is so imperative to correctly execute all phases of your kick in order to minimize the risks to you, and to maximize the effectiveness of your kick upon your opponent.

Improper pivoting on the base foot when kicking, especially on turning and spinning kicks, is the number one cause of knee and hip injuries for martial artists. Train hard, but train smart!

Front Leg Wheel Kick:

1. You and your opponent are facing each other in what is commonly referred to as an Open Position, meaning that Ron and I both have the front of our bodies facing the same direction. In this case, the front of both Ron and I's bodies are basically facing towards the camera.

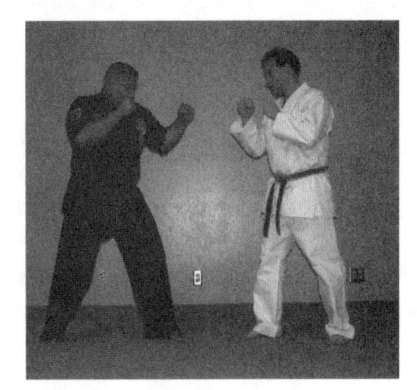

2. Sensing his impending attack, you begin to execute the kick. Remember to maintain eye contact with your attacker.

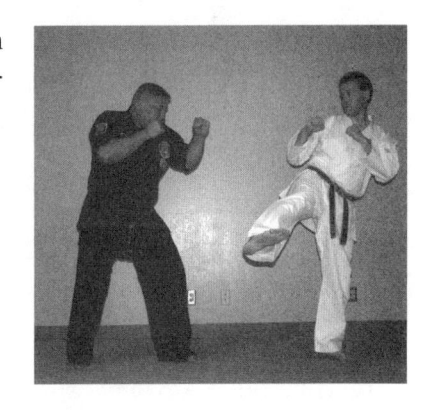

3. Execute the kick. Once again you want to strike your opponent when he is midway through his committed technique. Or as seen in this example, before he even initiates it. Notice how the leaning over of the body during the execution of the kick increases the distance between your head and upper body, and your opponents intended attack. However, now your kicking leg is the closest part of you to your opponent, and the easiest for him to reach. Remember, don't leave your leg in the air or your opponent will grab it!

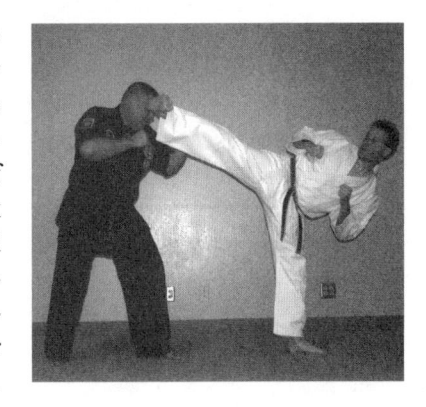

Did you notice anything wrong or improper in this series of photographs?

Take another look. See them now?

Look at photograph number three; once again, notice how my base leg foot is not in the correct position as my kicking foot initially strikes my opponent. I can not stress enough the utmost importance of correctly pivoting on the base leg foot throughout the entire execution of not only a Wheel Kick, but **all other kicks as well**. Although this may seem like a minor detail, it is very important to the overall effectiveness of your kick. No matter how you add it up, ninety-nine pennies do not add up to one dollar. All aspects of a properly executed kick are much like pennies in a dollar. Every one of the one hundred pennies must be present in order to have a complete dollar, just like every aspect of a kick must be performed correctly in order to have a proper kick.

Switch Wheel Kick:

1. Once again, you and your opponent are facing each other in an Open Position. Your opponent begins to throw a punch with his left hand towards your head.

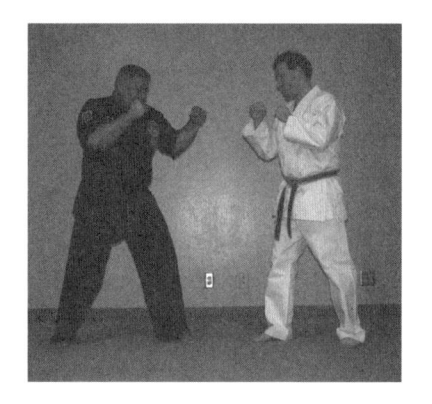

2. As you sense your opponent's impending attack, you switch your feet utilizing a scissors type motion, which now puts you and your opponent into a Closed Position.

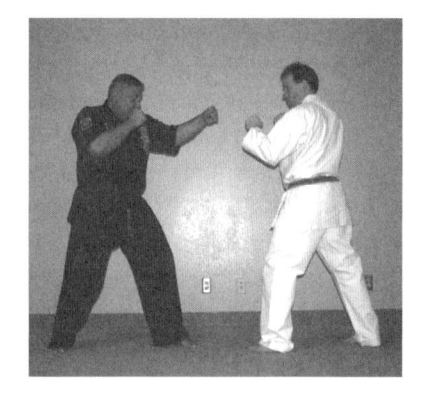

3. Begin to execute the kick. Remember to maintain eye contact with your opponent.

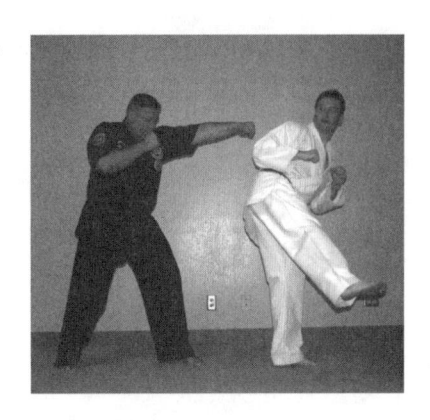

4. Execute the kick.

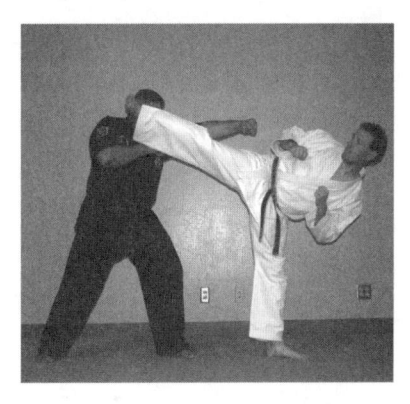

Did you notice anything wrong or improper in this series of photographs? Take another look. See them now?

Look at photograph number two; ideally I should have already struck Ron with my Wheel Kick instead of just switching my feet as seen in this photograph. The best time to strike your opponent is when he is midway through his committed technique, or just before he initiates it. If you look at photograph number three; you see that Ron has already full extended his punch, and yet my back is still turned towards him with my kicking foot barely off the ground. This is way too slow on my part, and I have left myself in an extremely vulnerable position! Now if you look at photograph number four; it may look like a perfectly executed kick. However, if you look closely, you will see that I have struck Ron not with the back of my heel, but with the back of my Achilles Tendon and calf muscle. Not exactly the preferred striking implement with any kick, let alone the Wheel Kick. **Always** strike the target area on your opponent with the correct striking implement. This not only maximizes the effectiveness of your kick, but it also minimizes the possibility of injury to you.

Remember that when executing the Switch Wheel Kick, the actual switch and kick is performed as a single fluid movement. However, you can separate the two techniques in order to confuse your opponent. If you do this, you are actually executing a switching of your feet followed by a Turning Wheel Kick, not a Switch Wheel Kick. They may look the same, but they aren't.

Off-Setting Wheel Kick:

1. You and your opponent are facing each other in a Closed Position. In this case, the front of my body is basically facing toward the camera, while the front of Ron's body is facing away from the camera.

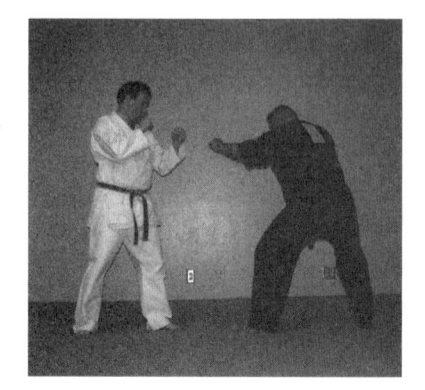

2. Your opponent begins to initiate his attack.

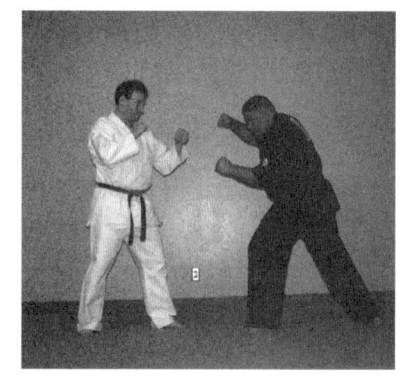

3. As you sense your opponent's impending attack, you begin to offset his attack by moving your right foot to the right and at a 45-degree angle to your opponent. Which you immediately follow with...

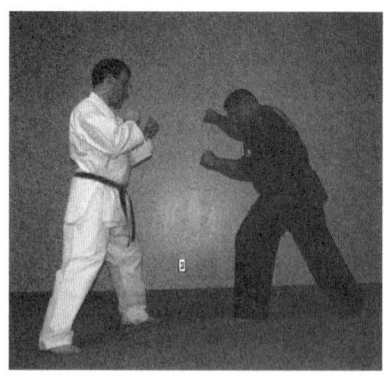

4. ...moving your left leg to the right, which will effectively move your body out of the line of attack. Remember to keep your hands up and protect yourself at all times. Don't get lazy! As soon as your left foot moves into position...

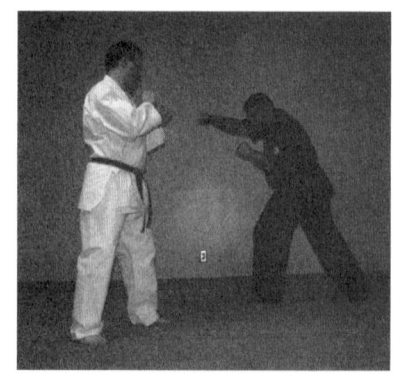

5. ...begin to execute the kick. Remember to maintain eye contact with your attacker at all times.

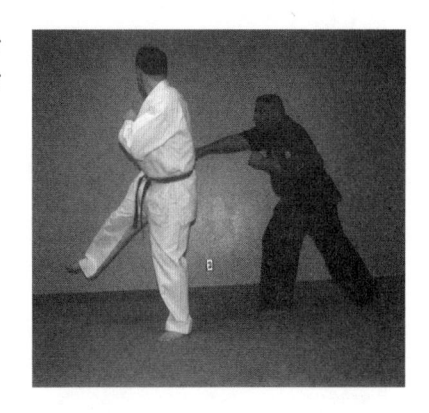

6. Execute the kick. Ideally you want to strike your attacker while he is off balance. As seen in this picture. Notice how Ron's body is leaning too far forward, while his entire body weight is over his left leg. Not only is this position very unstable, but it also leaves Ron very vulnerable to attack. Bad for Ron, but great for me! This kick would have been even more effective if I had my base leg foot in the proper position.

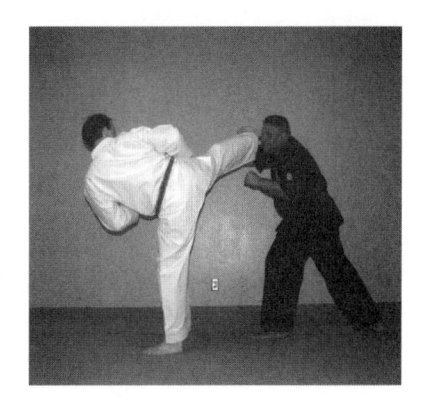

Did you notice anything wrong or improper in this series of photographs? Take another look. See them now?

If you look closely at photograph number two; you will see that Ron has already initiated his attack, yet I still haven't moved in response to his attack. **This is not only incorrect, but also very dangerous!** As soon as I sensed Ron's impending attack, in photograph number one, I should have off-set immediately as I have demonstrated in photograph number four. Now look closely at photographs number three, four, and five; in photographs number three and four, I still have not begun to execute my kick, even though I have already off-set Ron, who's punch is almost at full extension. Now when you take a look at photograph number five; you see Ron's punch at full extension and I have just turned and begun my Wheel Kick.

The position of my body in photograph number five, should actually be in photograph number three, while the execution of the kick depicted in photograph number six should actually be in photograph number four.

This response from me in this series of photographs is so slow, that Ron could almost sit down at a table and enjoy a healthy lunch before my kick would come anywhere near him. You must constantly strive to have your kicks so fast, that neither you nor your opponent knows that you have thrown the kick, until after it strikes your opponent.

Back Leg Wheel Kick:

1. You and your opponent are facing each other in a Closed Position.

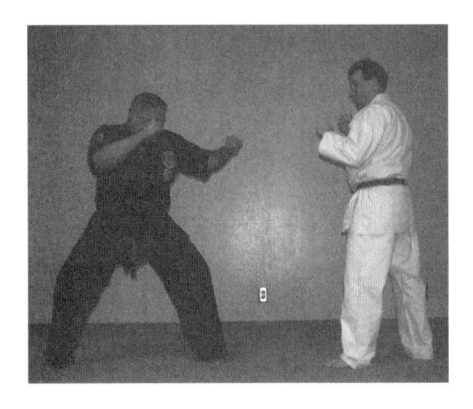

2. Sensing your opponent's impending attack, you begin to initiate your kick by bringing your leg in front of, and across your body.

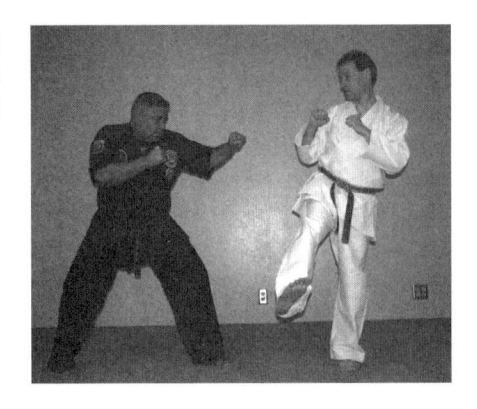

3. Execute the kick.

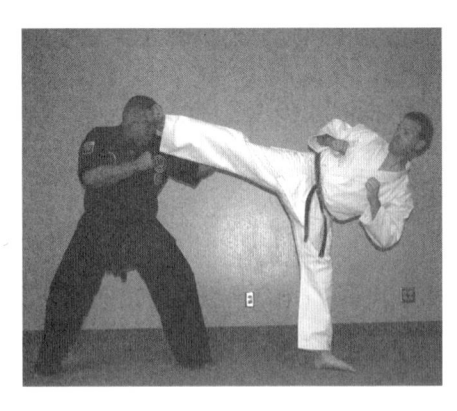

Did you notice anything wrong or improper in this series of photographs? Take another look. See them now?

If you look closely in photograph number three; you will see that once again my base leg foot is in the improper position upon impact with my opponent. As I have stated before, improper pivoting on the ball of the base leg foot when kicking, is the single greatest cause of knee and hip injuries. **Always utilize proper technique when executing your kicks!** This can not be stressed enough!

Step-Back Wheel Kick:

1. You and your opponent are facing each other in an Open Position. As you can see in this photograph, Ron and I are too close together for me to effectively execute a Wheel Kick. Although, we are in effective punching range. Ron begins to initiate his attack.

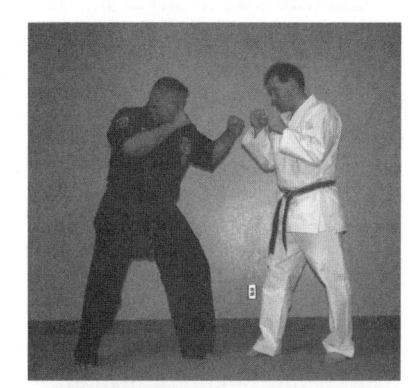

2. Keeping your hand up, step back with your kicking leg. This will increase the distance between you and your opponent, which will allow you the opportunity to execute your kick. As soon as your kicking leg steps back…

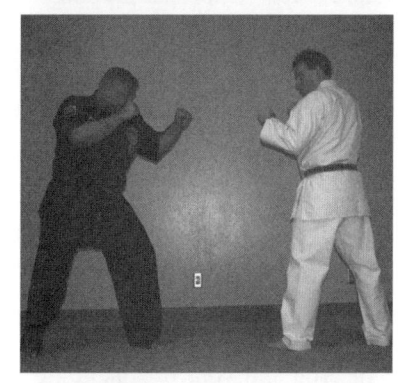

3. …begin to execute the kick. Remember that you never want to sacrifice technique for speed.

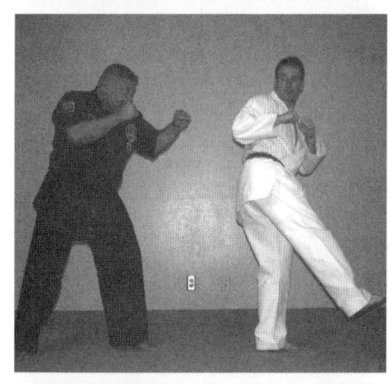

4. Execute the kick.

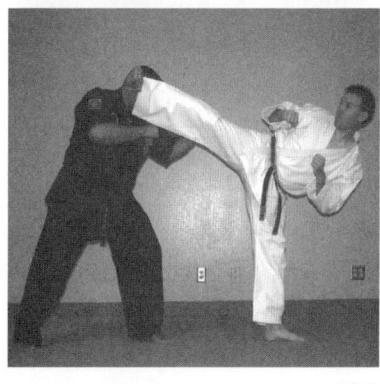

Did you notice anything wrong or improper in this series of photographs? Take another look. See them now?

Take a look at photograph number four; if you look closely, you can see that I struck Ron with my Achille's Tendon and the back of my calf muscle rather than the back of my heel. This is incorrect! No matter how perfectly you execute your kick, if you strike your intended target with the wrong part of your foot, or in this case your leg, you are going to have a far less effective kick. **You should constantly strive to improve the accuracy of your kicks until you can hit an area the size of a dime, with the correct part of your foot, every time you kick.**

Now look at the position of my base leg foot, you will see that once again my base leg foot is in the improper position upon impact with my opponent. As I have stated before, improper pivoting on the ball of the base leg foot when kicking, is not only the single greatest cause of knee and hip injuries, but it is also the single biggest mistake that is made when executing any kick, not just a Wheel Kick. **Always utilize proper technique when executing your kicks!** This can not be stressed enough!

Spinning Wheel Kick:
1. You and your opponent are facing each other in a Closed Stance.

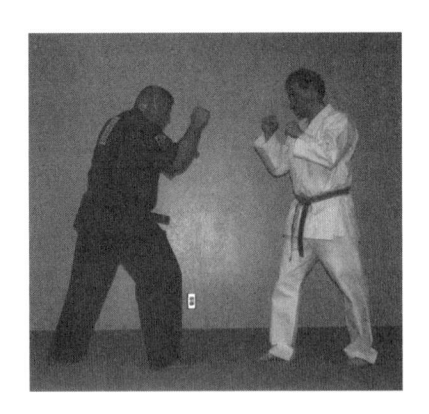

2. Your opponent steps back creating an Open Position, and increasing the distance between you and him.

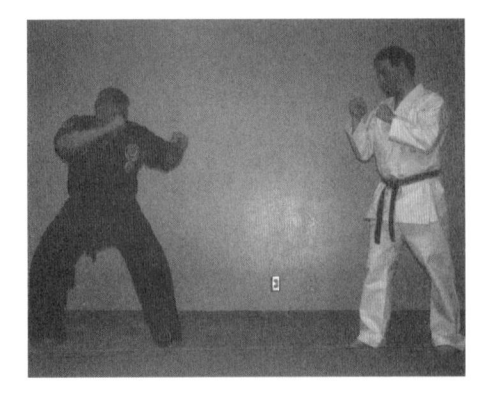

3. You step forward in order to close the distance, which will enable you to execute your kick. As soon as you step down with your foot, you should begin turning in order to execute a Wheel Kick.

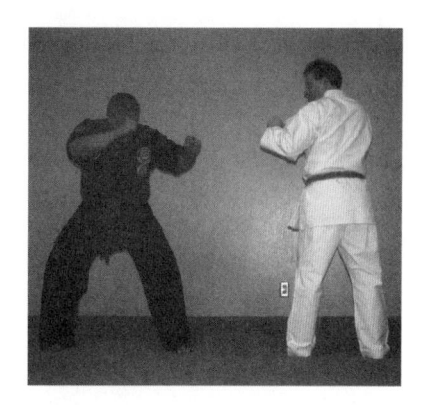

4. Begin to execute the kick.

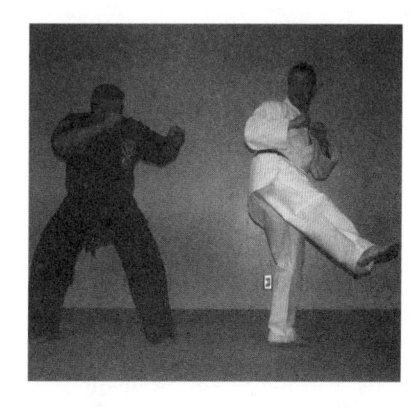

5. Execute the kick.

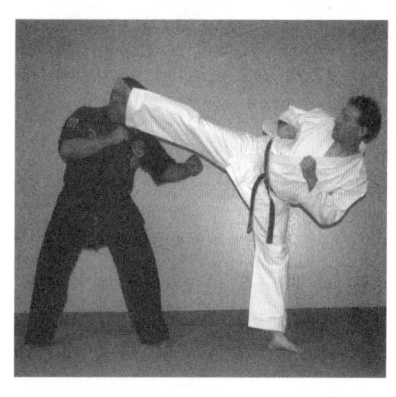

Did you notice anything wrong or improper in this series of photographs? Take another look. See them now?

If you look closely at photograph number two; you can see that I have not changed positions, even though Ron has moved away from me. As Ron moved back, I should have moved forward with him. Now take a look at photograph number five; once again I have pivoted improperly on the ball of my base leg foot during the "Impact" phase of this kick. I am saying it again, improper pivoting on the ball of the base leg foot when kicking, is not only the single greatest cause of knee and hip injuries, but it is also the single biggest mistake that is made when kicking.

Hopping/Sliding Forward Wheel Kick:

1. You and your opponent are facing each other in a Closed Position. However, at the moment, your opponent is just out of kicking range.

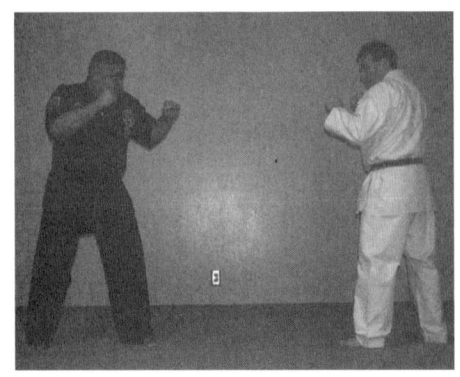

2. You begin to hop/slide forward in preparation for executing your kick. You can cover anywhere from a few inches to two feet with a correctly executed hop or slide. The exact distance will vary from application to application, but one factor remains. You must be exact in judging the correct distance or your kick will not attain its maximum effectiveness.

3. After you hop/slide forward, turn and begin to execute the kick.

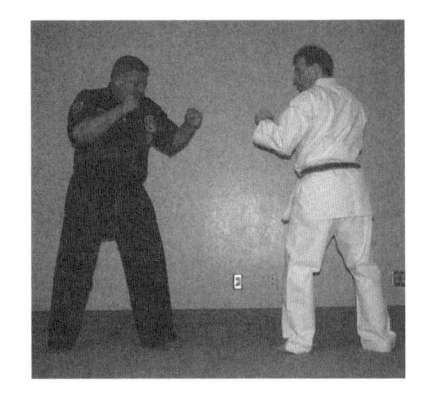

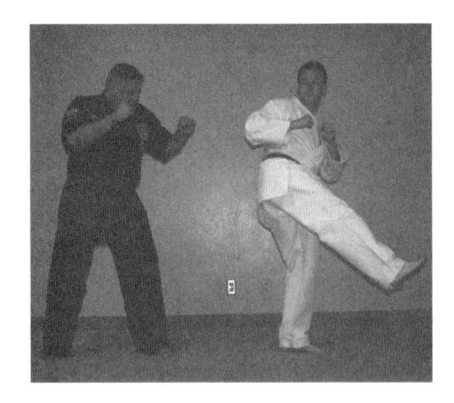

Note: When executing any circular kicks, such as a Wheel Kick, you want to make sure that you hop/slide prior to beginning the execution of your kick. Do not attempt to begin executing your kick and then hopping/sliding either forward or backward. It is not effective and is potentially very dangerous. The only time you can hop/slide either forward or backward after beginning to execute your kick, is when executing a straight line kick, such as a Back Kick.

4. Execute the kick.

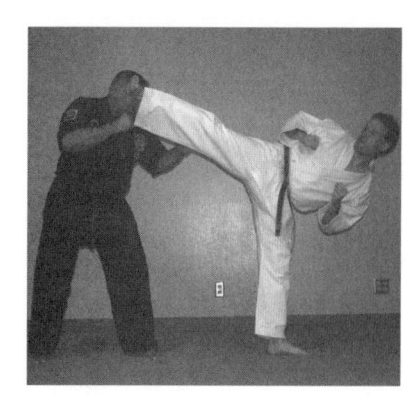

Did you notice anything wrong or improper in this series of photographs? Take another look. See them now?

Look closely at photograph number four; notice how once again, my base leg foot is in the wrong position upon impact with my target. I can not stress enough the importance of pivoting on the ball of your base foot correctly throughout the entire execution of not only a Wheel Kick, but all other kicks as well.

Remember, the number one cause of knee and hip injuries when kicking, is the improper pivoting on the ball of the base leg foot.

Hopping/Sliding Backward Wheel Kick:

1. You and your opponent are facing each other in a Closed Position. However at the moment your opponent is too close to you.

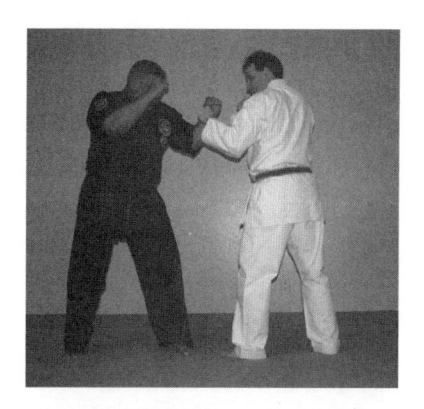

2. Hop/slide backward just enough to put you into an effective kicking range. As with the Hop/Slide Forward Wheel Kick, you can cover anywhere from a few inches to two feet with a correctly executed hop or slide. The exact distance will vary from application to application, but one factor remains. You must be exact in judging the correct distance or your kick will not attain its maximum effectiveness.

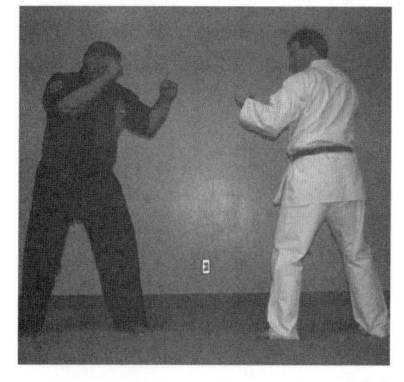

3. Immediately after hopping or sliding backward, turn and begin to execute your kick.

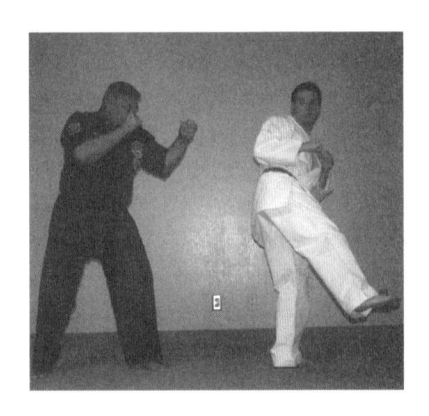

4. Execute the kick.

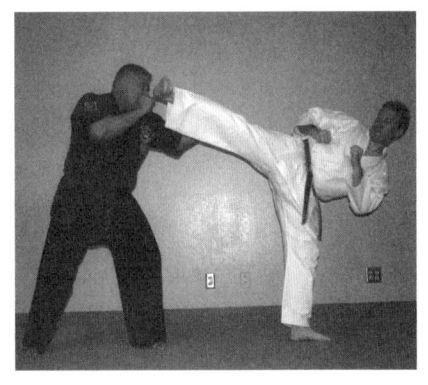

Did you notice anything wrong or improper in this series of photographs? Take another look. See them now?

First look closely at photograph number two; I misjudged the distance between Ron and I when I utilized the hop/slide backward movement. Remember, you have to be able to create the correct kicking distance between yourself and your opponent by adjusting your hop/slide backward (or forward), from a few inches up to 2 feet. This will come into play in a big way in just a moment. Now lets take a look at photograph number four; there are two big mistakes made in this photograph. Number one, is the obvious fact that I have missed Ron entirely with my kick due to the incorrect distance created in photograph number two when I utilized the hop/slide motion. And finally, number two; once again I have pivoted incorrectly on the ball of my base leg foot, resulting in my base leg foot being in the incorrect position during the moment of impact with my target.

Perhaps the best way to get my point across on this matter is through the use of an analogy. Imagine that your lower leg from the knee down is a pop bottle, with your knee being the bottle cap, and the rest of your body from the knee up is a hand on the bottle cap. Now if the bottle moves along with the twisting action of the hand on the bottle cap, what happens? Absolutely nothing! Now if the other hand grasps the bottom of the bottle and holds it firmly in place while the other hand twists on the bottle cap, what happens? The bottle cap twists right off the bottle, so will your knee!

Jump Turning Wheel Kick:

1. You and your opponent are facing each other in a Open Position.

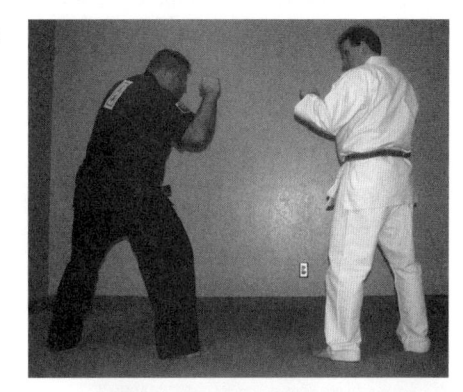

2. As your opponent starts to initiate his attack, you jump straight up into the air.

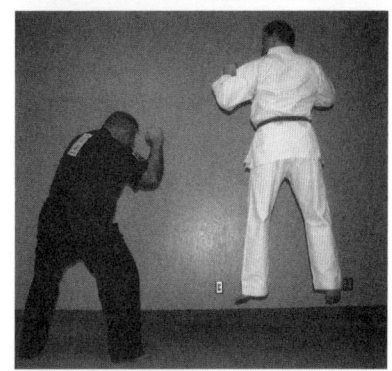

3. While you are jumping up into the air, you start to turn, bringing your kicking leg around in preparation for executing your kick.

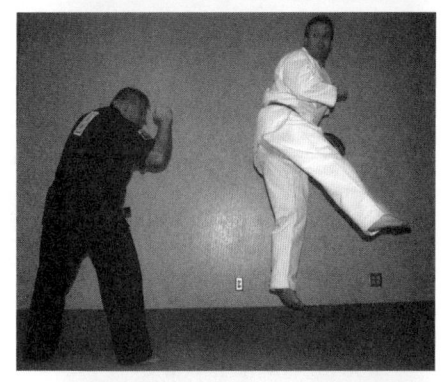

4. Ideally you would execute the kick at the peak of your jump while still in the air. However most individuals seem to strike their opponent when their non-kicking foot is already back down on the ground. This is not correct. Even though you may be proficient in kicking while one foot remains on the ground, that does not mean that you will automatically transfer

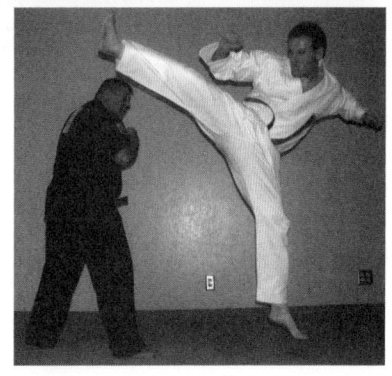

that skill over to the execution of aerial kicks. Aerial kicking is an art form unto itself and needs to be practiced diligently.

Did you notice anything wrong or improper in this series of photographs? Take another look. See them now?

In photograph number four I have committed perhaps one of the biggest mistakes made when executing this type of aerial kick, kicking over the opponents head rather than correctly kicking the selected vulnerable point within a specific target area. When executed correctly, and at the proper time, aerial kicking can be a very effective technique to have in your kicking arsenal.

540 Degree Jumping Wheel Kick:

1. You and your opponent are facing each other in an Closed Position.

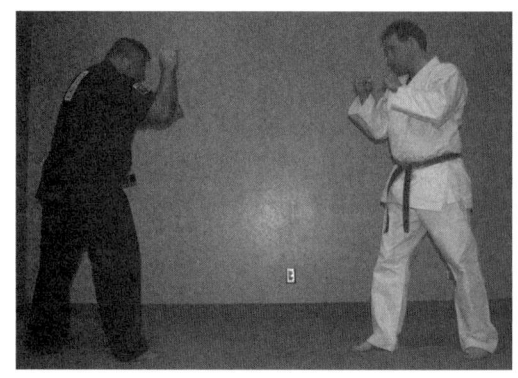

2. Bring your back leg knee up and around as if you were preparing to throw a Roundhouse Kick at your opponent.

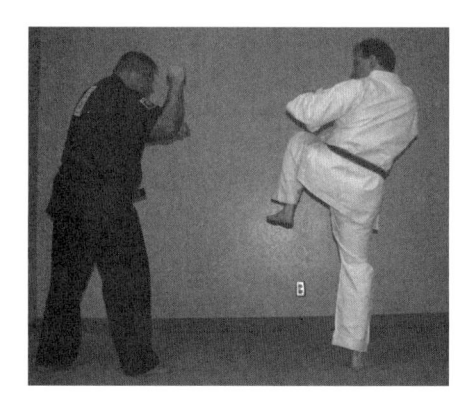

3. As your knee comes around to the front of your body, jump up and turn, bringing your kicking leg around in preparation for executing your kick.

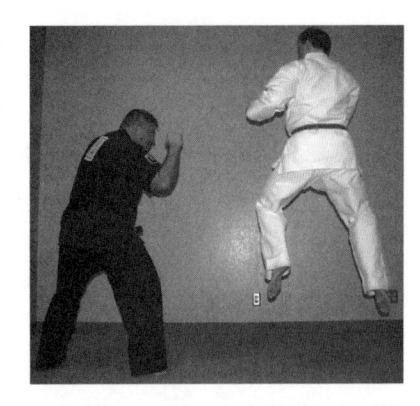

4. At the peak of your jump, execute the kick. As with the Jump Turning Wheel Kick, most individuals seem to strike their opponent when their non-kicking foot is already back down on the ground. This is incorrect! Remember, aerial kicking is an art form unto itself and needs to be practiced only after you have become very proficient at executing your primary kicks.

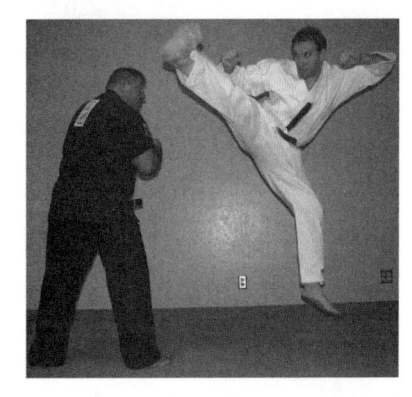

Did you notice anything wrong or improper in this series of photographs? Take another look. See them now?

If you look closely at photograph number four, you can see that I have executed my kick improperly and that instead of hitting Ron at the peak of my kick (at the "Impact" position), I will instead be hitting him towards the end of trajectory near the "Follow Through" position. This is generally caused by not turning the body enough prior to kicking, and also initiating your kick too soon.

Now you may be asking yourself, "What is the best way to improve my aerial kicking skills?" If you are, then you need to immediately go back to page number nine and read it again!

Awards & Accomplishments

This is a picture of the first world record certificate that I received from the Guinness Book of World Records for performing 10,502 High Kicks in 5 hours and 30 minutes on September 27, 1986 in Butte, Montana USA.

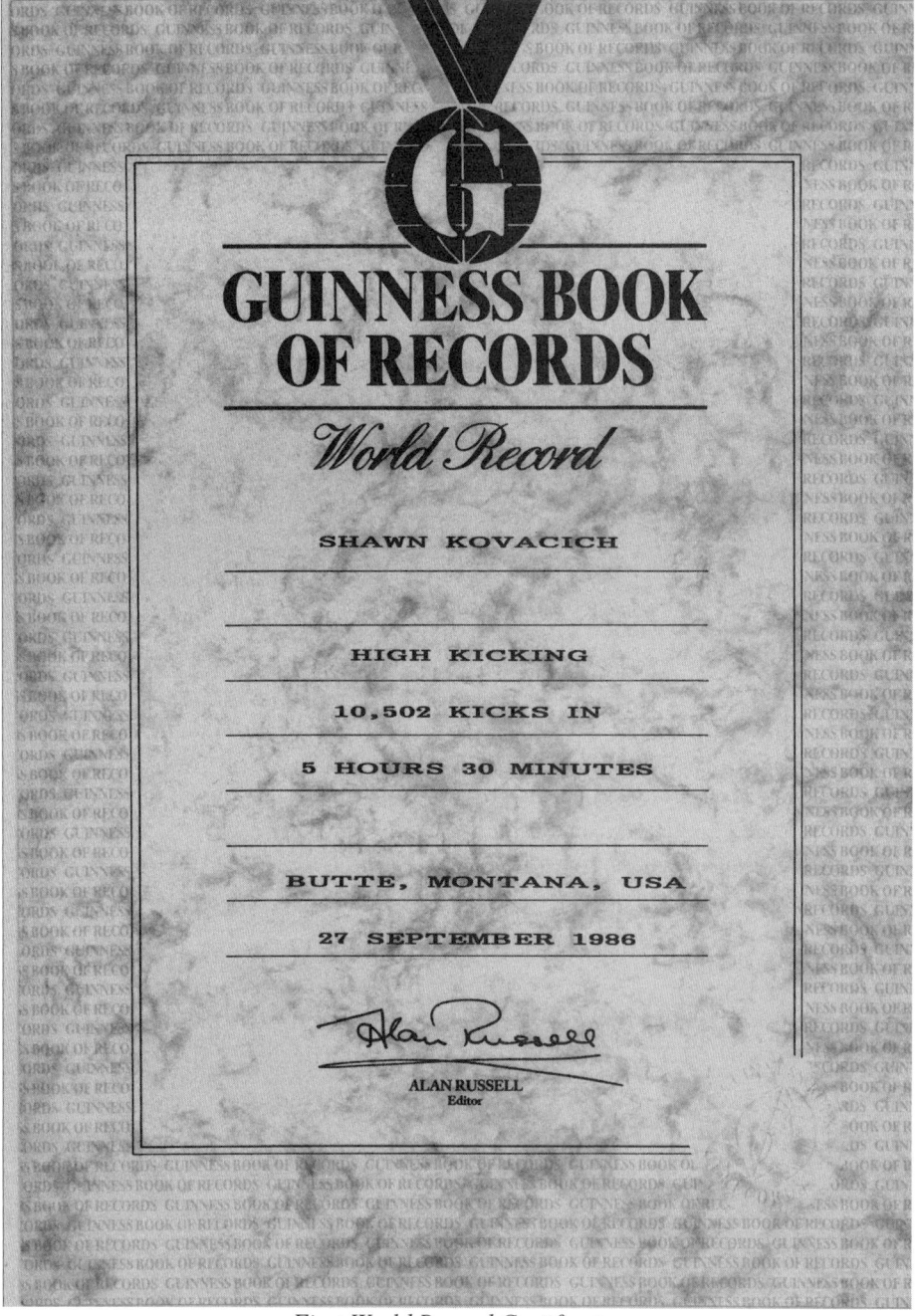

First World Record Certificate

This is a picture of the second world record certificate that I received from the Guinness Book of World Records for performing 11,000 High Kicks in 5 hours 18 minutes and 43 seconds on January 21, 1989 in Anaconda, Montana USA.

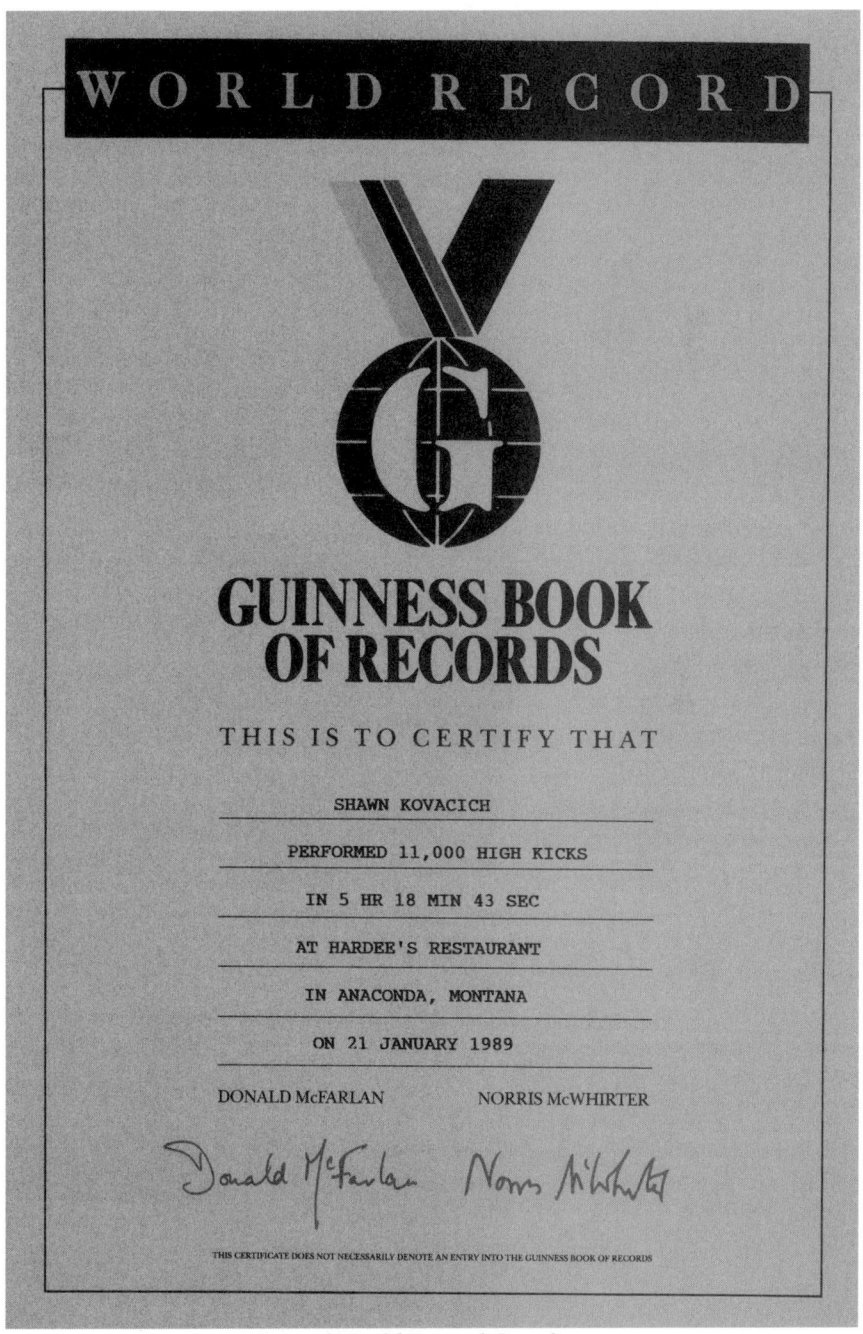

WORLD RECORD

GUINNESS BOOK OF RECORDS

THIS IS TO CERTIFY THAT

SHAWN KOVACICH

PERFORMED 11,000 HIGH KICKS

IN 5 HR 18 MIN 43 SEC

AT HARDEE'S RESTAURANT

IN ANACONDA, MONTANA

ON 21 JANUARY 1989

DONALD McFARLAN   NORRIS McWHIRTER

THIS CERTIFICATE DOES NOT NECESSARILY DENOTE AN ENTRY INTO THE GUINNESS BOOK OF RECORDS

Second World Record Certificate

Sneak Preview

Achieving Kicking Excellence; Volume Three: Axe Kick

Preview of Volume Three: Axe Kick

The Axe Kick is one of the ten primary kicks associated mainly with Karate and Tae Kwon Do. This kicked is delivered with a semi-circular type motion and relies more on speed and flexibility, along with a downward trajectory (gravity) for power, rather than actual physical strength. The striking surface utilized in the delivery of this kick is the back of the heel or calcaneus, although some instructors teach that you can also use the sole and/or ball of the foot. However, the effects of an Axe Kick are greatly reduced when any other part of the foot, other than the heel, is utilized.

The Axe Kick is used almost exclusively to an opponent's head, neck and shoulders, and is rarely if ever used to strike the body. The primary target areas for the Axe Kick are the top of the skull, nose, shoulder joint, and the collarbone. Although there are several major factors involved in the correct execution of an Axe Kick, one of the most important is the proper "coiling" of the kicking leg prior to execution of the kick. Many a student has succumbed to unnecessary injuries and wasted effort, due to a lack of understanding and improper technique when executing the Axe Kick.

The Axe Kick can be a very fast and effective kick when executed correctly. However, due to the increased distance it must travel before being ready to strike its target, it is better suited as a finishing technique after your opponent has already been set-up by another technique. The Axe Kick relies on strong flexibility not only of the entire leg, but also of the lower back and hips in order to obtain the extreme height needed to execute the kick correctly.

In order to obtain the maximum amount of impact potential in the Axe Kick, your kicking leg, hips and upper body have to be utilized correctly during the kicking sequence.

Pictorial Overview: Out-to-In Axe Kick

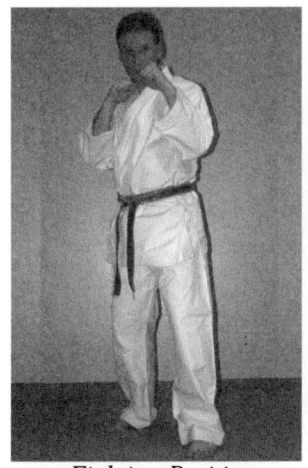

Fighting Position

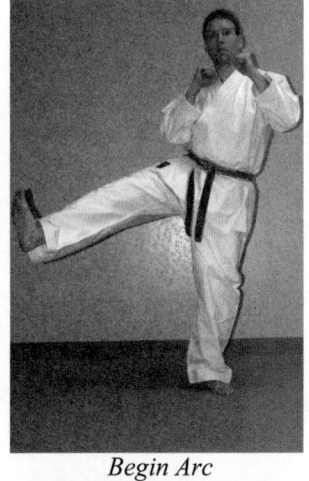

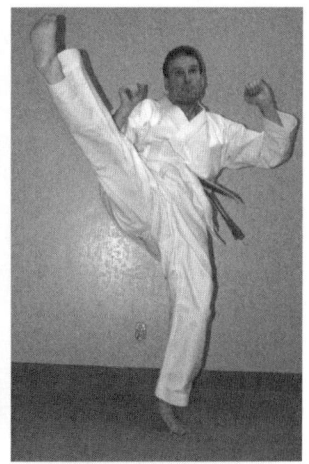

Begin Arc

3/4 to Peak of Arc

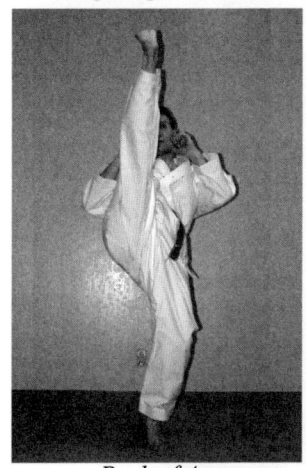

Peak of Arc

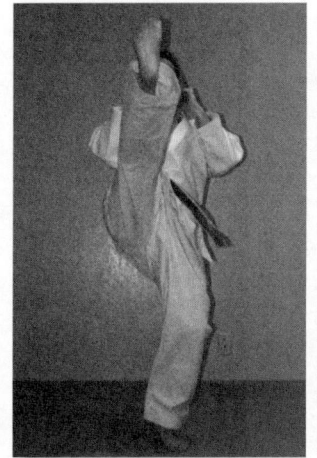

Impact

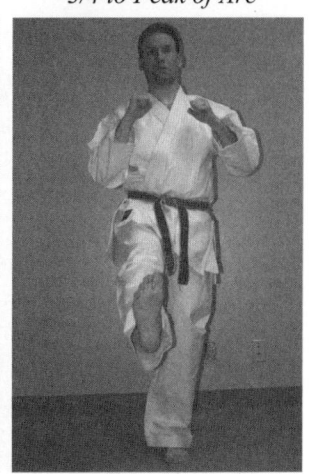

Follow Through

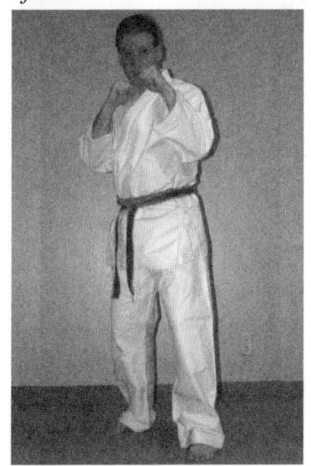

Position #1

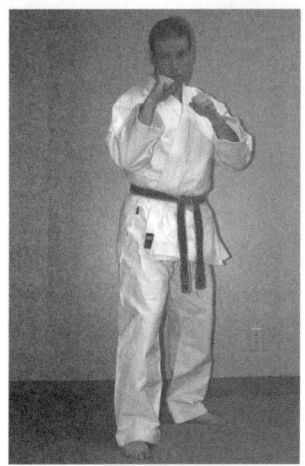

Position #2

Pictorial Overview: In-to-Out Axe Kick

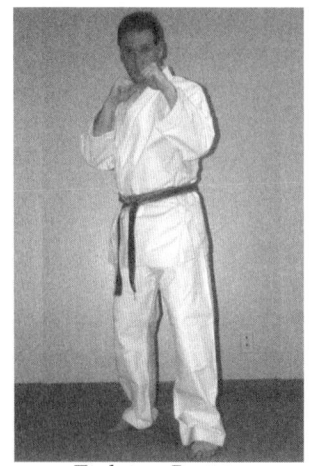

Fighting Position

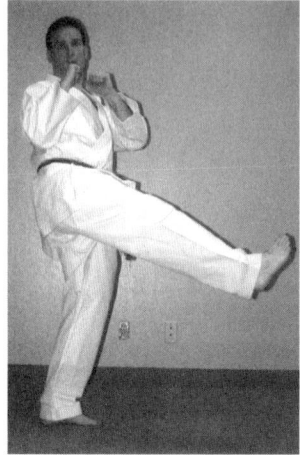

Begin Arc

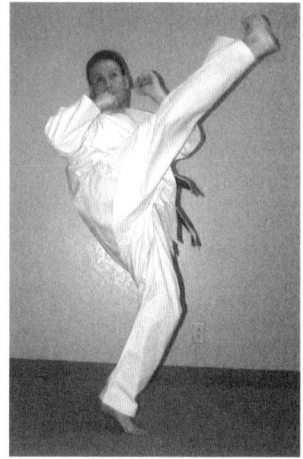

3/4 to Peak of Arc

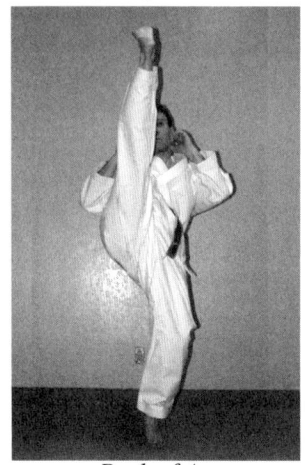

Peak of Arc

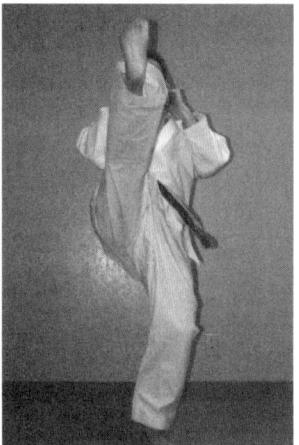

Impact

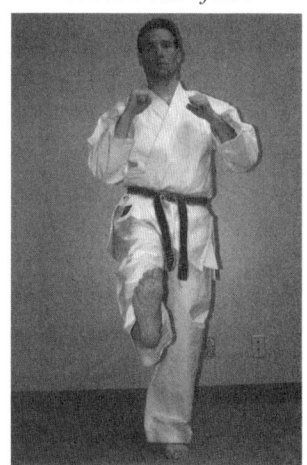

Follow Through

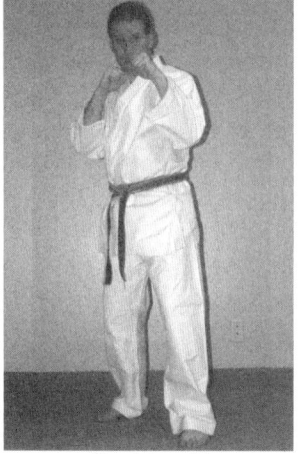

Position #1

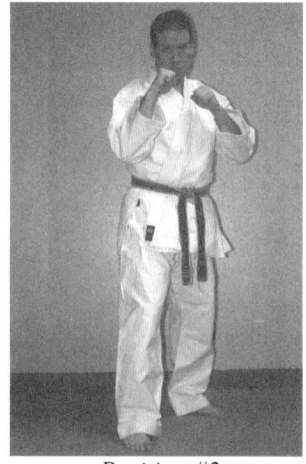

Position #2

Recommended Reading

Basic Anatomy of the Back Kick

1. Rasch, Philip J. Ph.D. & Burke, Roger K. Ph.D., Kinesiology and Applied Anatomy, (Lea & Febiger, Philadelphia, Pennsylvania, 1978)
2. Gray, Henry F.R.S., Gray's Anatomy, (Running Press, Philadelphia, Pennsylvania, 1974)

Warm Up and Stretching

1. Anderson, Bob, Stretching, (Shelter Publications, Inc., Bolinas, California, 1980)

Basic Principles of Kicking Movement

1. Fixx, James E., Maximum Sports Performance, (Random House, Inc., New York and Toronto, 1985)
2. Loehr, James E., Ed.D., Mental Toughness Training for Sports, (Stephen Greene Press, Inc., 1986)
3. Mashiro, N., Ph.D., Black Medicine: The Dark Art of Death, (Paladin Press, Boulder, Colorado, 1978)
4. Brancazio, Peter J., Sport Science, (Touchstone/Simon & Schuster, Inc., New York, New York, 1985)
5. Adams, Brian, Deadly Karate Blows: The Medical Implications, (Unique Publications, Burbank, California, 1985)
6. Hibbard, Jack, Karate Breaking Techniques: with Practical Applications, (Charles E. Tuttle Company, Inc., Tokyo, Japan, 1981)

Training and Practice Methods

1. Urquidez, Benny "The Jet", Training and Fighting Skills, (Unique Publications, Inc., Burbank, California, 1981)
2. Derse, Ed, Explosive Power-Plyometrics for Bodybuilders, Martial Artists & other Athletes, (Health for Life, Los Angeles, California, 1993)

3. Secrets of Advanced Body Builders, (Health For Life, Los Angeles, California, 1985)
4. Simon, Ilene Caryn, Mind Gains, (Health For Life, Los Angeles, California, 1995)
5. Robinson, Jerry & Carrino, Frank, Max 02 The Complete Guide To Synergistic Aerobic Training, (Health For Life, Los Angeles, California, 1993)
6. The Human Fuel Handbook, (Health For Life, Los Angeles, California, 1988)

Martial Arts & Self-Defense

1. Oyama, Masutatsu, This Is Karate, (Japan Publications, Inc., Tokyo, Japan, 1973)
2. Musashi, Miyamoto, A Book of Five Rings, (The Overlook Press, Woodstock, New York, 1974)
3. Chun, Richard, Tae Kwon Do: The Korean Martial Art, (Harper & Row, Publishers, Inc., New York, New York, 1976)
4. Westbrook, A., and Ratti, O., Aikido and the Dynamic Sphere, (Charles E. Tuttle Co., Inc., Boston, Massachusetts, 1970)
5. Lee, Joo Bang, The Ancient Martial Art of Hwarang Do, Vol. 1, (JL Publications, Inc., Downey, California, 1978)
6. Lee, Joo Bang, The Ancient Martial Art of Hwarang Do, Vol. 2, (JL Publications, Inc., Downey, California, 1978)
7. Lee, Joo Bang, The Ancient Martial Art of Hwarang Do, Vol. 3, (JL Publications, Inc., Downey, California, 1978)

INDEX

A

Ace in the Hole, 6
accuracy, 31
aerial kick, 146
alignment, 30
anatomy, 11-22
angle of attack, 138
angle of impact, 139
ankle weights, 165, 176
apple, 78, 88, 96, 104, 112, 122
automobile engine, 23, 70
axe kick, 202-204
axis point, 146

B

baby, 8, 10
balance, 30
barefoot, 84
basic prinicples of kicking, 25-34
base of support, 29
begin trajectory, 42-44
bicep femoris, 14-22
bird, 146
blink, 103
blueprint, 63
board, 26, 106, 141
bob & weave, 102
bobblehead, 102
bones, 11-14
bounce, 24
boxer, 35, 102
boxing, 28, 128
breathing, 32
bulldozer, 32-33
bullet, 32, 33, 78, 88, 96, 104, 112, 118, 119, 122
bullet casing, 118
bullet trajectory, 78, 88, 96, 104, 112, 122

C

cable machine leg raises, 170

calf machine, seated, 168
calcaneus, 11-14, 25
caliber, .22, 31
caliber, .45, 176
cats, 24
cement, 28
center of gravity, 28-30
chair practice, 164-165
clock, 36, 39, 45, 49, 52, 55, 61, 142
concrete, 63
conditioning, 32
coordination, 31
cuboid, 11-14
cuneiform, 11-14

D

Darden, Ellington Dr., 166
De LaHoya, Oscar, 28
deception, 120, 155
degree, "270", 158, 159
degree, "360", 49, 66, 146, 159
dimes, three, 162
direction of force, 140
distance, 33
doctor, 8
Do's and Don'ts, 24
drunken sailor, 8
Dunlap, Ron, 183-199
dynamic tension, 32

E

Eight Directions of Attack, 129
elbow techniques, 87, 151
end of trajectory, 55-57
equilibrium, 28
excessive force, 27
extensor digitorum longus, 14-22
extensor hallucis longus, 14-22
external oblique, 14-22
eye contact, 31, 36, 65

F

facial area, 27
femur, 11-14
femur, head of the, 11-14
fibula, 11-14
Fields, Joe, 34
fighting stance, 35-38
fighting position, 35-38
figure skater, 28
firing pin, 118
flashlight, 31, 36
flexibility, 23, 24
flexor digitorum longus, 14-22
follow through, 33, 52-54
footwork, 95, 133
force bag, 178
force=mass x acceleration, 178
Foreman, George, 28
foundation, 63
Front Leg Wheel Kick, 100

G

gastrocnemius, 14-22
gears, 135
gemelli, 14-22
glabella, 27
gluteus maximus, 14-22
gluteus medius, 14-22
golf club, 7, 147, 148
golfball, 7, 147
golfer, 7, 147
gracilis, 14-22
grappling, 29, 87, 151
gravel, 28
Guinness Book of World Records, 5, 200, 201
gunpowder, 118, 119

H

hack squat machine, 166-167
hammer, 26, 106
hammering, 26
hand techniques, 87, 151
high section, 94, 132
Hop/Slide Backward Wheel Kick, 91

Hop/Slide Forward Wheel Kick, 82
house, 63
human factor, 26
Hunn, Ben, 5

I

ice, 28
illiotibial tract, 14-22
iliopsoas, 20
impact, 33, 48-51
innate response, 86

J

jam, 33
jaw, 27, 139
joint techniques, 87, 93, 151
Jump Turning Wheel Kick, 136
Jumping Turning Wheel Kick, 540-Degree, 144

K

Karate, 202
Kiaa, 111
kicking paddle, 178-179
Knechtges, Brian, 5
knee, 11-14
knee joint, 11-14
knee strikes, 87
Kovacich, Shawn, 5

L

Lamborghini, 32-33
Lee, Bruce, 4, 24
left leg, 7, 153
leg curls, seated, 171
long range, 87
low section, 94

M

mathematical level, 9
metatarsals, 11-14
mid range, 87
midsection, 94
mirror, 162
mouth, 27
muscles, 14- 22

muscular control, 31
mushroomed, 88

N

nail, 26, 106, 141
navicular, 11-14nose, 27
Nurmi, Paavo, 34

O

Off-Setting Wheel Kick, 125
optimum level, 176
orbital bones, 27
over-extend, 95

P

patella, 11-14
Path of Trajectory, 31, 46-47, 56, 119, 123, 142
peak of trajectory, 45-47
pavement, 28
pectineus, 14-22
pelvic girdle, 11-14
pelvis, 11-14
pelvis, acetabulum of the, 11-14
penetrating impact, 26, 97
penetrating strike, 97
peripheral vision, 31, 36peroneus brevis, 14-22
peroneus longus, 14-22
peroneus tertius, 14-22
phalanges, 11-14
philtrum, 27
pivot, 67-70, 114
plantaris, 20
plyometrics, 174-175
pocketwatch, 135
point of chin, 27
popliteal region, 20
practice, 10, 31, 162-165, 176-177
pressure per square inch, 11, 25, 26
primary kick, 10, 35
primer, 118
proper practice, 10, 162, 177
punching, 28, 87, 93
push, 26

Q

quadriceps, 21
quality supervision, 10
quick draw, 176
Quinn, Michael, 166

R

reaching, 95
rectus femoris, 14-22
relaxation and tension, 32-33, 179
return to fighting position, 58-60
Reverse Crescent Kick, 110
rifle, 31, 118
ringing out, 114, 121
Rome, 24
rule-of-thumb, 10, 34, 63
running, 179
running stairs, 179

S

Sabaki Challenge, 5,
saw, 106
self-discipline, 7
semimembranosus, 14-22
semitendinosus, 14-22
Sesame Street, 5
shoes, 84
short range, 87
Shidokan, Team USA, 5
Shidokan, U.S. Open, 5
side-to-side squats, 169, 172-173
ski jumps, 174-175
Slide/Hop Backward Wheel Kick, 91
Slide/Hop Forward Wheel Kick, 82
soleus, 14-22
speed, 32, 176
Spinning Wheel Kick, 73, 153
squats, 166, 169, 172
stability, 28
Step-Back Wheel Kick, 63
strength, 32
strength training, 166
stretching, 9, 23, 24
strike into, 96
strike through, 97, 104, 113, 119, 128, 132

striking surface, 25
surface strike, 26, 79, 89, 97
Switch Wheel Kick, 116

T

Tae Kwon Do, 202
talus, 11-14
target areas, 26-27
tee, 7, 147
telegraphing, 31
temple, 27
tensor fascia latae, 14-22
throwing techniques, 93, 151
tibia, 11-14
tibialis anterior, 14-22
tibialis posterior, 22
timing, 33
top, 146
towel, 114, 121
training partner, 162
trigger, 118
trouble shooting, 180-182
turning, 39
Turning Wheel Kick, 35

U

USTU, 5

V

variations, 63
vastus medialis, 14-22
vastuslateralis, 14-22
visualization, 34
vital point, 26-27
vulnerable point, 26-27

W

wagon wheel, 75, 142
wall practice, 163
warm-up, 9, 23, 24
water training, 177
weak leg, 160
weight, 28
weight lifting belt, 166
weight lifting gloves, 166

Wheel Kick applications, 183-199
wobble, 146
wood, 26, 106

Y

Y, 149

Notes:

Notes:

Notes:

Notes:

Notes:

Notes:

Notes:

Notes:

Notes:

Notes: